Current Topics in Microbiology and Immunology

Volume 351

Current Topics in Microbiology and Immunology

Previously published volumes

Further volumes can be found at www.springer.com

Vol. 325: **Shenk, Thomas E.; Stinski, Mark F. (Eds.)**:
Human Cytomegalovirus. 2008.
ISBN 978-3-540-77348-1

Vol. 326: **Reddy, Anireddy S. N.; Golovkin, Maxim (Eds.)**:
Nuclear pre-mRNA processing in plants. 2008
ISBN 978-3-540-76775-6

Vol. 327: **Manchester, Marianne; Steinmetz Nicole F. (Eds.)**:
Viruses and Nanotechnology. 2008.
ISBN 978-3-540-69376-5

Vol. 328: **van Etten, (Ed.)**:
Lesser Known Large dsDNA Viruses. 2008.
ISBN 978-3-540-68617-0

Vol. 329: **Griffin, Diane E.; Oldstone, Michael B. A. (Eds.)**: Measles. 2009
ISBN 978-3-540-70522-2

Vol. 330: **Griffin, Diane E.; Oldstone, Michael B. A. (Eds.)**:
Measles. 2009.
ISBN 978-3-540-70616-8

Vol. 331: **Villiers, E. M. de (Ed.)**:
TT Viruses. 2009. ISBN 978-3-540-70917-8

Vol. 332: **Karasev A. (Ed.)**:
Plant produced Microbial Vaccines. 2009.
ISBN 978-3-540-70857-5

Vol. 333: **Compans, Richard W.; Orenstein, Walter A. (Eds.)**:
Vaccines for Pandemic Influenza. 2009.
ISBN 978-3-540-92164-6

Vol. 334: **McGavern, Dorian; Dustin, Micheal (Eds.)**:
Visualizing Immunity. 2009.
ISBN 978-3-540-93862-0

Vol. 335: **Levine, Beth; Yoshimori, Tamotsu; Deretic, Vojo (Eds.)**:
Autophagy in Infection and Immunity. 2009.
ISBN 978-3-642-00301-1

Vol. 336: **Kielian, Tammy (Ed.)**:
Toll-like Receptors: Roles in Infection and Neuropathology. 2009.
ISBN 978-3-642-00548-0

Vol. 337: **Sasakawa, Chihiro (Ed.)**:
Molecular Mechanisms of Bacterial Infection via the Gut. 2009.
ISBN 978-3-642-01845-9

Vol. 338: **Rothman, Alan L. (Ed.)**:
Dengue Virus. 2009.
ISBN 978-3-642-02214-2

Vol. 339: **Spearman, Paul; Freed, Eric O. (Eds.)**:
HIV Interactions with Host Cell Proteins. 2009.
ISBN 978-3-642-02174-9

Vol. 340: **Saito, Takashi; Batista, Facundo D. (Eds.)**:
Immunological Synapse. 2010.
ISBN 978-3-642-03857-0

Vol. 341: **Bruserud, Øystein (Ed.)**:
The Chemokine System in Clinical and Experimental Hematology. 2010.
ISBN 978-3-642-12638-3

Vol. 342: **Arvin, Ann M. (Ed.)**:
Varicella-zoster Virus. 2010.
ISBN 978-3-642-12727-4

Vol. 343: **Johnson, John E. (Ed.)**:
Cell Entry by Non-Enveloped Viruses. 2010.
ISBN 978-3-642-13331-2

Vol. 344: **Dranoff, Gelnn (Ed.)**:
Cancer Immunology and Immunotherapy. 2011.
ISBN 978-3-642-14135-5

Vol. 345: **Simon, M. Celeste (Ed.)**:
Diverse Effects of Hypoxia on Tumor Progression. 2010.
ISBN 978-3-642-13328-2

Vol. 346: **Christian Rommel; Bart Vanhaesebroeck; Peter K. Vogt (Ed.)**:
Phosphoinositide 3-kinase in Health and Disease. 2010.
ISBN 978-3-642-13662-7

Vol. 347: **Christian Rommel; Bart Vanhaesebroeck; Peter K. Vogt (Ed.)**:
Phosphoinositide 3-kinase in Health and Disease. 2010.
ISBN 978-3-642-14815-6

Vol. 348: **Lyubomir Vassilev; David Fry (Eds.)**:
Small-Molecule Inhibitors of Protein-Protein Interactions. 2011.
ISBN 978-3-642-17082-9

Vol. 349: **Michael Kartin (Ed.)**:
NF-kB in Health and Disease. 2011.
ISBN: 978-3-642-16017-2

Vol. 350: **Rafi Ahmed; Tasuku Honjo (Eds.)**
Negative Co-receptors and Ligands. 2011.
ISBN: 978-3-642-19545-7

Marcel B. M. Teunissen
Editor

Intradermal Immunization

Responsible series editor: Richard W. Compans

Springer

Marcel B. M. Teunissen, Ph.D
Department of Dermatology
Academic Medical Center
University of Amsterdam
Meibergdreef 9
1105 AZ Amsterdam
The Netherlands
e-mail: m.b.teunissen@amc.uva.nl

ISSN 0070-217X
ISBN 978-3-642-23689-1 e-ISBN 978-3-642-23690-7
DOI 10.1007/978-3-642-23690-7
Springer Heidelberg Dordrecht London New York

Library of Congress Control Number: 2011937253

Cover design: Deblik, Berlin

Printed on acid-free paper

Springer is part of Springer Science+Business Media (www.springer.com)

Preface

Intradermal Immunization: More than Just Skin-Deep

Vaccination is one of the most powerful interventions to effectively reduce mortality and morbidity caused by infectious diseases. It originated in 1796 when Jenner inoculated cowpox virus into the skin to render individuals resistant to subsequent infection with the potentially lethal smallpox virus. Since then, numerous vaccines have been developed against many bacteria and viruses, leading to eradication (smallpox) or control of prevailing infectious diseases (such as mumps, measles, rabies, yellow fever, influenza, and several others). Despite the impressive success of current vaccine programs, there remains a need to improve the effectiveness of current vaccines. A more powerful and longer lasting immune response induced by smaller and fewer doses of vaccine is an exciting challenge and necessary to reduce costs and to avoid vaccine shortages during pandemic epidemics. Improvement of effectiveness also enables induction of protective immunity in populations that respond poorly to vaccination, for example elderly or immunocompromised individuals. Furthermore, for some devastating infectious diseases (such as AIDS and malaria) effective vaccines have not been successfully developed. The rapidly expanding knowledge on the cellular and molecular mechanisms involved in and controlling protective immune responses will ultimately lead to better vaccines. According to the generally accepted dogma, dendritic cells have a crucial role in up taking antigens (e.g. vaccine) and priming the required type of T cell response for protective immunity. In addition, ample evidence proves that triggering pattern recognition receptors (such as Toll-like receptors) on dendritic cells boosts the immunostimulatory function of these cells.

Although the pioneering work of Jenner demonstrated that administration of pathogens as a vaccine in the skin provided protection, nowadays the vast majority of the vaccines are applied as subcutaneous and intramuscular injection. There is no scientific evidence to show that these routes are optimal for vaccination. The skin harbors a widespread network of dendritic cells and contains a well-developed immune system with a good connection to regional lymphatic tissues. Therefore, the skin forms an attractive site for efficient immunization. It may very well be that intradermal vaccination is superior to the conventional intramuscular or subcutaneous methods. The reviews in this volume of Current Topics in Microbiology and Immunology cover diverse topics related to intradermal immunization. The volume starts with a basic overview of murine and human skin dendritic cell network, respectively, and their role in immunity, as well as an extensive description of the immunobiology of the skin. The next chapter describes the state-of-the-art on delivery systems especially designed for intradermal vaccination. The remaining chapters highlight the effectiveness of intradermal immunization in experimental animal models or in clinical practice, all supporting the view that intradermal immunization is at least as good as other immunization routes. Keeping in mind that current vaccines are not specially designed for intradermal immunization, but show comparable efficiency even at reduced dosages, this underlines the great potential for the skin as a vaccination site and suggests that the efficacy can be further improved. Hopefully, the overview in this volume will encourage vaccine designers to focus on this promising immunization route, and in addition, to inspire them to develop a cocktail of antigen, adjuvant and formulation that is especially optimized for intradermal immunization.

Finally, I would like to thank Professor Richard W. Compans at Emory University School of Medicine (Atlanta, GA, USA) for inviting me to edit this volume, all the authors for their expert contributions, and Anne Clauss for her patience and taking care of organizing the process of publication.

Amsterdam, The Netherlands Marcel B. M. Teunissen

Contents

Contributors

M. P. Collin Institute of Cellular Medicine, Newcastle University, Newcastle upon Tyne, NE2 4HH, UK

T. D. de Gruijl Department of Medical Oncology, VU University Medical Center, De Boelelaan 1117, 1081 HV, Amsterdam, The Netherlands

S. Ebner Department of Dermatology and Venereology, Innsbruck Medical University, Anichstrasse 35, 6020, Innsbruck, Austria

V. Flacher Department of Dermatology and Venereology, Innsbruck Medical University, Anichstrasse 35, 6020, Innsbruck, Austria

L. B. S. Gelinck Department of Internal Medicine, Medisch Centrum Haaglanden, P.O. Box 432, 2501 CK, The Hague, The Netherlands

F. Ginhoux Singapore Immunology Network (SIgN), Agency for Science, Technology and Research (A*STAR), 8A Biomedical Grove, Immunos, Biopolis, Singapore 138648, Singapore

J. B. A. G. Haanen Division of Immunology, The Netherlands Cancer Institute, Plesmanlaan 121, 1066 CX, Amsterdam, The Netherlands

B. N. Hangalapura Department of Medical Oncology VU University Medical Center, De Boelelaan 1117, 1081 HV, Amsterdam, The Netherlands

M. Haniffa Institute of Cellular Medicine, Newcastle University, Newcastle upon Tyne, NE2 4HH, UK

C. Jarrahian PATH, Seattle, WA, 98121, USA

Y. C. Kim School of Chemical and Biomolecular Engineering, Georgia Institute of Technology, Atlanta, GA, 30332, USA

M. Merad Department of Gene and Cell Medicine and the Immunology Institute, Mount Sinai School of Medicine, 1425 Madison Avenue, New York, NY, 10029, USA

S. Mitragotri Department of Chemical Engineering, University of California Santa Barbara, Santa Barbara, CA, 93106, USA

L. G. Ng Singapore Immunology Network (SIgN), Agency for Science, Technology and Research (A*STAR), 8A Biomedical Grove, Immunos, Biopolis, Singapore 138648, Singapore

D. Oosterhoff Department of Medical Oncology, VU University Medical Center, De Boelelaan 1117, 1081 HV, Amsterdam, The Netherlands

K. Oosterhuis Division of Immunology, The Netherlands Cancer Institute, Plesmanlaan 121, 1066 CX, Amsterdam, The Netherlands

M. R. Prausnitz School of Chemical and Biomolecular Engineering, Georgia Institute of Technology, Atlanta, GA, 30332, USA

N. Romani Department of Dermatology and Venereology, Innsbruck Medical University, Anichstrasse 35, 6020, Innsbruck, Austria

A. H. E. Roukens Department of Infectious Diseases, Suite C5-P, Leiden University Medical Centre, Albinusdreef 2, 2333 ZA, Leiden, The Netherlands

T. N. Schumacher Division of Immunology, The Netherlands Cancer Institute, Plesmanlaan 121, 1066 CX, Amsterdam, The Netherlands

B. J. R. Sluijter Department of Surgical Oncology, VU University Medical Center, De Boelelaan 1117, 1081 HV, Amsterdam, The Netherlands

F. Sparber Department of Dermatology and Venereology Innsbruck Medical University, Anichstrasse 35, 6020, Innsbruck, Austria

P. Stoitzner Department of Dermatology and Venereology, Innsbruck Medical University, Anichstrasse 35, 6020, Innsbruck, Austria

M. B. M. Teunissen Department of Dermatology, Academic Medical Center, University of Amsterdam, Meibergdreef 9, 1105 AZ, Amsterdam, The Netherlands

C. H. Tripp Department of Dermatology and Venereology, Innsbruck Medical University, Anichstrasse 35, 6020, Innsbruck, Austria

J. H. van den Berg Division of Immunology, The Netherlands Cancer Institute, Plesmanlaan 121, 1066 CX, Amsterdam, The Netherlands

L. G. Visser Department of Infectious Diseases, Suite C5-P, Leiden University Medical Centre, Albinusdreef 2, 2333 ZA, Leiden, The Netherlands

M. J. Warrell Oxford Vaccine Group, Centre for Clinical Vaccinology and Tropical Medicine, Churchill Hospital, University of Oxford, Oxford, OX3 7LJ, UK

D. Zehrung PATH Seattle, WA, 98121, USA

Understanding the Murine Cutaneous Dendritic Cell Network to Improve Intradermal Vaccination Strategies

F. Ginhoux, L. G. Ng and M. Merad

Abstract Dendritic cells (DCs) form a heterogeneous group of antigen presenting cells that play different roles in tissue immunity. Recent studies have revealed the presence of distinct DC populations in murine skin, highlighting the complexity of the cutaneous DC network. In this review, we will define the major DC subsets that populate the different layers of the skin, focusing on their origin and the mechanisms controlling their homeostasis. We will also review recent evidence underlining the functional specialization of dermal DC subsets and its relevance in the design of novel vaccine approaches.

Contents

F. Ginhoux (✉) and L. G. Ng
Singapore Immunology Network (SIgN), Agency for Science, Technology and Research (A*STAR), 8A Biomedical Grove, Immunos, Biopolis, Singapore 138648, Singapore
e-mail: florent_ginhoux@immunol.a-star.edu.sg

M. Merad
Department of Gene and Cell Medicine and the Immunology Institute, Mount Sinai School of Medicine, 1425 Madison Avenue, New York, NY 10029, USA

Current Topics in Microbiology and Immunology (2012) 351: 1–24
DOI: 10.1007/82_2010_115

Published Online: 6 November 2010

1 Introduction

Dendritic cells (DCs) are a heterogeneous population of rare hematopoietic cells found in most tissues, including both lymphoid and non-lymphoid organs. The main role of DCs is to induce specific immunity against invading pathogens while maintaining tolerance to self-antigens (Banchereau et al. 2000; Steinman et al. 2003).

Several subsets of DCs have been described in mice and humans. Anatomically, DCs can be divided into those that reside in lymphoid tissues and those present in non-lymphoid tissues. Lymphoid tissue DCs are further categorized into two groups: the plasmacytoid DCs (pDCs) and the conventional DCs (cDCs), the latter including both $CD8\alpha^+$ and $CD8\alpha^-$ DC populations (Shortman and Naik 2007). Non-lymphoid organ DCs are found in all peripheral tissues in steady-state. DCs that populate the outer epidermal layer of stratified epithelia are often called Langerhans cells (LCs), while DCs in connective tissues such as the dermis or lamina propria, are called interstitial DCs. These tissue-resident DCs are also referred to as migratory DCs due to their ability to constitutively migrate to the draining lymph node (LN) (Kelly et al. 1978; Drexhage et al. 1979; Hemmi et al. 2001), a process strongly increased under inflammatory conditions (reviewed in (Randolph et al. 2008). Finally, in the inflamed tissue itself, two additional subsets of DCs can be found: a DC population derived from blood monocytes (Leon and Ardavin 2008) and pDCs (Liu 2005; Nestle et al. 2009).

As the first line of defense against a broad array of pathogens, the skin is equipped with a sophisticated immune surveillance system involving a rich network of DCs that are present throughout the different layers of the skin (Merad et al. 2008). Owing to its accessibility and its abundance in DCs, the skin represents an ideal site for vaccine delivery, allowing the induction of strong immune responses at much lower doses of antigen than intramuscular vaccines (Kenney et al. 2004). Recently, several studies have highlighted the complexity and the functional specialization of the cutaneous DC network, showing that as in the lymphoid organs, multiple subsets of DCs coexist in the dermis, and that skin DC subsets exhibit specific immune functions. In this review, we will define the origin, homeostasis, and functions of each cutaneous DC compartment and discuss the potential implications of these studies in the development of novel vaccine strategies.

2 The Skin Dendritic Cell Network

Phenotypically, the murine cutaneous DC population can be identified by the constitutive expression of both the integrin CD11c and major histocompatibility complex class II (MHCII) molecules. However, several studies have now established that this definition is too broad and that this population in fact includes several distinct DC subsets, each with a specific phenotype, origin, and function.

2.1 Langerhans Cells

Langerhans cells constitute the specific subset of DCs that populate the epidermal layer of the skin. Through their extended dendrites, LCs form a continuous cellular network that detects pathogens breaching the skin, thus providing the first immunological barrier to the external environment. Epidermal LCs account for 3–5% of all nucleated cells in the murine epidermis, with approximately 700 LCs per mm^2, which are arranged in a network occupying the interstices between neighboring keratinocytes (Merad et al. 2008). In addition to the hematopoietic marker CD45, CD11c and MHCII molecules, murine LCs constitutively express the lectin receptor langerin (Takahara et al. 2002), the sialoglycoprotein CD24 (Stutte et al. 2008) and the adhesion molecules E-cadherin (Tang et al. 1993) and epithelial-cell adhesion molecule (EpCAM or gp40) (Borkowski et al. 1996b), which anchors LCs to neighboring keratinocytes. LCs also express the lectin CD205 (DEC-205) implicated in antigen capture and antigen processing (Inaba et al. 1995; Jiang et al. 1995) (Table 1). In addition, LCs express several macrophage markers, including the integrin CD11b, the transmembrane protein F4/80 and the tyrosine-protein phosphatase non-receptor type substrate 1 SIRPα, but not the fractalkine receptor CX3CR1 (Table 1) (Ginhoux et al. 2009).

2.2 Dermal DC Subsets in Steady-State

Dermal DCs have been much less studied than LCs due to the difficulty of isolating these cells. DCs in the dermis include dermal resident DCs and migratory LCs on their way to the LNs (Merad et al. 2008). Murine dermal resident DCs were thought to form a homogenous population easily distinguishable from

Table 1 Phenotype of the murine cutaneous DC subsets

	Langerhans cells	Dermal $CD103^+$ DC	Dermal $CD11b^+$ DC	Dermal DN DC	Inflammatory $CD11b^+$ DC	Dermal macrophage
CD45	+	+	+	+	+	+
CD11c	++	++	++	+	++	−/+
MHC II	+	+	+	++	+	−/+
Langerin	++	+	−	−	−	−
CD103	−	+	−	−	−	−
CD24	++	++	+/++	−/+	ND	−/+
CD11b	+	−	++	−	++	++
EpCAM	++	−/+	−	−	ND	−
F4/80	+	−	+	−/+	+	+
CX3CR1	−	−	+	−/+	+	−/+
SIRPα	+	−	++	+	+	+

migratory LCs based on their lack of langerin expression (Valladeau and Saeland 2005). However, recent studies in mice showed that dermal $langerin^+$ cells comprise both LCs and a novel population of DCs (Table 1) (Bursch et al. 2007; Ginhoux et al. 2007; Poulin et al. 2007).

The classical $langerin^-$ dermal DCs represent the majority (up to 70%) of the dermal DC pool and express high levels of the integrin CD11b and several macrophage markers such as F4/80, CX3CR1, and SIRPα (Ginhoux et al. 2009). Interestingly, their expression of CD24 is heterogeneous, suggesting that dermal $langerin^-$ DCs might not represent a homogeneous subset of DCs, either in origin or in maturation status (Table 1) (Henri et al. 2009). The recently identified $langerin^+$ DC population represents 10–20% of the total dermal DC pool. In contrast to LCs, dermal $langerin^+$ DCs express the integrin $\alpha E\beta 7$ (CD103) (Cepek et al. 1994), although not homogenously (Henri et al. 2009). Dermal $langerin^+$ DCs express the same high level of CD24 as LCs, but do not express CX3CR1, F4/80, and SIRPα and express low levels of CD11b and EpCAM (Ginhoux et al. 2009) (Table 1). Importantly, similar DC subsets expressing CD103 or CD11b have also been identified in other non-lymphoid tissues, such as the lung (Sung et al. 2006), the liver, the kidney, and the pancreatic islets (Ginhoux et al. 2009). The phenotype of these DC populations is similar to that of the dermal DC subsets, although langerin expression is variable between tissues and totally absent from pancreatic islet $CD103^+$ DCs (Ginhoux et al. 2009). Therefore, the two dermal resident DC populations will be referred to as $CD103^+$ DCs and $CD11b^+$ DCs throughout this review. Finally, besides these two DC subsets, a remaining $MHCII^+CD11c^+$ $CD103^-langerin^-CD11b^-$ subset has also been identified in the dermis (Shklovskaya et al. 2008; Ginhoux et al. 2009; Henri et al. 2009). These cells express low level of CD24 and EpCAM, but do express bimodal levels of F4/80, SIRPα, and CX3CR1 (Table 1), suggesting again that this cell population might not be homogeneous, either in origin or in maturation status. Its further characterization is also hampered by the lack of a positive marker that clearly delineates it from the other DC subsets.

2.3 Localization of Dermal DC Subsets

While a detailed phenotype of the various dermal DC subsets is available, much less is known about their specific anatomical localization in the dermis. Confocal analysis of frozen skin sections from the CX3CR1-GFP mouse (Jung et al. 2000), combined with MHCII and CD103 staining, allow the visualization of both CD103$^+$ DCs (MHCII$^+$CD103$^+$CX3CR1-GFP$^-$) and CD11b$^+$ DCs (MHCII$^+$CD103$^-$CX3CR1-GFP$^+$) in the dermis (Fig. 1). CD103$^+$ DCs are present in the upper dermis in proximity to CD11b$^+$ DCs, just under the epidermal-dermal junction and are also associated with hair follicles (Bursch et al. 2007). Although it remains to be established whether CD103$^+$ DCs represent the only perifollicular DC subset, it is interesting to note that hair follicles constitute a point of entry in the skin, as seen upon topical application of naked DNA to the skin surface (Fan et al. 1999).

2.4 Inflammatory Dermal DC Subsets

Upon skin inflammation, the composition of the cutaneous DC population changes. Depending on the type and the degree of inflammation, tissue-resident DCs are either absent or reduced from injured sites, due to their death or their migration to the LNs and replaced by newly recruited blood-derived DCs. As mentioned above, two additional DC subsets are found in the inflamed skin. These are the

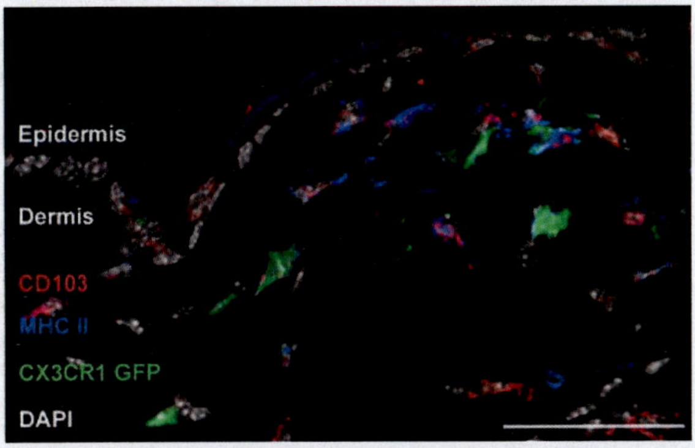

Fig. 1 The dermal dendritic cell network. Back skin cross-section isolated from C57BL/6 CX3CR1/EGFP (*green*) mouse was stained with anti-CD103 (*red*) and anti-MHCII (*blue*) monoclonal antibodies. Nuclei were counterstained with DAPI (*white*). Bar, 50 μm. CD11b$^+$ DCs (CX3CR1/GFP$^+$, MHCII$^+$) appear in *green*, while CD103$^+$ DCs (CD103$^+$, MHCII$^+$) appear in *pink*. Dermal T cells known to express CD103 appear in *red*. Image from Dr Michal Abel

pDCs and blood monocytes-derived DCs (reviewed in (Helft et al. 2010)). Monocyte-derived DCs arise from inflammatory Ly6C^{hi} monocytes that are recruited from the blood to the inflamed dermis (Leon and Ardavin 2008). Phenotypically, monocyte-derived DCs are very similar to steady-state resident CD11b^{+} DCs. Although Ly6C^{hi} monocytes express Ly6C, once recruited and differentiated into DCs in the inflamed tissue, they will downregulate Ly6C, rendering them indistinguishable from the CD11b^{+} DCs (Table 1).

3 Homeostasis of Cutaneous DCs

The homeostasis of lymphoid organs DC populations depends on a dynamic balance between cell division, death, and replenishment by blood circulating precursors (Liu et al. 2007, 2009). Homeostasis of cutaneous DCs will also depend on their migratory ability since they constitutively sample antigens and migrate through the afferent lymphatics to the T-cell areas of LNs (Randolph et al. 2008). In addition, there is no evidence of any associated cutaneous DC death in situ in steady-state. We will first review the different aspects of dermal DCs homeostasis and then address the unique homeostasis of epidermal LCs.

3.1 Proliferation

Dendritic cells were thought to be terminally differentiated cells, with no proliferative capacity. However, recent studies assessing BrdU labeling, cell cycle and rate of DC replacement in bone marrow chimeric and parabiotic mice proved the contrary, showing that in lymphoid organs DCs actively proliferate in the steady-state (Kabashima et al. 2005; Liu et al. 2007). The mechanisms regulating DC proliferation in the steady-state are yet to be fully elucidated but involve at least lymphotoxin-β (for the CD11b^{+}CD8^{-} subset) (Kabashima et al. 2005), as well as the Fms-like tyrosine kinase 3 ligand (Flt3L) (Waskow et al. 2008). Although most of this work concerns lymphoid tissue-resident DCs, recent studies have characterized the turnover of DCs in the dermis and other non-lymphoid tissues (Ginhoux et al. 2009; Henri et al. 2009). All dermal DC subsets proliferate, although CD103^{+} DCs do so at a higher rate than the CD11b^{+} subset (Ginhoux et al. 2009; Henri et al. 2009). It remains to be understood whether this reflects an intrinsic property of the subsets, or is a result of contamination of the CD11b^{+} subset with non-proliferative monocytes or dermal macrophages, as their phenotypes may overlap (Table 1).

3.2 Migration

The chemokine receptor CCR7 controls the constitutive migration of all cutaneous DCs to the skin draining LNs (Forster et al. 1999; Ohl et al. 2004).

Upon inflammation, tissue DC migration to the draining LNs markedly increases (Jakubzick et al. 2008). Interestingly, cutaneous DC subsets differentially migrate to the draining LNs in response to contact sensitizing agents. Migration of CD11b$^+$ and CD103$^+$ dermal DCs peaked after 1 day, followed by LCs at 4 days post-skin sensitization (Kissenpfennig et al. 2005; Shklovskaya et al. 2008). However, in a herpes simplex virus (HSV) skin infection model, epidermal LCs emigrated from the epidermis at earlier time points (Eidsmo et al. 2009). It is also important to note that cutaneous DCs undergo phenotypic changes upon migration from the skin to the LNs (Henri et al. 2009). Consequently, some markers used to identify them in the skin are not available for their characterization in the LNs, for example, CD11b or EpCAM (Henri et al. 2009).

3.3 *Origin of Cutaneous DCs*

In contrast to LCs (Merad et al. 2002), dermal DCs have a limited lifespan and are continually replaced by circulating blood DC precursors (Liu et al. 2007). Indeed, although all dermal DC subsets proliferate, their proliferation does not compensate for their loss due to their migration to the LNs. This was clearly demonstrated by the presence of DCs of dual origin in both lymphoid and non-lymphoid organs of parabiotic mice (Bogunovic et al. 2006; Liu et al. 2007; Ginhoux et al. 2009), which are surgically attached mice sharing the same blood circulation but separate organs for long periods of time (Wright et al. 2001).

The identity of the circulating precursors that contribute to steady-state DC replenishment has recently been elucidated, establishing the existence of a DC-restricted lineage that originates from the bone marrow to give rise to all DCs (for review, Geissmann et al. 2010). The circulating precursors of DCs, named pre-DCs, migrate through the blood from the BM to the lymphoid (Liu et al. 2009) and non-lymphoid (Ginhoux et al. 2009) organs, where they differentiate into DCs. Upon adoptive transfer, pre-DCs were able to give rise to both CD103$^+$ and CD11b$^+$ DC subsets in the liver and the kidney, while monocytes contributed only to the CD11b$^+$ DC subset (Ginhoux et al. 2009). Unfortunately, it was not possible to assess the presence of pre-DCs as well as pre-DCs-derived DCs in the dermis upon adoptive transfer, owing to the low number of events, due to the low yield of recovery of dermal cells. While there is no reason to expect that the dermis should be different to the liver or kidney, a genetic tagging model of the pre-DC progeny should help to prove this formally.

3.4 *Differentiation Program of Cutaneous DC Subsets*

The key cytokines shown to play a role in DC development in mice and humans include Flt3L, granulocyte/macrophage colony stimulating factor (GM-CSF), macrophage colony stimulating factor (M-CSF), and transforming growth factor-beta 1 (TGF-β1). Here, we review the evidence indicating that each cutaneous DC subset is regulated by specific cytokines (Table 2), which control their proliferation, differentiation, and likely influence their immune functions.

Flt3L and its receptor (Flt3) play an instructive role in the commitment of hematopoietic progenitors into the DC-restricted lineage and their development, and also regulate the homeostasis of tissue CD103$^+$ DCs. Flt3L is ubiquitously secreted by multiple tissue stromal and endothelial cells and by activated T cells (Lyman et al. 1995; Lyman and Jacobsen 1998), while the expression of Flt3 is restricted to the DC lineage. Mice that are deficient in Flt3 and Flt3L have reduced numbers of pDCs and cDCs in lymphoid organs (McKenna et al. 2000; Waskow et al. 2008). In the non-lymphoid tissues of mice lacking Flt3, CD103$^+$ DCs were absent, and CD11b$^+$ DCs were partially reduced (Ginhoux et al. 2009). Intriguingly, DC defects are much more severe in mice that lack Flt3L compared to mice lacking Flt3, suggesting the presence of an alternative Flt3L receptor (Waskow et al. 2008; Ginhoux et al. 2009).

Granulocyte/macrophage colony stimulating factor is a key cytokine for the differentiation of hematopoietic progenitors (Caux et al. 1992; Inaba et al. 1992) and monocytes (Sallusto and Lanzavecchia 1994) into DCs in vitro in mice and humans. Surprisingly, GM-CSF does not play a role in the development of DCs in lymphoid organs in the steady-state, as mice lacking GM-CSF or its receptor do not exhibit clear DC defects in lymphoid organs (Vremec et al. 1997). In contrast, GM-CSF seems to fulfill a crucial role in the development of DCs in lymphoid organs during inflammation (Naik et al. 2006). These observations led to the suggestion that GM-CSF mainly controls the development of inflammatory DCs, although this also remains to be clearly established. In the skin, the absence of GM-CSF slightly compromises the development of dermal CD11b$^+$ DCs but not CD11b$^-$ DCs (Kingston et al. 2009). Interestingly, a lack of both Flt3L and GM-CSF leads to an additional reduction in the dermal CD11b$^+$ DC subset (Kingston et al. 2009), whereas the CD11b$^-$ DC subset is primarily affected by Flt3L deficiency (Ginhoux et al. 2009; Kingston et al. 2009). Altogether, these results suggest that each of the dermal DC subsets has differential cytokine requirements.

Macrophage colony stimulating factor is known as a key cytokine for macrophage development. Mice deficient for M-CSF or its receptor M-CSFR lack

Table 2 Cytokine requirements of the murine cutaneous DC subsets

	Langerhans cells	Dermal CD103$^+$ DC	Dermal CD11b$^+$ DC	Dermal DN DC	Inflammatory CD11b$^+$ DC	Dermal macrophage
Flt3L	–	++	+	ND	ND	–
CSF-1	+	–	+/–	ND	ND	+
GM-CSF	–	–	+/–	ND	ND	ND
TGF-β1	+	–	–	ND	ND	ND

several macrophage populations and develop osteopetrosis due to the absence of osteoclasts (Yoshida et al. 1990; Dai et al. 2002). M-CSF is secreted by endothelial, stromal cells, osteoblasts, and macrophages, and is detectable in serum in the steady-state, and increases upon inflammation (Hamilton 2008). The M-CSFR is expressed by the different precursors of the DC lineage (Geissmann et al. 2008). Using a reporter mouse model in which GFP is expressed under the M-CSFR promoter, M-CSFR was also shown to be expressed by lymphoid organ DCs (Macdonald et al. 2005). A more detailed analysis of M-CSFR expression among DC subsets using a similar reporter mouse model (Burnett et al. 2004), showed that only the $CD11b^+$ DC subset expresses GFP in lymphoid and non-lymphoid organs, including the dermis (Ginhoux et al. 2009). However, the exact correlation between GFP levels and protein expression in these mice remains unclear. Although M-CSFR was initially thought to be dispensable for DC development (Takahashi et al. 1993; Witmer-Pack et al. 1993), recent data from our laboratory established that it regulates the development of $CD103^-CD11b^+$ DCs in several tissues including the dermis. Indeed, a partial reduction of this DC subset is observed in M-CSFR KO mice and M-CSFR KO mixed chimeric mice (Ginhoux et al. 2009). In contrast, M-CSFR is dispensable for the development of $CD103^+$ DCs in these tissues, correlating with the absence of M-CSFR expression by $CD103^+$ DCs. The exact role of M-CSFR in DC homeostasis remains to be fully appreciated. It is possible that, similar to macrophages, M-CSFR controls the proliferation and survival of DCs in situ. Alternatively, the reduction in $CD11b^+$ DCs in M-CSFR KO mice could simply reflect the role of M-CSFR in monocyte differentiation into DCs, since monocytes contribute only to the $CD11b^+$ DC subset in non-lymphoid organs upon adoptive transfer (Ginhoux et al. 2009).

3.5 The LC Exception

In contrast to most DCs, LCs maintain themselves throughout life locally and independently of any input from blood circulating precursor in the steady-state (Merad et al. 2002). The proliferative capacity of LCs was recognized over 20 years ago (for a complete review, see Merad et al. 2008). About 1–2% epidermal LCs are actively proliferating at any given time, both in mice (Ginhoux unpublished data) and humans (Haniffa et al. 2009), although LCs are not as proliferative as their dermal DC counterparts which divide at the rate of 5% (Liu et al. 2007; Ginhoux et al. 2009).

The steady-state mechanisms governing local LC homeostasis and differentiation, as well as the precise nature of the LC progenitors, are yet to be fully elucidated; however, it seems clear that LCs are regulated differently to the rest of the DC lineage. Epidermal LCs develop normally in Flt3 and Flt3L-deficient mice (Ginhoux et al. 2009), as well as in GM-CSF and GM-CSF receptor deficient mice, according to flow cytometric data from our own laboratory (Ginhoux unpublished data). In contrast, Kingston et al. reported a slight decrease of LC numbers in Flt3L or GM-CSF KO mice using immunofluorescence microscopy (Kingston et al. 2009). In addition, as for dermal $CD11b^+$ DCs, M-CSFR is also required for the development of LCs, as mice that lack M-CSFR lack epidermal LCs (Ginhoux et al. 2006). Again, in contrast to other dermal DCs (Nagao et al. 2009), in vivo LC development is uniquely dependent on TGF-β1 (Borkowski et al. 1996a). In the skin, keratinocytes are a source of TGF-β1, and it has been assumed that exogenous TGF-β1 was critical for LC development (Borkowski et al. 1997). Recent data, however, have challenged this view, as mice in which only LCs are TGF-β1 deficient, are devoid of LCs (Kaplan et al. 2007), suggesting that an autocrine source of TGF-β1 controls LC development.

Langerhans cell homeostasis in inflamed skin depends on the type and strength of inflammation. In severe inflammatory injuries, such as ultraviolet (UV) light exposure (Merad et al. 2002) and cutaneous graft-versus-host disease (Merad et al. 2004), LCs are replaced by circulating blood precursors. These were shown to be Gr-1^{hi} blood monocytes in the case of UV irradiation (Ginhoux et al. 2006). In contrast, in the case of less severe injuries that lead to moderate LC loss, preserve the epidermal-dermal barrier integrity and are not accompanied by the release of the inflammatory chemokines that recruit blood monocytes, the remaining LCs have the potential to repopulate themselves locally and achieve complete recovery in 1–4 weeks following tissue injury. Local LC repopulation was first identified in minor skin injuries induced by exposure to skin sensitizers and to X-ray irradiation (Merad et al. 2002). Similar results were recently obtained in a mouse model of atopic dermatitis, in which LC proliferation is controlled by keratinocyte-derived signals (Chorro et al. 2009). Interestingly, LC loss in the absence of inflammation, as in the case of diphtheria toxin (DT)-mediated ablation in langerin-DT receptor (DTR) mice, leads to a much slower LC repopulation. This suggests that inflammatory signals may control the dynamics of LC proliferation. Such examples represent extreme scenarios, and it is conceivable that during common skin injuries, LC repopulation occurs from both local and blood-derived precursors. This is supported by data from a mouse model of HSV skin infection, which causes limited LC depletion in the infected dermatome and perhaps provides a more physiological scenario for understanding LC repopulation (Eidsmo et al. 2009). Whether Gr-1^{hi} monocyte-derived LCs are equivalent to steady-state LCs, in terms of homeostasis and function remains to be established.

Altogether, these data suggest that the development of each cutaneous DC subset is regulated by specific cytokine requirements. The extent to which ontogeny governs functional specialization is not precisely known, but a better understanding of the homeostasis of each DC population will provide the means to develop new vaccination approaches targeting the DC subsets most relevant for the induction of a protective immune response. The implications for the development of new vaccine strategies will be discussed later in the review.

4 Functional Specialization of Cutaneous DC Subsets

As described in the previous section, DCs form a heterogeneous population of cells that reside in both lymphoid and non-lymphoid tissues. Emerging evidence suggests that each individual DC subset may be associated with distinct or potentially overlapping functions in both tolerance and immunity. Several studies have already established the functional diversity of DC populations in the spleen. $CD4^+$ and $CD8\alpha^+$ spleen DC subsets express different toll-like receptors, lectin receptors, and phagocytic receptors (Edwards et al. 2003; Dudziak et al. 2007; Sancho et al. 2009) and possess distinct antigen processing and presentation machinery (Dudziak et al. 2007; Bougneres et al. 2009; Sancho et al. 2009; Savina et al. 2009). Spleen $CD4^+$ DCs interact preferentially with $CD4^+$ T cells, while $CD8\alpha^+$ DCs are specialized in the cross-presentation of cell-associated antigens to $CD8^+$ T cells (den Haan et al. 2000; Iyoda et al. 2002). In contrast to lymphoid organ DCs, the heterogeneity of DCs in non-lymphoid tissue has only been recently established. More importantly, accumulating evidence suggests that similar to lymphoid organ DCs, cutaneous DCs are functionally specialized and play different roles in skin immunity. In this section, we will provide an overview of the current understanding of the functional role of cutaneous DC subsets.

4.1 Challenging the LC Paradigm

Owing to their prominent localization at the interface with the environment, epidermal LCs were considered prototypic sentinel DCs and have long been thought to play a major role in the induction of skin immunity. However, studies showing that during HSV-1 infection of the skin, epidermal LCs are unable to present viral antigens to $CD8^+$ T cells in the draining LNs (Allan et al. 2003), together with studies showing that vaginal LCs do not induce $CD4^+$ T cell responses upon vaginal HSV-2 infection (Zhao et al. 2003), have challenged this view. In the HSV-1 study, only $CD8\alpha^+$ DCs isolated from skin draining LNs but not skin migratory DCs, were able to prime naïve virus-specific TCR transgenic T cells in an ex vivo DC/T-cell co-culture assay (Allan et al. 2003), leading to the hypothesis that the main role of skin migratory DCs is to transport and deliver antigens to LN $CD8\alpha^+$ DCs. However, upon skin injection of a non-cytolytic lentiviral vector, cutaneous migratory DCs are indeed able to present antigens to $CD8^+$ T cells (He et al. 2006). Therefore, it has been proposed that the inability of LCs to present HSV antigens could be due to the cytopathic properties of this virus.

4.2 Lessons from Animal Models

The development of mouse models expressing the Diphtheria toxin receptor (DTR), under the control of the murine langerin promoter (langerin-DTR/EGFP)

(Bennett et al. 2005; Kissenpfennig et al. 2005) have helped to address the role of langerin$^+$ DCs in skin immunity. In this model, administration of Diphtheria Toxin (DT) leads to the swift elimination of all langerin-expressing cells (LCs and CD103$^+$ DCs), without affecting the langerin$^-$ DC compartment and without skin or systemic toxicity (Bennett et al. 2005; Kissenpfennig et al. 2005). A model with constitutive LC depletion was also created, consisting of a transgenic mouse expressing the diphtheria toxin A under the control of the human langerin promoter (Kaplan et al. 2005). In this model, LCs are absent from birth while dermal CD103$^+$langerin$^+$ DCs remain unaffected because the human langerin promoter is not functional in these cells (Kaplan et al. unpublished data). Altogether, data collected from these studies, notably in the model of hapten-induced contact hypersensitivity responses, have provided evidence that the immunogenic potential of LCs in vivo depends on the dose and localization of the antigen. Overall, it seems that LCs are required to induce immune responses against epidermal antigens while dermal DCs are required to induce immune responses against dermal antigens (for review, Helft et al. 2010; Merad et al. 2008). Using a different approach, consisting of a BM chimera model in which MHCII molecule IE is either restricted to host LCs or donor derived dermal DCs and circulating DCs, it was demonstrated that both migratory epidermal DCs and dermal DCs can stimulate CD4$^+$ T-cell responses, although LCs were always less efficient (Shklovskaya et al. 2008).

More recently, the role of cutaneous DC subsets was revisited again in a HSV-1 skin infection model. In contrast to previous findings emphasizing the small contribution of cutaneous DCs to the presentation of viral antigens to CD8$^+$ T cells, recent results from the same group revealed that migratory CD103$^+$ DCs isolated from the skin draining LNs during the second wave of HSV-1 infection, were the most potent DC subset for the presentation of viral antigens to CD8$^+$ T cells (Bedoui et al. 2009b). The reasons for the discrepancy in the CD103$^+$ DC involvement between the first and second wave of infection remains unclear, but may be a reflection of the limitations of ex vivo co-culture assays that do not assess the contribution of DCs to the induction of antigen-specific immune responses in vivo. In contrast, all migratory DCs including LCs, dermal CD11b$^+$ DCs and CD103$^+$ DCs were able to present viral antigens to CD4$^+$ T cells in ex vivo culture assays, although CD11b$^+$ DCs were the major activators (Bedoui et al. 2009b), as shown previously (Zhao et al. 2003). These results suggest that although the three cutaneous DC populations acquire viral antigens, only CD103$^+$ DCs are able to present viral antigens to CD8$^+$ T cells. Whether CD103$^+$ DC interaction with CD8$^+$ T cells ex vivo results from direct presentation of viral antigens or cross-presentation of infected epithelial cells remains unclear.

In addition, dermal CD103$^+$ DCs were potent presenters of skin antigens in a transgenic mouse model expressing the model antigen ovalbumin under the keratinocyte K5 promoter (Bedoui et al. 2009b). This was confirmed in a later study by Henri et al. (2009). The preferential ability of CD103$^+$ DCs to interact with CD8$^+$ T cells was also observed in lung immunization models (del Rio et al. 2007; Kim and Braciale 2009), as well as in a model of cutaneous Leishmaniasis

(Brewig et al. 2009). In the latter study, depletion of langerin$^+$ DCs (including dermal DCs and skin draining LN resident CD8α^+ DCs) in langerin-DTR transgenic mice impaired the priming of CD8$^+$ T cells, while the CD4$^+$ T-cell response remained intact (Brewig et al. 2009). Similarly, Batf3$^{-/-}$ mice, which lack lymphoid organ CD8α^+ DCs but not CD11b$^+$CD4$^+$ DCs, are unable to mount efficient anti-viral CD8$^+$ T-cell responses during subcutaneous infection with West Nile virus. This failure in response was attributed to the absence of lymphoid organ CD8α^+ DCs (Hildner et al. 2008). However, dermal CD103$^+$ DCs are also absent in these mice and their exact contribution (relative to the LN resident CD8α^+ DCs) into the control of the infection remains to be examined. Altogether, these studies suggest that CD103$^+$ DCs play a crucial role in the priming of CD8$^+$ T cells, but the molecular mechanisms underlying this ability remain to be clearly established.

While the quest to identify the best cross-presenting dermal DC subset is the major focus of investigation, little is known about the control of the skin humoral response. A recent study from Udey's group, using the langerin-DTR mice coupled with gene gun immunizations, demonstrates that LCs and CD103$^+$ DCs have distinct roles in humoral responses to antigens delivered in the skin. This study showed that dermal langerin$^+$ DCs were required for optimal induction of humoral responses and production of IgG2a/c and IgG2b, while LCs were required for maximal IgG1 responses (Nagao et al. 2009).

In contrast to dermal CD103$^+$ DCs, dermal CD11b$^+$ DCs play a critical role in the local expansion of effector and regulatory T cells (McLachlan et al. 2009). Upon skin immunization with incomplete Freund's adjuvant to mimic chronic skin inflammation, dermal CD11b$^+$ DCs were shown to regulate cytokine production by CD4$^+$ effector T cells and regulatory T cells that infiltrated the inflamed skin (McLachlan et al. 2009). Whether these dermal CD11b$^+$ DCs derive from circulating monocytes or are tissue-resident DCs that present antigens for prolonged periods of time, as found in chronic inflamed lung (Julia et al. 2002) remains to be examined. In line with the monocytic origin of CD11b$^+$ DCs during skin inflammation, recent evidence suggests that CD11b$^+$ DCs recruited to the inflamed tissue efficiently stimulate memory CD8$^+$ T cells, while migratory DCs are inefficient in this respect (Wakim et al. 2008). In addition, these blood-derived DCs that accumulate in the dermis upon inflammation participate in tissue immunity. Monocyte-derived DCs were essential for the efficient priming of CD8$^+$ T cells and their differentiation into cytolytic effectors after skin immunization (Le Borgne et al. 2006; Leon et al. 2007), as well as the induction of protective T helper 1 responses against Leishmania (Leon et al. 2007).

In conclusion, it appears that CD103$^+$ DCs are involved in the priming of CD8$^+$ T cells, while CD11b$^+$ DCs, whether resident or inflammatory, play a key role at the site of the inflammation or infection. In addition, the role of LCs remains controversial. A system allowing the ablation of each DC subset in vivo with high specificity, but leaving the remaining subsets intact would help to establish the exact contribution of each individual dermal DC subset as well as lymphoid organ DCs in the induction of immune responses.

5 Perspectives: Implications for Vaccination

The strength of the immune responses to vaccination depends essentially on the vaccine type and dose, the use of adjuvant, and the route of administration. Indeed, all these parameters directly affect the appropriate targeting of cutaneous DCs and their activation, which in turn controls the initiation of an effective immune response. In this last section, we will discuss these parameters with regard to the recently appreciated complexity of the cutaneous DC network, as described earlier.

5.1 Antigen Delivery

Antigen may be delivered topically by stripping or chemical modification, transcutaneous immunization (TCI) or "vaccine patch," gene gun technology and intradermal injection, as reviewed extensively elsewhere in this special volume on intradermal immunization (Kim et al. 2011). Epicutaneous immunization primarily targets LCs although dermal DCs are also involved, while intradermal immunization mainly reaches dermal DCs (Flacher et al. 2009). Upon intradermal immunization with DNA-encoded antigens, dermal DCs were shown to be required for T-cell priming in vivo, though epidermal LCs were dispensable (Bedoui et al. 2009a). In addition, intradermal delivery of recombinant lentiviral vectors also induced potent and durable primary and memory T-cell immunity involving cutaneous migratory DCs (He et al. 2006). Interestingly, lentiviral vectors are able to efficiently transduce non-dividing cells, including DCs (He and Falo 2007), making them a potentially valuable tool. However, it is still unknown if lentiviral vectors transduce preferentially one or another skin DC subsets.

Gene gun delivery consists of plasmid DNA coated onto gold particles that are "bombarded" under helium pressure, allowing transepidermal immunization (Williams et al. 1991). Upon gene gun delivery, cutaneous DCs take up DNA-coated beads and migrate within 24 h to the LNs to induce immunity (Condon et al. 1996; Porgador et al. 1998). Using gene gun delivery combined with a genetic tagging strategy (transfer of plasmid encoding CRE recombinase in a loxP target mouse model), Garg et al. showed that the main population of skin DCs targeted by gene gun expressed langerin and reasonably identified them as LCs (Garg et al. 2003). However, dermal langerin$^+$CD103$^+$ DCs were not described at this time. A careful reevaluation of the skin DC subsets targeted by gene gun and their contribution to the immune responses needs to be performed, since in the langerin-DTR model, LCs were shown to be dispensable for the humoral and cell-mediated immunity elicited by gene gun immunization (Stoecklinger et al. 2007).

Transcutaneous immunization is a novel immunization strategy by which antigen and associated adjuvant are applied topically to intact and hydrated skin (Glenn et al. 1998a, b). TCI induces potent systemic immune responses that are protective against mucosal live virus challenge in mice (Glenn et al. 1998a, b; Belyakov et al. 2004) and in humans (Glenn et al. 2000). It is assumed that the cutaneously applied antigens are taken up by epidermal LCs but the precise nature of the DC subset that carries the antigen to the LNs and subsequently initiates adaptive immune responses remains elusive. Interestingly, in a murine model of sublingual TCI, the induction of the immune response was dependent on DCs, but independent of langerin$^+$ DCs, as depletion of langerin$^+$ cells did not abrogate the immune priming (Song et al. 2009). Moreover, although migratory DCs carried the antigen from the sublingual mucosa, both migratory DCs and resident CD8α^+ DCs were required to prime CD4$^+$ T cells in the LNs (Song et al. 2009).

5.2 DC Targeting

The functional specialization of DC subsets argues that subset targeting holds the key to the development of more effective intradermal immunization strategies. DC subsets in lymphoid organs differentially express toll-like receptors, lectin receptors, and endocytic/phagocytic receptors, which can be targeted to stimulate efficient antigen presentation. Antigen targeting to DCs can be achieved using chimeric monoclonal antibodies recognizing specific endocytic DC receptors, such as DEC-205 or 33D1, fused to antigens of interest (Hawiger et al. 2001; Bonifaz et al. 2002; Dudziak et al. 2007). Anti-DEC205-mediated antigen targeting allows efficient antigen processing and presentation into the MHC class I and II compartments and the induction of more potent antigen-specific T-cell immune responses (Hawiger et al. 2001; Bonifaz et al. 2002) compared to immunization with antigens alone (Bonifaz et al. 2004). Consistently, the use of DEC-205 specific HIV gag fusion antibody vaccine led to protective CD4$^+$ T-cell immunity in mice (Trumpfheller et al. 2006). Similarly, such strategy can improve the efficacy of DNA vaccines, which are weak when delivered alone. Indeed, DNA vaccines encoding antigens fused to single chain antibody fragment specific for DEC-205 or CD11c exhibit enhanced immunogenicity (Demangel et al. 2005; Nchinda et al. 2008).

Much less is known regarding the endocytic receptors that could be used for DC subset targeting in the dermis. However, since CD103$^+$ DCs appear to be developmentally and functionally related to CD8α^+ DCs (Bedoui et al. 2009b; Ginhoux et al. 2009), it is possible that they share similar endocytic receptor patterns. LCs and CD103$^+$ DCs express high DEC-205 levels and were more efficiently targeted than CD11b$^+$ DCs upon epicutaneous immunization with DEC-205 antibody (Flacher et al. 2009). This protocol required tape-stripping and so the preferential targeting of CD103$^+$ DCs over CD11b$^+$ DCs may have been influenced by their proximity to the epidermis. When anti-DEC-205 antibody was delivered intradermally, antigen was delivered to both dermal DCs and LCs (Flacher et al. 2010).

Other candidate receptors include the lectin CLEC9A, which is expressed by splenic CD8α^+ but not CD4$^+$ DCs and recently found to be required for the cross-presentation of necrotic cell-associated antigens to CD8$^+$ T cells (Sancho et al. 2009). CLEC9A is specifically expressed on dermal CD103$^+$ DCs but not CD11b$^+$ DCs (Helft et al. unpublished data) and could be potentially used to target this population. Consistently, CLEC9A targeting appears to be a promising strategy to enhance the efficiency of vaccines, even in the absence of adjuvant (Caminschi et al. 2008). The C-type lectin CLEC12A shares a similar profile of expression in lymphoid organs DCs and is also a candidate for targeting, although it has a greater requirement for adjuvant than CLEC9A (Lahoud et al. 2009). The precise expression profile of CLEC12A in dermal DC subsets is yet to be tested.

Finally, based on recent experimental data, it appears that migratory DC subsets inefficiently stimulate memory CD8$^+$ T cells, while inflammatory DCs are crucial for this process (Wakim et al. 2008). Therefore, optimization of vaccination schedules might demand different targeting during the initial prime and subsequent boost phases. Inflammatory DCs might play a specific role in promotion of durable memory responses, although a specific molecular target for these inflammatory DCs remains to be identified.

5.3 DC Poietins as Adjuvants

Adjuvants are used to potentiate the immune response and may function to gather and slowly release antigen at or near the site of administration or to directly or indirectly activate DCs to achieve effective antigen processing and/or presentation. The cytokines involved in DC homeostasis can also be used as molecular adjuvants as they influence the differentiation and maturation of specific DC subsets. Injection of mice with Flt3L leads to massive expansion of cDCs in lymphoid and non-lymphoid organs (Maraskovsky et al. 1996), including the dermis albeit at a lower magnitude (Ginhoux unpublished data). Induction of CD8$^+$ immune responses was significantly increased in mice pre-treated with Flt3L before immunization with anti-DEC-205 targeted antigen (Bozzacco et al. 2010). Similarly, Flt3L-treated mice developed significantly higher immune responses to a model antigen following TCI (Baca-Estrada et al. 2002), supporting the use of Flt3L to enhance vaccine efficacy in vivo.

Injection of GM-CSF is used in clinical studies to attract or generate DCs at disease sites (Dranoff et al. 1993; Simons et al. 1999). Intramuscular administration of a plasmid coding for GM-CSF, concomitantly to a plasmid coding for a rabies virus glycoprotein, enhanced the antibody response to the viral antigen (Xiang and Ertl 1995). This effect was observed only if both plasmids were injected simultaneously, reflecting the localized activity of the cytokine on DCs. Topical application of GM-CSF (as a protein adjuvant) can enhance TCI-mediated protective immunity in a model of genital and respiratory tract chlamydial infections (Hickey et al. 2005), however, it remains unclear which DC subset participates in the process.

5.4 *Visualization of DC Function: A Systematic Approach for Better Vaccines*

Over the past few years, our knowledge about DC function has increased dramatically. However, there is still limited temporal resolution to our understanding of the behavior of DC subsets during infections or after vaccination. Filling these gaps will permit a better appreciation of the sequence of events that lead to protective immunity in the natural in vivo microenvironment. Imaging of DCs by multiphoton microscopy has much promise in this regard.

Using transgenic CD11c-YFP mice, in which enhanced yellow fluorescent protein expression is driven by CD11c promoter (Lindquist et al. 2004), it is possible to perform intravital imaging of skin DCs over relatively long periods of time (>4 h) (Ng et al. 2008; Roediger et al. 2008). Using this model of multiphoton microscopy, it was shown that LCs are relatively sessile at resting state (Kissenpfennig et al. 2005; Nishibu et al. 2006), but remain capable of elongating their dendrites directly into epidermal tight junctions to sample external antigens (Kubo et al. 2009). In contrast, dermal DCs are highly motile and crawl extensively through extracellular spaces within the dermis, phagocytosing a prototypic skin pathogen, Leishmania major, through extension of their pseudopods (Ng et al. 2008).

These data reveal the orchestration of immunity through a complex interplay of specific DC functions. Notably, several novel features of LCs have been uncovered, such as the ability to act as sensors of external antigens located at epidermal tight junctions; to serve as reservoirs for concentrating external antigens and to provide instructing signals for other DCs through secretion of soluble factors or direct cell–cell interactions. Further insight into skin DC biology and new avenues for vaccine development are likely to follow.

6 Conclusion

Better understanding of the generation of immunity through DC biology continues to make an important impact in the field of vaccine science. Prominent among recent achievements is the unraveling of DC ontogeny and the deepening appreciation of DC functional specialization. The next challenge is to translate these discoveries into improved human vaccine strategies. A key step in this direction is to identify parallel DC subsets in human skin and to confirm as far as possible that the functional predictions from mice can be extrapolated between species. This will pave the way for the next generation of vaccines to induce directed immune responses of high potency and specificity.

References

Allan RS, Smith CM, Belz GT, van Lint AL, Wakim LM, Heath WR, Carbone FR (2003) Epidermal viral immunity induced by CD8alpha$^+$ dendritic cells but not by Langerhans cells. Science 301:1925–1928

Baca-Estrada ME, Ewen C, Mahony D, Babiuk LA, Wilkie D, Foldvari M (2002) The haemopoietic growth factor, Flt3L, alters the immune response induced by transcutaneous immunization. Immunology 107:69–76

Banchereau J, Briere F, Caux C, Davoust J, Lebecque S, Liu YJ, Pulendran B, Palucka K (2000) Immunobiology of dendritic cells. Annu Rev Immunol 18:767–811

Bedoui S, Davey GM, Lew AM, Heath WR (2009a) Equivalent stimulation of naive and memory CD8 T cells by DNA vaccination: a dendritic cell-dependent process. Immunol Cell Biol 87:255–259

Bedoui S, Whitney PG, Waithman J, Eidsmo L, Wakim L, Caminschi I, Allan RS, Wojtasiak M, Shortman K, Carbone FR, Brooks AG, Heath WR (2009b) Cross-presentation of viral and self antigens by skin-derived CD103$^+$ dendritic cells. Nat Immunol 10:488–495

Belyakov IM, Hammond SA, Ahlers JD, Glenn GM, Berzofsky JA (2004) Transcutaneous immunization induces mucosal CTLs and protective immunity by migration of primed skin dendritic cells. J Clin Invest 113:998–1007

Bennett CL, van Rijn E, Jung S, Inaba K, Steinman RM, Kapsenberg ML, Clausen BE (2005) Inducible ablation of mouse Langerhans cells diminishes but fails to abrogate contact hypersensitivity. J Cell Biol 169:569–576

Bogunovic M, Ginhoux F, Wagers A, Loubeau M, Isola LM, Lubrano L, Najfeld V, Phelps RG, Grosskreutz C, Scigliano E, Frenette PS, Merad M (2006) Identification of a radio-resistant and cycling dermal dendritic cell population in mice and men. J Exp Med 203:2627–2638

Bonifaz L, Bonnyay D, Mahnke K, Rivera M, Nussenzweig MC, Steinman RM (2002) Efficient targeting of protein antigen to the dendritic cell receptor DEC-205 in the steady state leads to antigen presentation on major histocompatibility complex class I products and peripheral CD8$^+$ T cell tolerance. J Exp Med 196:1627–1638

Bonifaz LC, Bonnyay DP, Charalambous A, Darguste DI, Fujii S, Soares H, Brimnes MK, Moltedo B, Moran TM, Steinman RM (2004) In vivo targeting of antigens to maturing dendritic cells via the DEC-205 receptor improves T cell vaccination. J Exp Med 199:815–824

Borkowski TA, Letterio JJ, Farr AG, Udey MC (1996a) A role for endogenous transforming growth factor beta 1 in Langerhans cell biology: the skin of transforming growth factor beta 1 null mice is devoid of epidermal Langerhans cells. J Exp Med 184:2417–2422

Borkowski TA, Nelson AJ, Farr AG, Udey MC (1996b) Expression of gp40, the murine homologue of human epithelial cell adhesion molecule (Ep-CAM), by murine dendritic cells. Eur J Immunol 26:110–114

Borkowski TA, Letterio JJ, Mackall CL, Saitoh A, Wang XJ, Roop DR, Gress RE, Udey MC (1997) A role for TGFbeta1 in Langerhans cell biology. Further characterization of the epidermal Langerhans cell defect in TGFbeta1 null mice. J Clin Invest 100:575–581

Bougneres L, Helft J, Tiwari S, Vargas P, Chang BH, Chan L, Campisi L, Lauvau G, Hugues S, Kumar P, Kamphorst AO, Dumenil AM, Nussenzweig M, MacMicking JD, Amigorena S, Guermonprez P (2009) A role for lipid bodies in the cross-presentation of phagocytosed antigens by MHC class I in dendritic cells. Immunity 31:232–244

Bozzacco L, Trumpfheller C, Huang Y, Longhi MP, Shimeliovich I, Schauer JD, Park CG, Steinman RM (2010) HIV gag protein is efficiently cross-presented when targeted with an antibody towards the DEC-205 receptor in Flt3 ligand-mobilized murine DC. Eur J Immunol 40:36–46

Brewig N, Kissenpfennig A, Malissen B, Veit A, Bickert T, Fleischer B, Mostbock S, Ritter U (2009) Priming of CD8$^+$ and CD4$^+$ T cells in experimental leishmaniasis is initiated by different dendritic cell subtypes. J Immunol 182:774–783

Burnett SH, Kershen EJ, Zhang J, Zeng L, Straley SC, Kaplan AM, Cohen DA (2004) Conditional macrophage ablation in transgenic mice expressing a Fas-based suicide gene. J Leukoc Biol 75:612–623

Bursch LS, Wang L, Igyarto B, Kissenpfennig A, Malissen B, Kaplan DH, Hogquist KA (2007) Identification of a novel population of Langerin^{+} dendritic cells. J Exp Med 204:3147–3156

Caminschi I, Proietto AI, Ahmet F, Kitsoulis S, Shin Teh J, Lo JC, Rizzitelli A, Wu L, Vremec D, van Dommelen SL, Campbell IK, Maraskovsky E, Braley H, Davey GM, Mottram P, van de Velde N, Jensen K, Lew AM, Wright MD, Heath WR, Shortman K, Lahoud MH (2008) The dendritic cell subtype-restricted C-type lectin Clec9A is a target for vaccine enhancement. Blood 112:3264–3273

Caux C, Dezutter-Dambuyant C, Schmitt D, Banchereau J (1992) GM-CSF and TNF-alpha cooperate in the generation of dendritic Langerhans cells. Nature 360:258–261

Cepek KL, Shaw SK, Parker CM, Russell GJ, Morrow JS, Rimm DL, Brenner MB (1994) Adhesion between epithelial cells and T lymphocytes mediated by E-cadherin and the alpha E beta 7 integrin. Nature 372:190–193

Chorro L, Sarde A, Li M, Woollard KJ, Chambon P, Malissen B, Kissenpfennig A, Barbaroux JB, Groves R, Geissmann F (2009) Langerhans cell (LC) proliferation mediates neonatal development, homeostasis, and inflammation-associated expansion of the epidermal LC network. J Exp Med 206:3089–3100

Condon C, Watkins SC, Celluzzi CM, Thompson K, Falo LD Jr (1996) DNA-based immunization by in vivo transfection of dendritic cells. Nat Med 2:1122–1128

Dai XM, Ryan GR, Hapel AJ, Dominguez MG, Russell RG, Kapp S, Sylvestre V, Stanley ER (2002) Targeted disruption of the mouse colony-stimulating factor 1 receptor gene results in osteopetrosis, mononuclear phagocyte deficiency, increased primitive progenitor cell frequencies, and reproductive defects. Blood 99:111–120

Del Rio ML, Rodriguez-Barbosa JI, Kremmer E, Forster R (2007) CD103^{-} and CD103^{+} bronchial lymph node dendritic cells are specialized in presenting and cross-presenting innocuous antigen to CD4^{+} and CD8^{+} T cells. J Immunol 178:6861–6866

Demangel C, Zhou J, Choo AB, Shoebridge G, Halliday GM, Britton WJ (2005) Single chain antibody fragments for the selective targeting of antigens to dendritic cells. Mol Immunol 42:979–985

Den Haan JM, Lehar SM, Bevan MJ (2000) CD8(+) but not CD8(−) dendritic cells cross-prime cytotoxic T cells in vivo. J Exp Med 192:1685–1696

Dranoff G, Jaffee E, Lazenby A, Golumbek P, Levitsky H, Brose K, Jackson V, Hamada H, Pardoll D, Mulligan RC (1993) Vaccination with irradiated tumor cells engineered to secrete murine granulocyte-macrophage colony-stimulating factor stimulates potent, specific, and long-lasting anti-tumor immunity. Proc Natl Acad Sci USA 90:3539–3543

Drexhage HA, Mullink H, de Groot J, Clarke J, Balfour BM (1979) A study of cells present in peripheral lymph of pigs with special reference to a type of cell resembling the Langerhans cell. Cell Tissue Res 202:407–430

Dudziak D, Kamphorst AO, Heidkamp GF, Buchholz VR, Trumpfheller C, Yamazaki S, Cheong C, Liu K, Lee HW, Park CG, Steinman RM, Nussenzweig MC (2007) Differential antigen processing by dendritic cell subsets in vivo. Science 315:107–111

Edwards AD, Chaussabel D, Tomlinson S, Schulz O, Sher A, Reis e Sousa C (2003) Relationships among murine CD11c(high) dendritic cell subsets as revealed by baseline gene expression patterns. J Immunol 171:47–60

Eidsmo L, Allan R, Caminschi I, van Rooijen N, Heath WR, Carbone FR (2009) Differential migration of epidermal and dermal dendritic cells during skin infection. J Immunol 182:3165–3172

Fan H, Lin Q, Morrissey GR, Khavari PA (1999) Immunization via hair follicles by topical application of naked DNA to normal skin. Nat Biotechnol 17:870–872

Flacher V, Sparber F, Tripp CH, Romani N, Stoitzner P (2009) Targeting of epidermal Langerhans cells with antigenic proteins: attempts to harness their properties for immunotherapy. Cancer Immunol Immunother 58:1137–1147

Flacher V, Tripp CH, Stoitzner P, Haid B, Ebner S, Del Frari B, Koch F, Park CG, Steinman RM, Idoyaga J, Romani N (2010) Epidermal Langerhans cells rapidly capture and present antigens from C-type lectin-targeting antibodies deposited in the dermis. J Invest Dermatol 130:755–762

Forster R, Schubel A, Breitfeld D, Kremmer E, Renner-Muller I, Wolf E, Lipp M (1999) CCR7 coordinates the primary immune response by establishing functional microenvironments in secondary lymphoid organs. Cell 99:23–33

Garg S, Oran A, Wajchman J, Sasaki S, Maris CH, Kapp JA, Jacob J (2003) Genetic tagging shows increased frequency and longevity of antigen-presenting, skin-derived dendritic cells in vivo. Nat Immunol 4:907–912

Geissmann F, Auffray C, Palframan R, Wirrig C, Ciocca A, Campisi L, Narni-Mancinelli E, Lauvau G (2008) Blood monocytes: distinct subsets, how they relate to dendritic cells, and their possible roles in the regulation of T-cell responses. Immunol Cell Biol 86:398–408

Geissmann F, Manz MG, Jung S, Sieweke MH, Merad M, Ley K (2010) Development of monocytes, macrophages, and dendritic cells. Science 327:656–661

Ginhoux F, Tacke F, Angeli V, Bogunovic M, Loubeau M, Dai XM, Stanley ER, Randolph GJ, Merad M (2006) Langerhans cells arise from monocytes in vivo. Nat Immunol 7:265–273

Ginhoux F, Collin MP, Bogunovic M, Abel M, Leboeuf M, Helft J, Ochando J, Kissenpfennig A, Malissen B, Grisotto M, Snoeck H, Randolph G, Merad M (2007) Blood-derived dermal langerin$^+$ dendritic cells survey the skin in the steady state. J Exp Med 204:3133–3146

Ginhoux F, Liu K, Helft J, Bogunovic M, Greter M, Hashimoto D, Price J, Yin N, Bromberg J, Lira SA, Stanley ER, Nussenzweig M, Merad M (2009) The origin and development of nonlymphoid tissue CD103$^+$ DCs. J Exp Med 206:3115–3130

Glenn GM, Rao M, Matyas GR, Alving CR (1998a) Skin immunization made possible by cholera toxin. Nature 391:851

Glenn GM, Scharton-Kersten T, Vassell R, Mallett CP, Hale TL, Alving CR (1998b) Transcutaneous immunization with cholera toxin protects mice against lethal mucosal toxin challenge. J Immunol 161:3211–3214

Glenn GM, Taylor DN, Li X, Frankel S, Montemarano A, Alving CR (2000) Transcutaneous immunization: a human vaccine delivery strategy using a patch. Nat Med 6:1403–1406

Hamilton JA (2008) Colony-stimulating factors in inflammation and autoimmunity. Nat Rev Immunol 8:533–544

Haniffa M, Ginhoux F, Wang XN, Bigley V, Abel M, Dimmick I, Bullock S, Grisotto M, Booth T, Taub P, Hilkens C, Merad M, Collin M (2009) Differential rates of replacement of human dermal dendritic cells and macrophages during hematopoietic stem cell transplantation. J Exp Med 206:371–385

Hawiger D, Inaba K, Dorsett Y, Guo M, Mahnke K, Rivera M, Ravetch JV, Steinman RM, Nussenzweig MC (2001) Dendritic cells induce peripheral T cell unresponsiveness under steady state conditions in vivo. J Exp Med 194:769–779

He Y, Falo LD Jr (2007) Lentivirus as a potent and mechanistically distinct vector for genetic immunization. Curr Opin Mol Ther 9:439–446

He Y, Zhang J, Donahue C, Falo LD Jr (2006) Skin-derived dendritic cells induce potent CD8(+) T cell immunity in recombinant lentivector-mediated genetic immunization. Immunity 24:643–656

Helft J, Ginhoux F, Bogunovic M, Merad M (2010) Origin and functional heterogeneity of non-lymphoid tissue dendritic cells in mice. Immunol Rev 234:55–75

Hemmi H, Yoshino M, Yamazaki H, Naito M, Iyoda T, Omatsu Y, Shimoyama S, Letterio JJ, Nakabayashi T, Tagaya H, Yamane T, Ogawa M, Nishikawa S, Ryoke K, Inaba K, Hayashi S, Kunisada T (2001) Skin antigens in the steady state are trafficked to regional lymph nodes by transforming growth factor-beta1-dependent cells. Int Immunol 13:695–704

Henri S, Poulin LF, Tamoutounour S, Ardouin L, Guilliams M, de Bovis B, Devilard E, Viret C, Azukizawa H, Kissenpfennig A, Malissen B (2009) CD207$^+$ CD103$^+$ dermal dendritic cells cross-present keratinocyte-derived antigens irrespective of the presence of Langerhans cells. J Exp Med 207(1):189–206

Hickey DK, Bao S, Ikeda LT, Carey AJ, Beagley KW (2005) Induction of anti-chlamydial mucosal immunity by transcutaneous immunization is enhanced by topical application of GM-CSF. Curr Mol Med 5:599–605

Hildner K, Edelson BT, Purtha WE, Diamond M, Matsushita H, Kohyama M, Calderon B, Schraml BU, Unanue ER, Diamond MS, Schreiber RD, Murphy TL, Murphy KM (2008) Batf3 deficiency reveals a critical role for CD8alpha^{+} dendritic cells in cytotoxic T cell immunity. Science 322:1097–1100

Inaba K, Inaba M, Romani N, Aya H, Deguchi M, Ikehara S, Muramatsu S, Steinman RM (1992) Generation of large numbers of dendritic cells from mouse bone marrow cultures supplemented with granulocyte/macrophage colony-stimulating factor. J Exp Med 176:1693–1702

Inaba K, Swiggard WJ, Inaba M, Meltzer J, Mirza A, Sasagawa T, Nussenzweig MC, Steinman RM (1995) Tissue distribution of the DEC-205 protein that is detected by the monoclonal antibody NLDC-145. I. Expression on dendritic cells and other subsets of mouse leukocytes. Cell Immunol 163:148–156

Iyoda T, Shimoyama S, Liu K, Omatsu Y, Akiyama Y, Maeda Y, Takahara K, Steinman RM, Inaba K (2002) The CD8^{+} dendritic cell subset selectively endocytoses dying cells in culture and in vivo. J Exp Med 195:1289–1302

Jakubzick C, Bogunovic M, Bonito AJ, Kuan EL, Merad M, Randolph GJ (2008) Lymph-migrating, tissue-derived dendritic cells are minor constituents within steady-state lymph nodes. J Exp Med 205:2839–2850

Jiang W, Swiggard WJ, Heufler C, Peng M, Mirza A, Steinman RM, Nussenzweig MC (1995) The receptor DEC-205 expressed by dendritic cells and thymic epithelial cells is involved in antigen processing. Nature 375:151–155

Julia V, Hessel EM, Malherbe L, Glaichenhaus N, O'Garra A, Coffman RL (2002) A restricted subset of dendritic cells captures airborne antigens and remains able to activate specific T cells long after antigen exposure. Immunity 16:271–283

Jung S, Aliberti J, Graemmel P, Sunshine MJ, Kreutzberg GW, Sher A, Littman DR (2000) Analysis of fractalkine receptor CX(3)CR1 function by targeted deletion and green fluorescent protein reporter gene insertion. Mol Cell Biol 20:4106–4114

Kabashima K, Banks TA, Ansel KM, Lu TT, Ware CF, Cyster JG (2005) Intrinsic lymphotoxin-beta receptor requirement for homeostasis of lymphoid tissue dendritic cells. Immunity 22:439–450

Kaplan DH, Jenison MC, Saeland S, Shlomchik WD, Shlomchik MJ (2005) Epidermal Langerhans cell-deficient mice develop enhanced contact hypersensitivity. Immunity 23:611–620

Kaplan DH, Li MO, Jenison MC, Shlomchik WD, Flavell RA, Shlomchik MJ (2007) Autocrine/paracrine TGFbeta1 is required for the development of epidermal Langerhans cells. J Exp Med 204:2545–2552

Kelly RH, Balfour BM, Armstrong JA, Griffiths S (1978) Functional anatomy of lymph nodes. II. Peripheral lymph-borne mononuclear cells. Anat Rec 190:5–21

Kenney RT, Frech SA, Muenz LR, Villar CP, Glenn GM (2004) Dose sparing with intradermal injection of influenza vaccine. N Engl J Med 351:2295–2301

Kim TS, Braciale TJ (2009) Respiratory dendritic cell subsets differ in their capacity to support the induction of virus-specific cytotoxic CD8^{+} T cell responses. PLoS One 4:e4204

Kim YC, Jarrahian C, Zehrung D, Mitragotri S, Prausnitz MR (2011) Delivery systems for intradermal vaccination. Curr Top Microbiol Immunol 351:77–112

Kingston D, Schmid MA, Onai N, Obata-Onai A, Baumjohann D, Manz MG (2009) The concerted action of GM-CSF and Flt3-ligand on in vivo dendritic cell homeostasis. Blood 114:835–843

Kissenpfennig A, Henri S, Dubois B, Laplace-Builhe C, Perrin P, Romani N, Tripp CH, Douillard P, Leserman L, Kaiserlian D, Saeland S, Davoust J, Malissen B (2005) Dynamics and function of Langerhans cells in vivo: dermal dendritic cells colonize lymph node areas distinct from slower migrating Langerhans cells. Immunity 22:643–654

Kubo A, Nagao K, Yokouchi M, Sasaki H, Amagai M (2009) External antigen uptake by Langerhans cells with reorganization of epidermal tight junction barriers. J Exp Med 206:2937–2946

Lahoud MH, Proietto AI, Ahmet F, Kitsoulis S, Eidsmo L, Wu L, Sathe P, Pietersz S, Chang HW, Walker ID, Maraskovsky E, Braley H, Lew AM, Wright MD, Heath WR, Shortman K, Caminschi I (2009) The C-type lectin Clec12A present on mouse and human dendritic cells can serve as a target for antigen delivery and enhancement of antibody responses. J Immunol 182:7587–7594

Le Borgne M, Etchart N, Goubier A, Lira SA, Sirard JC, van Rooijen N, Caux C, Ait-Yahia S, Vicari A, Kaiserlian D, Dubois B (2006) Dendritic cells rapidly recruited into epithelial tissues via CCR6/CCL20 are responsible for $CD8^+$ T cell crosspriming in vivo. Immunity 24:191–201

Leon B, Ardavin C (2008) Monocyte-derived dendritic cells in innate and adaptive immunity. Immunol Cell Biol 86:320–324

Leon B, Lopez-Bravo M, Ardavin C (2007) Monocyte-derived dendritic cells formed at the infection site control the induction of protective T helper 1 responses against Leishmania. Immunity 26:519–531

Lindquist RL, Shakhar G, Dudziak D, Wardemann H, Eisenreich T, Dustin ML, Nussenzweig MC (2004) Visualizing dendritic cell networks in vivo. Nat Immunol 5:1243–1250

Liu YJ (2005) IPC: professional type 1 interferon-producing cells and plasmacytoid dendritic cell precursors. Annu Rev Immunol 23:275–306

Liu K, Waskow C, Liu X, Yao K, Hoh J, Nussenzweig M (2007) Origin of dendritic cells in peripheral lymphoid organs of mice. Nat Immunol 8:578–583

Liu K, Victora GD, Schwickert TA, Guermonprez P, Meredith MM, Yao K, Chu FF, Randolph GJ, Rudensky AY, Nussenzweig M (2009) In vivo analysis of dendritic cell development and homeostasis. Science 324(5925):392–397

Lyman SD, Jacobsen SE (1998) c-kit ligand and Flt3 ligand: stem/progenitor cell factors with overlapping yet distinct activities. Blood 91:1101–1134

Lyman SD, James L, Escobar S, Downey H, de Vries P, Brasel K, Stocking K, Beckmann MP, Copeland NG, Cleveland LS et al. (1995) Identification of soluble and membrane-bound isoforms of the murine flt3 ligand generated by alternative splicing of mRNAs. Oncogene 10:149–157

Macdonald KP, Rowe V, Bofinger HM, Thomas R, Sasmono T, Hume DA, Hill GR (2005) The colony-stimulating factor 1 receptor is expressed on dendritic cells during differentiation and regulates their expansion. J Immunol 175:1399–1405

Maraskovsky E, Brasel K, Teepe M, Roux ER, Lyman SD, Shortman K, McKenna HJ (1996) Dramatic increase in the numbers of functionally mature dendritic cells in Flt3 ligand-treated mice: multiple dendritic cell subpopulations identified. J Exp Med 184:1953–1962

McKenna HJ, Stocking KL, Miller RE, Brasel K, De Smedt T, Maraskovsky E, Maliszewski CR, Lynch DH, Smith J, Pulendran B, Roux ER, Teepe M, Lyman SD, Peschon JJ (2000) Mice lacking flt3 ligand have deficient hematopoiesis affecting hematopoietic progenitor cells, dendritic cells, and natural killer cells. Blood 95:3489–3497

McLachlan JB, Catron DM, Moon JJ, Jenkins MK (2009) Dendritic cell antigen presentation drives simultaneous cytokine production by effector and regulatory T cells in inflamed skin. Immunity 30:277–288

Merad M, Manz MG, Karsunky H, Wagers A, Peters W, Charo I, Weissman IL, Cyster JG, Engleman EG (2002) Langerhans cells renew in the skin throughout life under steady-state conditions. Nat Immunol 3:1135–1141

Merad M, Hoffmann P, Ranheim E, Slaymaker S, Manz MG, Lira SA, Charo I, Cook DN, Weissman IL, Strober S, Engleman EG (2004) Depletion of host Langerhans cells before transplantation of donor alloreactive T cells prevents skin graft-versus-host disease. Nat Med 10:510–517

Merad M, Ginhoux F, Collin M (2008) Origin, homeostasis and function of Langerhans cells and other langerin-expressing dendritic cells. Nat Rev Immunol 8:935–947

Nagao K, Ginhoux F, Leitner WW, Motegi S, Bennett CL, Clausen BE, Merad M, Udey MC (2009) Murine epidermal Langerhans cells and langerin-expressing dermal dendritic cells are unrelated and exhibit distinct functions. Proc Natl Acad Sci USA 106:3312–3317

Naik SH, Metcalf D, van Nieuwenhuijze A, Wicks I, Wu L, O'Keeffe M, Shortman K (2006) Intrasplenic steady-state dendritic cell precursors that are distinct from monocytes. Nat Immunol 7(6):663–671

Nchinda G, Kuroiwa J, Oks M, Trumpfheller C, Park CG, Huang Y, Hannaman D, Schlesinger SJ, Mizenina O, Nussenzweig MC, Uberla K, Steinman RM (2008) The efficacy of DNA vaccination is enhanced in mice by targeting the encoded protein to dendritic cells. J Clin Invest 118:1427–1436

Nestle FO, Di Meglio P, Qin JZ, Nickoloff BJ (2009) Skin immune sentinels in health and disease. Nat Rev Immunol 9:679–691

Ng LG, Mrass P, Kinjyo I, Reiner SL, Weninger W (2008) Two-photon imaging of effector T-cell behavior: lessons from a tumor model. Immunol Rev 221:147–162

Nishibu A, Ward BR, Jester JV, Ploegh HL, Boes M, Takashima A (2006) Behavioral responses of epidermal Langerhans cells in situ to local pathological stimuli. J Invest Dermatol 126:787–796

Ohl L, Mohaupt M, Czeloth N, Hintzen G, Kiafard Z, Zwirner J, Blankenstein T, Henning G, Forster R (2004) CCR7 governs skin dendritic cell migration under inflammatory and steady-state conditions. Immunity 21:279–288

Porgador A, Irvine KR, Iwasaki A, Barber BH, Restifo NP, Germain RN (1998) Predominant role for directly transfected dendritic cells in antigen presentation to $CD8^+$ T cells after gene gun immunization. J Exp Med 188:1075–1082

Poulin LF, Henri S, de Bovis B, Devilard E, Kissenpfennig A, Malissen B (2007) The dermis contains $langerin^+$ dendritic cells that develop and function independently of epidermal Langerhans cells. J Exp Med 204:3119–3131

Randolph GJ, Ochando J, Partida-Sanchez S (2008) Migration of dendritic cell subsets and their precursors. Annu Rev Immunol 26:293–316

Roediger B, Ng LG, Smith AL, Fazekas de St Groth B, Weninger W (2008) Visualizing dendritic cell migration within the skin. Histochem Cell Biol 130:1131–1146

Sallusto F, Lanzavecchia A (1994) Efficient presentation of soluble antigen by cultured human dendritic cells is maintained by granulocyte/macrophage colony-stimulating factor plus interleukin 4 and downregulated by tumor necrosis factor alpha. J Exp Med 179:1109–1118

Sancho D, Joffre OP, Keller AM, Rogers NC, Martinez D, Hernanz-Falcon P, Rosewell I, Reis e Sousa C (2009) Identification of a dendritic cell receptor that couples sensing of necrosis to immunity. Nature 458:899–903

Savina A, Peres A, Cebrian I, Carmo N, Moita C, Hacohen N, Moita LF, Amigorena S (2009) The small GTPase Rac2 controls phagosomal alkalinization and antigen crosspresentation selectively in CD8(+) dendritic cells. Immunity 30:544–555

Shklovskaya E, Roediger B, Fazekas de St Groth B (2008) Epidermal and dermal dendritic cells display differential activation and migratory behavior while sharing the ability to stimulate $CD4^+$ T cell proliferation in vivo. J Immunol 181:418–430

Shortman K, Naik SH (2007) Steady-state and inflammatory dendritic-cell development. Nat Rev Immunol 7:19–30

Simons JW, Mikhak B, Chang JF, DeMarzo AM, Carducci MA, Lim M, Weber CE, Baccala AA, Goemann MA, Clift SM, Ando DG, Levitsky HI, Cohen LK, Sanda MG, Mulligan RC, Partin AW, Carter HB, Piantadosi S, Marshall FF, Nelson WG (1999) Induction of immunity to prostate cancer antigens: results of a clinical trial of vaccination with irradiated autologous prostate tumor cells engineered to secrete granulocyte-macrophage colony-stimulating factor using ex vivo gene transfer. Cancer Res 59:5160–5168

Song JH, Kim JI, Kwon HJ, Shim DH, Parajuli N, Cuburu N, Czerkinsky C, Kweon MN (2009) CCR7-CCL19/CCL21-regulated dendritic cells are responsible for effectiveness of sublingual vaccination. J Immunol 182:6851–6860

Steinman RM, Hawiger D, Nussenzweig MC (2003) Tolerogenic dendritic cells. Annu Rev Immunol 21:685–711

Stoecklinger A, Grieshuber I, Scheiblhofer S, Weiss R, Ritter U, Kissenpfennig A, Malissen B, Romani N, Koch F, Ferreira F, Thalhamer J, Hammerl P (2007) Epidermal Langerhans cells are dispensable for humoral and cell-mediated immunity elicited by gene gun immunization. J Immunol 179:886–893

Stutte S, Jux B, Esser C, Forster I (2008) CD24a expression levels discriminate Langerhans cells from dermal dendritic cells in murine skin and lymph nodes. J Invest Dermatol 128: 1470–1475

Sung SS, Fu SM, Rose CE Jr, Gaskin F, Ju ST, Beaty SR (2006) A major lung CD103 (alphaE)-beta7 integrin-positive epithelial dendritic cell population expressing Langerin and tight junction proteins. J Immunol 176:2161–2172

Takahara K, Omatsu Y, Yashima Y, Maeda Y, Tanaka S, Iyoda T, Clausen BE, Matsubara K, Letterio J, Steinman RM, Matsuda Y, Inaba K (2002) Identification and expression of mouse Langerin (CD207) in dendritic cells. Int Immunol 14:433–444

Takahashi K, Naito M, Shultz LD, Hayashi S, Nishikawa S (1993) Differentiation of dendritic cell populations in macrophage colony-stimulating factor-deficient mice homozygous for the osteopetrosis (op) mutation. J Leukoc Biol 53:19–28

Tang A, Amagai M, Granger LG, Stanley JR, Udey MC (1993) Adhesion of epidermal Langerhans cells to keratinocytes mediated by E-cadherin. Nature 361:82–85

Trumpfheller C, Finke JS, Lopez CB, Moran TM, Moltedo B, Soares H, Huang Y, Schlesinger SJ, Park CG, Nussenzweig MC, Granelli-Piperno A, Steinman RM (2006) Intensified and protective $CD4^+$ T cell immunity in mice with anti-dendritic cell HIV gag fusion antibody vaccine. J Exp Med 203:607–617

Valladeau J, Saeland S (2005) Cutaneous dendritic cells. Semin Immunol 17:273–283

Vremec D, Lieschke GJ, Dunn AR, Robb L, Metcalf D, Shortman K (1997) The influence of granulocyte/macrophage colony-stimulating factor on dendritic cell levels in mouse lymphoid organs. Eur J Immunol 27:40–44

Wakim LM, Waithman J, van Rooijen N, Heath WR, Carbone FR (2008) Dendritic cell-induced memory T cell activation in nonlymphoid tissues. Science 319:198–202

Waskow C, Liu K, Darrasse-Jeze G, Guermonprez P, Ginhoux F, Merad M, Shengelia T, Yao K, Nussenzweig M (2008) The receptor tyrosine kinase Flt3 is required for dendritic cell development in peripheral lymphoid tissues. Nat Immunol 9:676–683

Williams RS, Johnston SA, Riedy M, DeVit MJ, McElligott SG, Sanford JC (1991) Introduction of foreign genes into tissues of living mice by DNA-coated microprojectiles. Proc Natl Acad Sci USA 88:2726–2730

Witmer-Pack MD, Hughes DA, Schuler G, Lawson L, McWilliam A, Inaba K, Steinman RM, Gordon S (1993) Identification of macrophages and dendritic cells in the osteopetrotic (op/op) mouse. J Cell Sci 104(Pt 4):1021–1029

Wright DE, Wagers AJ, Gulati AP, Johnson FL, Weissman IL (2001) Physiological migration of hematopoietic stem and progenitor cells. Science 294:1933–1936

Xiang Z, Ertl HC (1995) Manipulation of the immune response to a plasmid-encoded viral antigen by coinoculation with plasmids expressing cytokines. Immunity 2:129–135

Yoshida H, Hayashi S, Kunisada T, Ogawa M, Nishikawa S, Okamura H, Sudo T, Shultz LD (1990) The murine mutation osteopetrosis is in the coding region of the macrophage colony stimulating factor gene. Nature 345:442–444

Zhao X, Deak E, Soderberg K, Linehan M, Spezzano D, Zhu J, Knipe DM, Iwasaki A (2003) Vaginal submucosal dendritic cells, but not Langerhans cells, induce protective Th1 responses to herpes simplex virus-2. J Exp Med 197:153–162

Insight into the Immunobiology of Human Skin and Functional Specialization of Skin Dendritic Cell Subsets to Innovate Intradermal Vaccination Design

M. B. M. Teunissen, M. Haniffa and M. P. Collin

Abstract Dendritic cells (DC) are the key initiators and regulators of any immune response which determine the outcome of $CD4^+$ and $CD8^+$ T-cell responses. Multiple distinct DC subsets can be distinguished by location, phenotype, and function in the homeostatic and inflamed human skin. The function of steady-state cutaneous DCs or recruited inflammatory DCs is influenced by the surrounding cellular and extracellular skin microenvironment. The skin is an attractive site for vaccination given the extended local network of DCs and the easy access to the skin-draining lymph nodes to generate effector T cells and immunoglobulin-producing B cells for long-term protective immunity. In the context of intradermal vaccination we describe in this review the skin-associated immune system, the characteristics of the different skin DC subsets, the mechanism of antigen uptake and presentation, and how the properties of DCs can be manipulated. This knowledge is critical for the development of intradermal vaccine strategies and supports the concept of intradermal vaccination as a superior route to the conventional intramuscular or subcutaneous methods.

M. B. M. Teunissen (✉)
Department of Dermatology, Academic Medical Center,
University of Amsterdam, Meibergdreef 9,
1105 AZ Amsterdam, The Netherlands
e-mail: m.b.teunissen@amc.uva.nl

M. Haniffa · M. P. Collin
Institute of Cellular Medicine, Newcastle University,
Newcastle upon Tyne, NE2 4HH, UK

Current Topics in Microbiology and Immunology (2012) 351: 25–76
DOI: 10.1007/82_2011_169

Published Online: 11 August 2011

Contents

1 Introduction

1.1 Skin as Defense Organ

The skin is the outermost peripheral tissue that covers the entire body surface. One of its major functions is to protect the interior from all kinds of dangers from the outside world. As these insults are highly diverse the skin is equipped with a variety of functional mechanisms to maintain homeostasis. The continuous growth and tightly-regulated differentiation of the epidermal layer of the skin establishes a solid physical barrier which precludes invasion by pathogens and penetration by chemical agents, but also avoids dehydration. The regeneration capacity maintains tissue integrity and the presence of melanin and other photoreceptors reduce the detrimental effects of ultraviolet radiation. The skin also harbors subtle systems such as temperature control and tactile sense, which are essential to prevent physical insults by excessive heat, cold, pressure, vibrations, electricity, etc. Remarkably, despite having evolved into a barrier to protect from microbial assaults, the skin serves as a niche for the commensal skin flora, mainly consisting of bacteria, thereby allowing close symbiosis of a myriad of potentially harmful microbes.

All delicate and complex defense functions are concomitantly operational in healthy skin and provide a permanent broad defense. However, the skin is vulnerable to damage as the protective barrier is easily disrupted by insults, like incisions, insect bites, aggressive chemicals, and burns, which allow the entry of hostile microbes. In order to resist the attack of an invading pathogen, the skin possesses a highly sophisticated immune system; an initial, rapid, and robust response in the form of pre-stored antimicrobials and inflammatory mediators which is followed by the generation of long-term memory cells that provide resistance to subsequent infection with that microbe. The latter situation can be mimicked by vaccination, whereby attenuated or dead microbes or microbial components are administered under controlled conditions.

1.2 Skin as Target for Vaccine Administration

The concept of using skin as a route for vaccination has been acknowledged for a long time. Back in 1796, Edward Jenner established variolation, implying inoculation of the related, but safer, vaccinia virus into the skin to generate protection against the potentially lethal variola virus, the etiologic agent of smallpox (Eyler 2003). The term vaccination is referring to this milestone event in the history of medicine. Variolation was based on Jenner's observation that milkmaids who had caught cowpox through contact with cowpox pustules became resistant to smallpox. At the end of the 1960s the World Health Organisation successfully launched a global program to extirpate smallpox and in 1980 the World Health Assembly officially announced that the disease was eradicated worldwide (Alcami et al. 2010). Variolation is performed by scarification with a special bifurcated needle, designed to adsorb a tiny droplet of the vaccine and to superficially damage the skin through firm scratching perpendicularly to the skin till traces of blood appear. Scarification as a method of vaccinia-virus vaccination appears to be superior to subcutaneous and intramuscular injection in the induction of vaccinia-virus-specific immune responses (McClain et al. 1997). Another important historical step was made in 1910 by Charles Mantoux who reported cutaneous delivery of tuberculin as a diagnostic test for tuberculosis. Mantoux (1910) introduced the technique for intradermal (ID) injection using a small conventional needle. Keeping the bevel upward the needle is pushed into the skin at a slight angle, almost parallel to the skin surface, till the bevel is completely inserted. Then, slowly, the vaccine can be administered into the dermis resulting in a local elevation of the skin, also referred to as wheal. To date this is still the most widely used technique for ID delivery of vaccines.

Although the proof of principle for immunization via the skin had been established more than two centuries ago, vaccine delivery via the skin has made very little progress. Only rabies and Bacille Calmette–Guérin (BCG) vaccines are currently licensed to be delivered via the ID route. To date, the majority of the vaccines are still administered by intramuscular injection, which is striking as conclusive scientific evidence that muscles are optimal targets for vaccination is lacking. Over the last few decades, significant advances in immunology have been made. A major discovery is the critical role for dendritic cells (DCs) in the generation of immunity and that the skin harbors a widespread network of these cells. Moreover the skin is an easily accessible organ and contains a well-developed immune system with extensive connections to regional lymphatic tissues. For these reasons the skin has gained recognition as an attractive target for immunization. In order to utilize the full potential of ID vaccination, a thorough understanding of cutaneous immunology, in particular the function of skin DCs is needed. To this end we summarize current views on human skin DC subsets, and for a better grasp of the subject, we first describe the basic organization and features of normal human skin, all in the context of ID vaccination.

2 Immunobiology of Human Skin

2.1 Functional Anatomy

The skin forms the boundary between the body and the external environment and encompasses three primary layers with different features and functions: epidermis, dermis and hypodermis (Fuchs and Raghavan 2002; Segre 2006; Proksch et al. 2008). The epidermis, which is renewed every 4 weeks, is the thinnest and outermost part consisting of stratified squamous epithelium and is devoid of blood and lymph vessels (Fig. 1a, b). Its thickness varies between 50–150 μm depending on the site of the body. The epidermis, comprised primarily of keratinocytes, is subdivided into the layers stratum basale, stratum spinosum, stratum granulosum, and stratum corneum, each corresponding to a distinct differentiation stage of a keratinocyte (Fuchs and Raghavan 2002; Segre 2006; Proksch et al. 2008). Progenitor keratinocytes (distinct to epidermal stem cells) present in the basal layer have a high potential to multiply and divide symmetrically or asymmetrically, the latter results in some daughter cells remaining proliferative while others undergo terminal differentiation (Clayton et al. 2007). The progenitor-derived keratinocytes are thought to be sufficient to renew the overlying epidermis under normal homeostatic conditions, but if the epidermis is destroyed by injury, stem cells from the hair follicle bulge may be recruited to reconstitute the tissue (Clayton et al. 2007; Ito et al. 2005). Keratinocytes progressively differentiate while slowly displacing outward. The stratum corneum (cornified layer) is the most superficial layer of the epidermis and is formed by terminally differentiated, flattened, dead keratinocytes (now called corneocytes) that have lost their nuclei and cytoplasmic organelles (Fuchs and Raghavan 2002; Segre 2006; Proksch et al. 2008). The tightly packed corneocytes are interconnected by corneodesmosomes

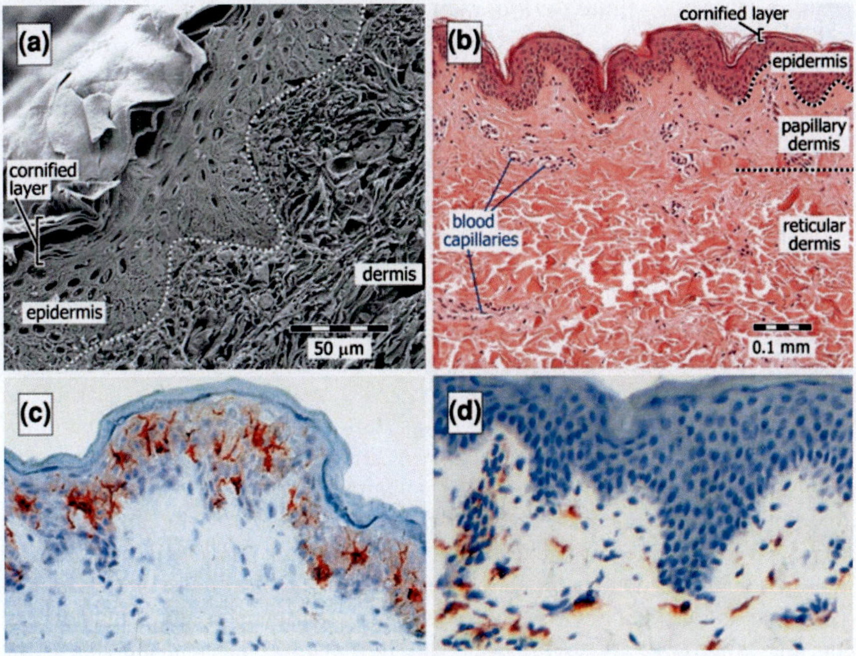

Fig. 1 **a** Transverse view of healthy human skin showing the squamous cornified layer, the epidermal layer of compact clustered keratinocytes and the abundance of collagen and elastin fibers in the dermis with potential space for ID vaccination. The basement membrane zone is marked with a *white dotted line*. Scanning electron micrograph by courtesy of Kristian Pfaller and Nikolaus Romani, Innsbruck Medical University. **b** Haematoxylin and eosin staining of normal human skin showing relative thickness of the epidermis to the dermis, which is only partially depicted. **c** LCs in a skin section are visualized as *red cells* by immunoperoxidase staining using anti-CD1a antibodies. **d** DC-SIGN staining of human skin identifying (in *red*) DCs and macrophages in the dermis

and surrounded by insoluble lipid bilayers, all together forming a virtually impermeable, highly hydrophobic physical barrier. Another crucial barrier in the epidermis is formed by the bicellular and tricellular tight junctions, which are present in the lateral membranes of keratinocytes in the stratum granulosum, composed of flattened living keratinocyte sheets (Brandner et al. 2002; Kubo et al. 2009). This tight junction-based intercellular sealing is indispensable to limit desiccation and to prevent transit of small molecules. The cornified layer together with the tight junctions make it hard for molecules larger than 500–600 Da to penetrate the skin (Bos and Meinardi 2000). These features are essential for survival, but limit the applicability of topical medicines for therapy or the possibilities of transdermal vaccination. In addition to keratinocytes, the living normal epidermis contains low but significant numbers of langerhans cells (LCs) (Fig. 1c) and melanin-producing melanocytes (only in the stratum basale). In contrast to the epidermis in mice, the human epidermis is sparsely populated with T cells.

The epidermis is firmly fixed to the basement membrane, which separates the epidermis from the underlying connective tissue called the dermis (Fuchs and Raghavan 2002; Segre 2006; Proksch et al. 2008). Because of the ridged shape of the epidermis, the dermo-epidermal junction has an undulating appearance in cross-sections of the skin (Fig. 1). The dermis varies in thickness (from 1 mm on the face to 4 mm on the back) and is mainly composed of a mucopolysaccharide gel held together by a collagen- and elastin- containing fibrous network rendering the tissue tough and resilient. The dermis has a rich blood supply, excellent lymph drainage, and also contains nerves and skin appendages like sweat glands, sebaceous glands, hair follicles, and arrector pili muscles that upon contraction cause hairs to stand on end (goose bumps). In addition, the homeostatic dermis harbors fibroblasts, mast cells, macrophages, DCs (Fig. 1d), natural killer (NK) cells, natural killer T (NKT) cells, and mainly $\alpha\beta$ T cells (i.e. T cells bearing the heterodimeric T-cell receptors (TCRs) consisting of an α and β chain), and rarely $\gamma\delta$ T cells (TCRs consist of $\gamma\delta$ chain heterodimers) as residents, but the number and composition of the cutaneous cell population substantially alter in pathologic conditions such as inflammation (Nestle et al. 2009). During inflammation, the phenotype and function of resident cells will change, a variety of new leukocytes (e.g. granulocytes, monocytes, and additional DCs and T cells) will be recruited via the capillaries which will be accompanied by an increase of cells emigrating from the skin via the lymph vessels. The third primary layer of the skin is the hypodermis, the subcutaneous adipose layer, which comprises connective tissue interspersed with lobules of fat cells, called adipocytes, but also contains fibroblasts, macrophages, small blood vessels, and nerve tissue (Kanitakis 2002; Eto et al. 2009). Remarkably, despite being the largest component of the skin, the hypodermis has received scant immunological attention. Adipocytes supply fatty acids to their microenvironment. The composition of fatty acids can alter during inflammation, thereby affecting the function of immune cells within the skin (e.g. DCs), which constantly sample lipids from their surrounding environment. Cytokines released by adipocytes may also modulate the surrounding immune cells. The role of adipocytes in modulating skin immune responses has been little explored.

A prerequisite for successful cutaneous delivery of vaccines is that the vaccine antigens can reach the skin DCs, as these cells are essential to initiate immunization (Steinman and Banchereau 2007). The DCs in the epidermis are located just above the stratum basale and are called LCs (Fig. 1c) (Teunissen 2005). For many years LCs were designated as the major antigen-presenting cells in the skin. Now it is clear that the dermal DCs (DDCs) are also important with some reports suggesting that DDCs (Fig. 1d) are more important than LCs in immunity. The dermis harbors several DC subsets and the complexity of all these subsets is just beginning to be understood (Teunissen 2005). A detailed description of all DC subsets in human skin will be provided in one of the following sections. Because the cornified layer and tight junctions limit the penetration of molecules larger than 500–600 Da, vaccines cannot simply be applied onto the skin. Both barriers need to be disrupted to enable vaccine antigens to enter the skin. Scratching with a bifurcated needle till bleeding is visible, as is done during variolation, is an old-school and rather crude though effective method. However, only a very limited volume of a vaccine (few μl) can be applied into this superficial wound and wound healing processes may interfere with vaccination efficiency. Delivery of the vaccine with a small needle directly into the dermis, following the Mantoux technique, provides not only a more suitable way for reproducible accurate dosage administration, it also permits administration of aliquots up to 200 μl into the interstitial space between the loosely intertwined collagen and elastin fibers. New technological developments in ID vaccination devices, such as micro-needles and nano-needles, provide a subtler, minimally destructive, and less painful way to get the vaccine into the skin. The drawback of this strategy is the small administrable volume. New developments in technologies for vaccine delivery into the skin are described in another review in this volume of current topics in microbiology and immunology (Kim et al. 2011).

2.2 *Skin-Associated Innate and Adaptive Immunology*

In the mid 1980s the concepts of "skin-associated lymphoid tissue" and "skin immune system" were launched, both describing the cutaneous content of immune cells and molecules that are in dynamic equilibrium with the systemic immune system. This equlibrium is maintained by a variety of immune cells, which circulate through blood vessels and emigrate via lymph vessels to the draining lymph nodes (Streilein 1983; Bos and Kapsenberg 1986). It is currently widely accepted that the skin comprises a well-organized regional immune system, which is responsible for the maintenance of tolerance and homeostasis in the steady state, though at the same time alert to potential danger and capable of exerting and regulating powerful defense responses. Both the innate and adaptive arms of the immune system are represented in the skin. Provision of quick non-specific resistance to pathogens is a hallmark of innate immunity. Mechanisms for this prompt protection include phagocytosis and secretion of special molecules, such as antimicrobial peptides, microbial-binding lectins, complement, and pro-inflammatory cytokines and chemokines, which stimulate and attract other immune cells. The principal phagocytes in the skin are the dermal-resident macrophages and the non-resident neutrophilic granulocytes, which can be rapidly recruited from the circulation. Both cell types can kill and degrade ingested pathogens in the endosome/lysosome pathway. DDCs can also take up particles like bacteria or parasites, although not as extensively as macrophages and granulocytes, whereas LCs have a limited phagocytic capacity. In response to infection, contact-allergens, ultraviolet radiation, or other kinds of perturbation of the epidermal homeostasis, keratinocytes produce large amounts of antimicrobial peptides, pro-inflammatory cytokines, and chemokines (Albanesi et al. 2005; Keller et al. 2008; Glaser et al. 2009; Lai and Gallo 2009). As an innate defense response DCs can produce large amounts of IL-12, TNF-α, and type I interferons

(IFNs). In addition (Blanco et al. 2008), DCs can attract and activate other innate lymphocytes, like NK cells NKT cells and $\gamma\delta$ T-cells (Degli-Esposti and Smyth 2005; Fujii et al. 2007). These innate lymphocytes then quickly release large quantities of IFN-γ and upregulate their cytotoxic activity towards cells that express foreign antigen or cells that lack or have down-regulated self-identifying MHC class I molecules, which are signatures induced by pathogens or transformation. IFN-γ amplifies the cytokine production of DCs and potentiates the intracellular killing of the phagocytes. The innate leukocytes present in normal skin will not only respond to pathogens but also to ID administered vaccines.

Specificity and memory are the hallmarks of adaptive immunity, aiming to protect the host from subsequent infections with the same microbe by means of faster and stronger responses and especially tailored to the type of pathogen. The key players in the adaptive immunity are a large variety of $\alpha\beta$ T cells and the immunoglobulin-producing B cells. T cells can be divided into two main subgroups, based on the expression of either CD4 or CD8. The latter group, the cytotoxic T cells, can kill infected or transformed target cells by production of granzyme and perforin. $CD4^+$ T cells encompass the families of T helper (Th) cells and regulatory T cells (Stockinger et al. 2006; Reiner et al. 2007; McGeachy and Cua 2008). There are different lineages of Th cells that are specialized to secrete distinct sets of cytokines to determine and enhance the effector functions of other innate and adaptive immune cells. So far Th1, Th2, Th17, Th22 cells, and T follicular helper cells (Tfh) have been described, but it is to be expected that more types will be defined. Th1 cells produce IFN-γ that enhances clearance of viruses and intracellular bacteria (Mosmann and Coffman 1989; Del Prete et al. 1991; Ansel et al. 2003); Th2 cells are characterized by production of IL-4, IL-5, and IL-13 that promote antibody-mediated immunity and clearance of extracellular parasites (Mosmann and Coffman 1989; Del Prete et al. 1991; Ansel et al. 2003); Th17 typically produce IL-17 (also known as IL-17A), often in combination with IL-22, and play a role in immunity against several extracellular bacteria and fungi (Harrington et al. 2005; Romagnani et al. 2009); Th22, which produce IL-22, but neither IL-17 nor IFN-γ, have only recently been described (Duhen et al. 2009; Trifari et al. 2009) and have been suggested to have a critical role in the maintenance of normal barrier homeostasis (antimicrobial immunity and tissue repair) (Sonnenberg et al. 2011); Tfh, which home in the lymph nodal follicles, produce IL-21 that is important not only in germinal center formation and induction of immunoglobulin production in B cells, but also for the development of Tfh themselves (King et al. 2008; Crotty 2011). All these types of Th, except for Tfh cells, can be observed in normal human skin. Of note, the distinction between different Th types is not a strict black and white situation, as it is clear that there are T-cell clones that simultaneously produce cytokines characteristic of two different lineages, for example T cells producing both IL-4 and IFN-γ (designated as Th0) or both IL-17 and IFN-γ (Sallusto and Lanzavecchia 2009). It may very well be that T cells committed to a certain lineage maintain the memory of the originally imprinted cytokine, but at the same time have the flexibility to acquire expression of additional cytokines if stimulated under appropriate polarizing conditions. The group of $CD4^+$ regulatory T cells comprises the naturally occurring $Foxp3^+CD25^{high}$ regulatory T cells and inducible regulatory T cells ($Foxp3^+CD25^{high}$ or IL-10-producing $Foxp3^-CD25^{medium}$), all of which are able to suppress effector functions of other T cells via secretion of suppressive cytokines TGF-β or IL-10 or by cell–cell contact in a cytokine-independent fashion (Sakaguchi et al. 2010; Campbell and Koch 2011). Regulatory T cells are thought to play a pivotal role in inhibiting autoimmune responses and preventing excessive immune responses. Analysis of skin-derived T cells revealed that approximately 20% display the phenotype of regulatory T cells ($CD4^+CD25^{high}CD69^-$) with functional regulatory activity (proliferation inhibition of $CD25^-$ T cells) (Clark et al. 2006). This figure is in line with immunohistochemical analysis of skin sections showing approximately 25% of $CD4^+CD25^+Foxp3^+$ cells within the cutaneous T-cell network (de Boer et al. 2007).

Normal human skin is devoid of B cells but does contain considerable numbers of T cells, usually around blood capillaries and skin appendages in the dermis and the majority expressing CD4. In contrast, in homeostatic epidermis the presence of T cells is rare and $CD8^+$ T cells outnumber $CD4^+$ T cells (Foster et al. 1990). It has been estimated that the entire skin of a healthy adult individual harbors a remarkable high number of approximately 2×10^{10} T cells, which is twice as many as the total number of T cells in the blood circulation (Clark et al. 2006). The TCR repertoire of skin-resident T cells is highly diverse and is only slightly less than that of peripheral blood T cells. Almost all skin-homing T cells express cutaneous lymphocyte-associated antigen (CLA), the chemokine receptors CCR4 and CCR6, and LFA-1 (CD11a/CD18), which are pivotal elements for selective migration into the skin, where their respective ligands E-selectin, chemokines CCL17 and CCL20, and ICAM-1 (CD54) are constitutively and inducibly expressed by endothelial cells of the post-capillary venules in the skin (Campbell et al. 2003; Schon et al. 2003; Kupper and Fuhlbrigge 2004). The migration of T cells into the skin is further supported by CCL17 and CCL20 derived from keratinocytes and dermal fibroblasts. Another important skin-homing element is CCR10, which is expressed by a subset of CLA^+ T cells only, and whose ligand CCL27 is preferentially produced by basal keratinocytes. CCL27 may be responsible for the retention of $CCR10^+$ T cells in or near the epidermis and can participate in (though is not required for) the extravasation of T cells from the venules into the dermis (Homey et al. 2002). Inflammatory conditions increase the production of these skin-homing-related chemokines causing enhancement of T-cell infiltration into the skin. Subsequently, cytokines derived from these recruited T cells can influence the local chemokine production. For example, IFN-γ can induce keratinocytes to produce CXCL9, CXCL10, and CXCL11 that promote the recruitment of T cells and other cell types that express CXCR3, the receptor for this chemokine triad. Skin-resident T cells universally express the memory T-cell marker CD45RO and approximately 20% co-express both CCR7 and CD62L (L-selectin) which are typical for central memory T cells, implicating that the majority of the T cells in the skin are effector memory T cells (Clark et al. 2006). The highly diverse population of T cells in the skin is thought to originate from a pool of naive T cells that reside in local lymphoid tissues that have been activated, polarized, and instructed to migrate to the skin by skin-derived DCs.

3 DCs are Key Regulators of Immune Responses

3.1 Detection of Danger

Recognition of bacteria, viruses, fungi, and parasites by DCs is a paramount first step in the induction of protective immune responses. DCs are equipped with an array of so-called pattern recognition receptors (PRRs), which can detect evolutionary-conserved pathogen-associated molecular patterns (PAMPs), including proteins, lipids, carbohydrates and nucleic acids that are essential for the life cycle of the pathogen, but are not expressed by the host (Medzhitov and Janeway 1997; Palm and Medzhitov 2009; Takeuchi and Akira 2010). The PRRs encompass the families of membrane-bound Toll-like receptors (TLRs) and C-type lectin receptors (CLRs), which survey the extracellular space and the endosomal/lysosomal compartments for signs of infection. The PRRs also include the families of NOD-like receptors (NLRs), RIG-I-like receptors (RLRs), and DNA receptors which scan the cytoplasm for danger. TLRs are considered to be the primary sensors of pathogens and are the most widely studied PRRs. Ten TLR family members have been identified in humans (Kawai and Akira 2010). TLR 1–6 are expressed on the cell surface and recognize extracellular PAMPs derived from bacteria, fungi and protozoa, whereas TLR3, 7–9 are expressed within endocytic compartments and primarily recognize nucleic acid (Kawai and Akira 2010; Barbalat et al. 2011). For example, TLR3 recognizes the viral replication intermediate dsRNA, TLR7 and TLR8 sense ssRNA, and TLR9 senses bacterial/viral genomic DNA rich in unmethylated CpG. The heterodimers TLR2/TLR1 and TLR2/TLR6 sense lipids and peptidoglycans, TLR5 senses bacterial flagellin, and TLR4 recognizes Lipid A of LPS, the major cell wall component of Gram-negative bacteria. TLRs signal via their cytoplasmic TIR domain and recruit adaptor molecules. All TLRs, except for TLR3, initiate MyD88-dependent signaling to activate NF-κB and MAP kinases to induce pro-inflammatory cytokines (Palm and Medzhitov 2009; Kawai and Akira 2010). TLR3 and TLR4 initiate TRIF-dependent signaling to activate NF-κB and IRF3 to induce production of pro-inflammatory cytokines and type I IFNs. TLR7/8 and TLR9 induce MyD88-dependent type I IFN production through activation of IRF7. The different DC subsets show differential TLR expression indicating that there may be specialization of different DC subsets to particular pathogens.

The CLRs have one or more domains that recognize mannose, fucose, and/or glucan carbohydrate structures present on most classes of human pathogens (Geijtenbeek et al. 2004). CLRs can be divided into two groups: group I CLRs belong to the mannose receptor family and group II CLRs belong to the asialoglycoprotein receptor family. Following pathogen binding, CLRs trigger distinct signaling pathways via ITAM-containing adaptor molecules or via activation of protein kinases or phosphatases and induce the expression of specific cytokines which influences the fate of T cell responses. Recognition by CLRs facilitates the internalization of the pathogen and affects its degradation and subsequent antigen presentation. The signaling of several CLRs is TLR-independent, but there is crosstalk between some of the CLR and TLR signaling pathways (Underhill 2007; Geijtenbeek and Gringhuis 2009; Kawai and Akira 2011). Some CLRs synergize with TLRs and co-stimulate the production of pro-inflammatory cytokines, whereas other CLRs antagonize TLR signaling. All human DC subsets have a diverse expression of multiple CLRs showing a broad distribution for some CLRs, whereas some CLRs are uniquely expressed by a single DC subset, as will be discussed in more detail below. NOD1 and NOD2 of the NLR family of cytoplasmic pathogen sensors recognize peptidoglycans, essential major components of Gram-positive bacteria, and activate NF-κB or MAP kinases to induce the production of inflammatory cytokines (Martinon and Tschopp 2005). As some TLRs also recognize these components, synergistic activation and pro-inflammatory cytokine production may occur. The NLR family also encompasses multiprotein-complexes, called inflammasomes, that sense a wide range of ligands within the cytoplasm of cells, including not only microbial PAMPs but also endogeneous host molecules and even environmental pollutants, such as silica and asbestos (Martinon et al. 2009). The NLRP3 inflammasome is the most widely studied inflammasome. Stimulation of DCs with microbial PAMPs initiates the assembly of the inflammasome protein complex, which converts procaspase-1 into active caspase-1, which, in turn, cleaves pro-forms of IL-1β, IL-18 and IL-33 thereby generating the bio-active forms of these key pro-inflammatory cytokines. Other members of the PRR family are the RLR family (RIG-I, MDA-5, and LGP2, recognizing the RNA from RNA viruses in the cytoplasm) and the cytosolic DNA sensors DAI and AIM2, all of which activate NF-κB and IRF3/IRF7 leading to the production of inflammatory cytokines and type I IFNs (Kawai and Akira 2010; Barbalat et al. 2011). Detailed information about differential expression of NLR, RLR, and cytoplasmic DNA sensors by distinct DC subsets is lacking.

Most studies on PAMP-induced activation of TLRs and other PRRs have been performed with single ligands and often using mouse models. However, these studies may not reflect the true picture of host–pathogen interactions in the context of human disease. Pathogens consist of manifold PAMPs that simultaneously activate multiple PRRs and various interconnected signaling pathways, resulting in complicated innate immune responses. The use of clinical isolates of pathogens instead of pure ligands may provide better insight into host–pathogen interaction. To extend our knowledge on the composite net result of innate responses against whole pathogens by DCs and how this determines T cell-polarization fates, will be helpful to enable the selection of an appropriate PRR-agonist combination to set the adaptive immune response for a required outcome. This knowledge may ultimately lead to improved potency and T-cell-polarization features of PAMP-based adjuvants. The usefulness of TLR agonists as an adjuvant is clearly established and some TLR agonists have even found their way to the clinic, for example the hepatitis B vaccine Fendrix that contains the TLR4 agonist MPL as an adjuvant (Mbow et al. 2010). It may also be worth exploring the usefulness of non-TLR agonist as candidate adjuvant.

Another issue that should be included in future studies is the contribution of the tissue-specific factors on the outcome of any immune response (Matzinger 2007; Matzinger and Kamala 2011). Although the direct effects of PAMPs on DC functions are of paramount importance in shaping adaptive immune responses, we know that pathogens also affect the local tissue microenvironment surrounding the DCs. In the skin for example, keratinocytes can respond to danger by releasing IL-1β and TNF-α, both important triggers for the emigration of LCs from the epidermis. Furthermore, tissue damage induced by microbial infection results in the release of intracellular molecules (e.g. heat shock proteins, S100 proteins and self-DNA) or extracellular matrix molecules (e.g. hyaluronic acid, which is broken down into oligosaccharides) that can act as damage or danger signals to which inflammatory responses are mounted (Rubartelli and Lotze 2007; Manfredi et al. 2009). These damage or danger signals are often referred to as damage-associated molecular patterns or danger-associated molecular patterns, or in short DAMPs, and activate a profile of cytokines and inflammatory responses analogous to that induced by PAMPs. DAMP receptors have not been thoroughly defined, but may include CD91, CD36, CD40, CD14, and some of the TLRs and inflammasomes (Chen and Nunez 2010). It is inevitable that administration of any vaccine in the dermis will cause local damage and induce the release of DAMPs. As DAMPs directly affect the function of DCs and modify the PAMP-induced activation of DCs, it is important to learn if and how much skin-derived DAMPs contribute to skin DC-mediated immune response and to utilize this knowledge in ID vaccination.

3.2 Uptake and Processing of Antigen

Extracellular antigens need to be internalized and processed into small fragments before they can be presented to T cells. Several types of endocytosis can be distinguished based on the cargo size and uptake mechanisms: phagocytosis for the uptake of particulate antigens such as pathogens, (macro)pinocytosis for the uptake of soluble antigens, receptor-mediated uptake (e.g. Fc receptors, CLRs, complement receptors, scavenger receptors, and many others), and clathrin-dependent or caveolin-dependent antigen internalization (Trombetta and Mellman 2005). Extracellular cargo is encapsulated by the plasma membrane during uptake, forming an intracellular vacuole termed phagosome or endosome and subsequently both undergo a series of regulated changes, such as progressive acidification and fusion with organelles containing proteolytic enzymes, in particular lysosomes. Early endosomes are not just one pool of common organelles, but comprise of distinct populations of early endosomes with different maturation kinetics: some show rapid transformation into late endosomes, whereas others are more stable (Lakadamyali et al. 2006). In late endosomes/lysosomes the antigenic peptides are loaded onto MHC class II molecules, upon HLA-DM catalyzed removal of CLIP from the peptide-binding groove, followed by transport of the complexes to the cell surface for presentation to CD4$^+$ T cells (Trombetta and Mellman 2005; Burgdorf and Kurts 2008). Exogenous antigens can also be presented by MHC class I molecules to CD8$^+$ T cells, a process referred to as cross-presentation to discriminate it from the conventional MHC class I-restricted presentation of endogenous cytosolic-derived proteins. Cross-presentation is essential for priming (in this case called cross-priming) naive CD8$^+$ T-cell responses to tumor cells and virus-infected cells (Lin et al. 2008). DC subsets differ in their ability to cross-present exogenous antigens. Mouse splenic CD8$^+$ DCs and their putative human equivalents, peripheral blood CD141$^+$ DCs are the most powerful cross-presenting cells (Jongbloed et al. 2010; Poulin et al. 2010; Bachem et al. 2010; Crozat et al. 2010a). The MHC class I-related pathway to process exogenous antigens is not entirely clear, but active alkalization of the phagosome is required to rescue internalized particulate antigen from rapid degradation (Savina et al. 2006). In addition, the phagocytosed exogenous antigens need to be degraded by proteasomes and therefore need to be translocated from the phagosome lumen into the cytoplasm, after which the peptide fragments are shuttled back into the lumen of probably the same phagosome by a TAP-dependent mechanism where the peptides are loaded onto MHC class I molecules (Guermonprez et al. 2003). The alkalization of phagosomes is transient however, permitting further degradation into peptides that can be loaded onto MHC class II molecules. This enables MHC class I-restricted and MHC class II-restricted processing of particulate antigens to occur sequentially (Burgdorf and Kurts 2008; Burgdorf et al. 2008).

Interestingly, some cell-surface receptors can route soluble antigen to different endosomal pathways thereby favoring MHC class I-restricted or MHC class II-restricted antigen presentation. For example, the mannose receptor (CD206) routes antigen to the mildly acidic stable early endosomes for exclusive presentation by MHC class I, whereas soluble antigen taken up by the scavenger receptor is directed rapidly toward lysosomes to be processed only for MHC class II presentation (Burgdorf et al. 2007). On the other hand, DEC-205 and Fc receptors can target antigens to both MHC class I and II loading. Heat shock proteins, which are capable of interacting with a broad range of peptides and act as molecular chaperones, have been shown to facilitate efficient CD8$^+$ T-cell responses by cross-presentation (Oura et al. 2011). Knowledge on receptor-controlled selection of the antigen-processing pathway can for instance be considered in vaccination strategies aimed at improving CD8$^+$ T-cell responses, like targeting antigen to the mannose receptor or heat shock protein in order to promote cross-presentation (Oura et al. 2011; Singh et al. 2011).

In addition to the mechanisms to process/present proteins via MHC class I and II molecules, DCs possess pathways to process exogenous and endogenous non-protein antigens (such as lipids, glycolipids, and lipopeptides), which are subsequently loaded into the binding groove of CD1 molecules (Cohen et al. 2009). Similar to the polymorphic transmembrane heavy chain of MHC class I molecules that are non-covalently associated with β2-microglobulin, non-polymorphic CD1 heavy chains also form heterodimeric complexes with β2-microglobulin. Based on sequence homology, the CD1 family has been classified into three groups: group 1 contains CD1a, CD1b, and CD1c, group 2 contains CD1d, and CD1e belongs to group 3. The human genome encodes for all five CD1 molecules, but mice only express CD1d. Newly synthesized CD1 molecules traffic to the cell surface first, and upon internalization they reach the endosomal compartments to get loaded. The different CD1 molecules are loaded with lipids or glycolipids in distinct compartments of the endocytic pathway and after recycling they appear on the cell surface again, enabling display of lipidic antigens to T cells (Cohen et al. 2009; Moody and Porcelli 2003). The different CD1 molecules are variably expressed on DC subsets. Human LCs appear to express high levels of CD1a, moderate levels of CD1c, but typically lack CD1b and CD1d; DDCs express CD1a, b, c, and d (Gerlini et al. 2001; Ochoa et al. 2008), whereas plasmacytoid DCs lack expression of CD1 molecules (Liu 2005). Differences in expression patterns of CD1a, b, c, and d may reflect functional differences between DC subsets.

Human T cells restricted to CD1d define a population of T cells known as NKT cells, which can be divided into a well-studied category that expresses a semi-invariant TCR consisting of Vα24 Jα18 with Vβ11 and a poorly characterized category with a much more diverse TCR repertoire. Upon activation, NKT cells may orchestrate immune responses through their rapid and diverse secretion of large quantities of both Th1- and Th2-type cytokines and they can influence the maturation process of DCs (Cohen et al. 2009; Bendelac et al. 2007). NKT cells have been considered to be innate-like lymphocytes based on the limited TCR diversity and the promptness of their response. They participate in immunity against a wide range of pathogens including bacteria, fungi, parasites, and viruses. The CD1a, b, and c-restricted T cells appear to be functionally like MHC-restricted adaptive Th1 T cells and CTL, but with specificity for recognition of lipids antigens rather than proteins (Cohen et al. 2009). CD1a-restricted blood T cells express skin-homing markers CLA, CCR6, CCR4, and CCR10, they can be isolated from the skin, and remarkably, they show a substantially enhanced production of IL-22, but no upregulation of either IFN-γ or IL-17, in response to the presentation of CD1a-lipid complexes by epidermal LCs (de Jong et al. 2010). The concept that T-cell reactivity is limited to peptides that bind MHC molecules is now considered obsolete. There is overwhelming evidence that T cell-mediated lipid antigen recognition is important in detection and clearance of pathogens as well. Therefore, future studies aimed at understanding the function and therapeutic potential of these unconventional CD1-restricted T-cell populations are warranted and may reveal new CD1-based vaccine strategies.

3.3 *Translation of Sensed Danger to Adequate T-cell Responses*

In peripheral tissues, such as skin, there is a permanent risk of pathogen entry and DCs continuously scan their microenvironment for invading pathogens. The literature often mentions that DCs in peripheral tissues are immature, a term reflecting their incapability to activate naive T cells. At this stage of their life cycle when the immature DCs reside in the peripheral tissues they are highly active at all forms of endocytosis to capture encountered pathogens or self antigens. The DCs are well-equipped with a variety of PRRs to recognize a myriad of PAMPs (as described above) and, in addition they express numerous cell-surface receptors that mediate or support the internalization of antigens. Recognition and uptake of pathogens, as well as activatory signals from the surrounding cells (such as TNF-α and IL-1β), initiate the exit of DCs from the tissue and trigger a program of DC maturation, leading to a dramatic phenotype and functional metamorphose to become potent effector DCs capable of activating naive T cells (Cella et al. 1997; Banchereau and Steinman 1998). The exodus of antigen-loaded DCs coincides with the downregulation of homing receptors (for example E-cadherin on LCs) and at the same time CCR7 is upregulated, making the DCs responsive to chemokines CCL19 and CCL21 that are selectively co-expressed in the T-cell zones in lymphoid organs, predominantly by the stromal cells (Luther et al. 2000). CCL19 and CCL21 attract CCR7^{+} DCs to the T-cell zones in the local lymph nodes, guiding the DCs to come in close contact with naive T cells for the initiation of immune responses (Sallusto et al. 1998). On their way to the lymph node, DCs decrease endocytic activity, enhance antigen-processing and presentation, increase cell-surface expression of MHC class I and II molecules that are loaded with microbial-derived peptides and co-stimulatory molecules such as CD40, CD80, and CD86 on the plasma membrane. Upon arrival in the lymph node migratory DCs are mature and endowed with the unique capacity to initiate antigen-specific activation of naive T cells (Cella et al. 1997; Banchereau and Steinman 1998). Thus, in short, peripheral tissue DCs are dedicated to capture soluble and particulate antigens and transport this cargo to the lymph node in order to display small fragments of antigen on their surface as MHC–peptide complexes or CD1–lipid complexes for presentation to naive T cells.

When a naive T-cell receptor recognizes the corresponding MHC–peptide complex on a DC (signal 1) it will only become activated if also simultaneously receives co-stimulatory triggers (signal 2) from the mature DC (Kalinski et al. 1999; Kapsenberg 2003). This leads to naive T-cell proliferation and differentiation into effector memory T-cells (CD45RO^{+}CCR7^{-}CD62L^{-}) which are capable of cytokine production and cytolysis or become long-lived central memory T cells (CD45RO^{+}CCR7^{+}CD62L^{+}) capable of providing rapid protective responses upon reinfection (Sallusto et al. 2004). Most importantly, mature DCs have the unique potential to orchestrate the development of distinct lineages of antigen-specific effector Th cells (Fig. 2), which is essential to combat the different classes of pathogens (e.g. Th1 cells for the clearance of intracellular pathogens and Th2 cells for the clearance of extracellular parasites). Mature DCs acquire this polarizing-imprinting potential during their immature stage and subsequent maturation program (Kapsenberg 2003; Lanzavecchia and Sallusto 2001). When immature DCs encounter and internalize microbes they receive a variety of signals via their PRRs (different types of pathogens provide different kinds of stimuli) and additional signals from surrounding tissue that also respond to the danger. During maturation, DCs integrate this pandemonium of information into relevant instructions for naive T cells to direct the development of the required effector T-cell type. This polarizing imprinting is regarded as the third signal that is delivered to naive T cells (Kalinski et al. 1999). For example, viruses programme DCs to express (among others) IL-12, a well-known factor to promote Th1 development. Intriguingly, some pathogens interfere with MHC class I antigen-presentation pathway or have adapted to abuse the polarizing mechanism to induce regulatory T cells and tolerance to evade eradication by the immune system (Sacks and Sher 2002; Engering et al. 2002; Hansen and Bouvier 2009). Furthermore, as a fourth signal, the mature DCs provide homing instructions to activated T cells in order to navigate the T cells to the tissue where the DCs originated from and where the infection is going on. The exact mechanism of this fourth signal is not clear, but upregulation of skin-targeting receptors CLA and CCR10 or gut-targeting receptors $\alpha4\beta7$ and CCR9 will endow T cells with specific tissue homing properties. It has been shown that DCs posses the enzymes to metabolize sunlight-induced vitamin D3 into the active form 1,25-dihydroxyvitamin D3, which induces CCR10 on T cells and concomitantly suppress gut-homing receptors $\alpha4\beta7$ and CCR9 (Sigmundsdottir et al. 2007). This linkage between ultraviolet B-induced vitamin in the outer layers of the skin and subsequent induction of epidermotropism in activated T cells is an example of how DCs interpret local circumstances and direct T cells to target tissues. In the context of ID vaccination the paradigm that DCs provide homing cues as a fourth signal to naive T cells poses a conundrum: if T cells are instructed go to the site of DC origin, how can ID vaccination be successful for immunization against non-skin pathogens? ID vaccination against for example influenza has already been proven successful, so instructions for T-cell homing is more complex than currently known.

From the moment immature DCs sense pathogens or urgent changes in the tissue homeostasis till the moment mature DCs provide a combination of instructions to naive T cells, a highly complex cascade of molecular remodeling takes place in the DCs that ultimately lead to an appropriate T-cell response for protective immunity or tolerance. It is clear that DC function and subsequent T-cell responses are modulated by the pathogen type. Understanding the mechanism how pathogens can manipulate the flavor and magnitude of the immune response, or even evade the immune system, is of crucial importance in the design of effective vaccines or microbial-based adjuvants, which for instance, offers the choice to induce either protective immunity or tolerance. Understanding the mechanism that regulates the MHC class II-related antigen-processing and presentation machinery can also innovate vaccine design because this can lead to improvement of the stability of MHC–peptide complexes and prolongation of the half-life of the MHC–peptide complexes on the DC surface.

One important element that has not been dealt with so far, although is critical in determining the outcome of T-cell responses is the heterogeneity of DC subsets. Human non-lymphoid tissue contains distinct DC subsets with different phenotypes and functions, and as a consequence, they differ in their ability to generate specific T cell responses. The forthcoming paragraphs will highlight the different human DC subsets, in particular the DC subsets in the human skin. There are differences between DC subsets in humans and mice. For a more in-depth review about murine DC subsets the reader is referred to a companion article by Ginhoux et al. (2010).

4 Human DC Subsets

4.1 Surface Markers

DCs were originally described in the murine lymphoid tissue based on morphological criteria (Steinman and Cohn 1973) and the ability to prime naive T-cell proliferation with approximately 100-fold greater efficiency than other ‘accessory’ populations such as adherent macrophages (Steinman and Cohn 1974). Subsequently, a universal definition of DCs included high expression of MHC class II together with lack of defined lineage markers to exclude monocytes (CD14), B cells (CD19), T cells (CD3), NK cells (CD56), and stem cells (CD34). In more recent years a number of DC-restricted positive markers have proven to be useful. The expression of integrin CD11c together with co-stimulatory molecules such as CD40, CD80, CD86, and CD83 has been widely used in mouse and human immunology. In addition, expression of the CD1 antigens has been very useful in humans and defines DC subsets in a number of tissues. The Blood Dendritic Cell Antigens (BDCA) that characterize human blood DCs include: CD1c (BDCA-1): CD303/CLEC4C (BDCA-2); CD141/thrombomodulin (BDCA-3) and CD304/neuropilin-1 (BDCA-4) (Dzionek et al. 2000; MacDonald et al. 2002). In recent years, lectins such as Langerin (CD207), DEC-205 (CD205), DC-SIGN (CD209), DCIR2 (33D1 antigen in mice), and CLEC9A have been shown to mark specific DC subsets (Bonifaz et al. 2004; Huysamen et al. 2008). The potential to target different DC subsets through antibodies to specific lectins is currently of great interest (Badiee et al. 2007; Kato et al. 2007). In human histopathology, stains for S100A, clotting factor XIIIa (FXIIIa), fascin, and ATPase are still routinely employed to identify DC populations, although these markers are also shared by macrophages. Furthermore, it has not always been clear how intracellular antigen staining relates to surface marker expression.

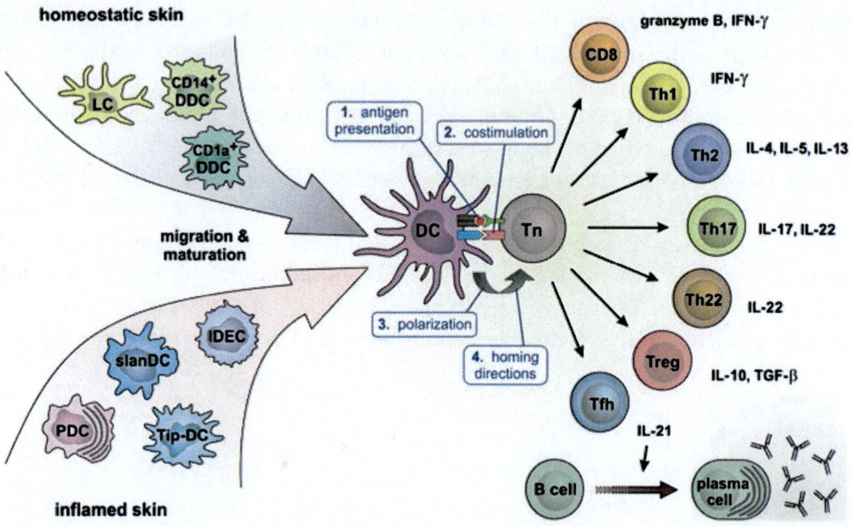

Fig. 2 DCs control the development of distinct T-cell responses. After internalization of environmental antigens, cutaneous DCs migrate to the skin-draining lymph node while undergoing a process of maturation to acquire the unique capacity to prime naive T cells (Tn). The different DC subsets in homeostatic skin and additional DC subsets in inflammatory conditions are indicated on the left site. The original antigenic stimulus and the local mediators from the neighboring cells at the site of infection are integrated by the DC into four signals (indicated in the *blue boxes*) that direct the development of the required type of effector T cell. A more extensive description is provided in Sect. 3.3

4.2 Human Blood DC Subsets

The MHC class II positive lineage negative (HLA-DR$^+$ lin$^-$) subset of human mononuclear cells has been intensively studied but different definitions based on flow cytometry gating strategies abound. HLA-DR$^+$ cells in human blood include: DCs, monocytes, CD34$^+$ precursors, B cells, activated T cells, and activated NK cells. Lineage marking with CD34, CD19/CD20, CD3, and CD56 will exclude the precursors and lymphoid cells, leaving DCs and monocytes. The separation of monocytes from DCs is a source of some confusion. CD14 and CD16 expression marks subsets of monocytes, but staining for both antigens is a smear (Passlick et al. 1989). Within CD16$^+$ cells there is a subset of 6-sulfo LacNAc (slan)$^+$ cells (Siedlar et al. 2000) thought to be a distinct population of DCs by some authors and called slanDCs (Schakel et al. 2002, 2006). Prior to the availability of antibodies for slan it was not possible to make proper distinction between slanDCs and CD16$^+$CD14^{low} monocytes. CD16$^+$ cells were variously referred to as either DCs (MacDonald et al. 2002; Lindstedt et al. 2005; Piccioli et al. 2007) or monocytes (Geissmann et al. 2003; Gordon and Taylor 2005; Ingersoll et al. 2010). Both CD14$^+$ monocytes and CD16$^+$ slan$^+$ DCs are CD11c$^+$. When CD14$^+$ and CD16$^+$ cells are both excluded, this leaves a population of HLA-DR$^+$ cells that contain the classical $CD123^+$ plasmacytoid DCs (PDCs) and $CD11c^+$ myeloid blood DCs. The PDC is $CD11c^-$ and co-expresses CD303 (BDCA-2) and CD304 (BDCA-4), while the $CD11c^+$ myeloid DCs expresses low levels of CD123 and may be further split into CD1c (BDCA-1) positive CD141 $(BDCA\text{-}3)^{low}$ and CD1c negative $CD141^{high}$ fractions (Dzionek et al. 2000; MacDonald et al. 2002). The latter also expresses CLEC9A (Huysamen et al. 2008), CLEC12A (Lahoud et al. 2009), and Nectin-like protein 2 (cell adhesion molecule 1: CADM1). A variety of phenotypic and functional observations and genomic comparison link human blood CD141 $(BDCA\text{-}3)^+$ cells with $CD8^+$ lymph node DCs in mice (Jongbloed et al. 2010; Poulin et al. 2010; Bachem et al. 2010; Crozat et al. 2010a; Robbins et al. 2008) and is reviewed by Shortman and Heath (2010) and Crozat et al. (2010b).

4.3 Human Lymphoid Tissue DC Subsets

Progress in the identification of human lymphoid DC subsets is much more limited than in the murine system. In human tonsil, it is possible to find a number of $HLA\text{-}DR^+$ lin^- populations, including $CD11c^+$ and $CD123^+$ fractions (Summers et al. 2001). An early study of superficial lymph nodes described $CD1a^+$ and $CD1a^-$ subpopulations (Takahashi et al. 1998). The population of $CD123^+$ PDCs is easier to understand in terms of functional correlates and has been studied in various pathological states including HIV, malignancy, and autoimmune disease (Farkas et al. 2001; Cox et al. 2005; Vermi et al. 2005; Sakuraba et al. 2009; Hochrein et al. 2001; Tanis et al. 2004; Faith et al. 2007; Nishikawa et al. 2009; Dillon et al. 2008).

DC subsets identified in tonsil and blood DCs by BDCA expression were compared by expression profiling and found to be reasonably parallel (Lindstedt et al. 2005). A further study identified two main groups of lymph node antigen-presenting cells by immunofluorescence staining that were either $CD14^+CD206^+CD209^+$ or $CD207^+CD208^+$ (Angel et al. 2009). By their location and phenotype these bear some correlation to the traditional categories of sub-capsular or medullary macrophages and paracortical interdigitating cells, respectively. Further functional insights were gleaned from studies of lymph node draining inflamed skin, in which expansion of a particular subset of $CD1a^+CD207^+$ immature DCs was revealed, presumed to be LC-derived (Geissmann et al. 2002) and documentation of the distribution of DC-SIGN (CD209) in normal and reactive nodes (Engering et al. 2004).

In human spleen $CD11c^+$ and $CD11c^-$ DCs may be found principally in the marginal zones, white pulp and peri-arteriolar sheath (McIlroy et al. 2001). Further clarification of their phenotype and localization was more recently achieved using antibodies to lectins (Pack et al. 2008) and BDCA molecules (Velasquez-Lopera et al. 2008). Phenotypically similar DC subsets in the human spleen and blood have been recently identified (Mittag et al. 2011).

5 DC Subsets in Human Skin

5.1 *Epidermal Langerhans cells*

There is reasonable consensus over the content of normal human skin DCs, being more accessible than lymph node populations, through the analysis of skin removed during plastic surgery (Valladeau and Saeland 2005). The outer epidermal layer of keratinocytes contains the most renown of all DCs, the LC, first described by Langerhans in 1868. This archetypical DC was subsequently shown to be a bone marrow-derived cell (Volc-Platzer et al. 1984) bearing Fc and complement receptors (Stingl et al. 1977) and MHC class II antigens (Stingl et al. 1980) and containing cytoplasmic Birbeck granules, which are rod-shaped structures with a zipper-like appearance at ultrastructural level, comprising CD1a and Langerin and presumed to be involved in antigen processing (Birbeck et al. 1961; Valladeau et al. 2000). The dendritic shape of LCs is best appreciated in epidermal sheet preparations, giving the impression that these cells form a regular, almost interconnected network with their protrusions forming a network (Fig. 3a). Multiple studies have focused on the quantification of epidermal LCs yielding a remarkable variety in results, reviewed in (Teunissen 2005). The following can be concluded from these studies (*i*) LCs constitute approximately 2% of the total epidermal cell population in normal healthy skin; (*ii*) a wide interindividual variation exists for the number of LCs per mm^2, likely due to the variation in thickness of the epidermis; (*iii*) on the average there are 1000–1200 LCs per mm^2 in normal adult human skin, and (*iv*) the density of LCs may vary at different anatomical regions, being the highest in the face and neck and the lowest in the foot sole. Given that an average adult (70 kg, 170 cm) has approximately 1.8 m^2 of skin surface area, according to the formula of Dubois (Burton 2008), it can be estimated that an average individual has $1.8–2.2 \times 10^9$ epidermal LCs. High accurate three-dimensional quantification revealed a remarkable constant ratio of one LCs to 53 other epidermal cells and that one LC can cover an area of as much as 554–1096 μm^2 thanks to their dendrites (Bauer et al. 2001).

LCs are in some way locked up by the surrounding keratinocytes that are tightly packed and firmly connected by desmosomal and tight junctions. Epidermal LCs are connected to the keratinocytes through homophilic adhesive interactions between E-cadherin molecules expressed on both cell types (Udey 1997). Taking into account that the different epidermal layers are continuously displacing outward slowly—because of the epidermal turnover by which new cells are generated at the base of the epidermis while the outermost surface flakes off at the same rate—LCs have to move slowly in the opposite direction to keep their position just above the basal layer of the epidermis. It is commonly assumed that it is impossible for microbes or molecules from the external environment to penetrate the skin without being noticed by the strategically positioned extensive network of LCs that are busy sampling antigens in the epidermis. However, it is hard for microbes or molecules to pass the cornified layer (stratum corneum) and tight

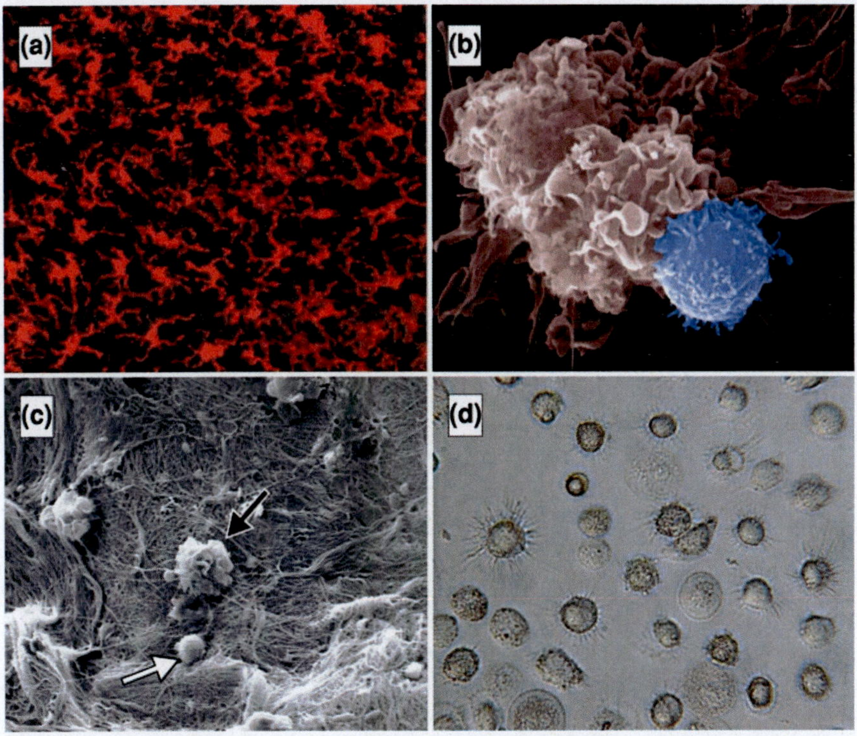

Fig. 3 **a** Epidermal sheet from normal human skin showing a tight network of LCs (in *red*) that are visualized by fluorescent-labeled anti-CD1a antibody. **b** *Pseudo-colored* scanning electron micrograph shows the intimate contact between a LC (taupe-colored) and a naive $CD8^+$ T-cell (*blue*). **c** Scanning electron micrograph of a 2-day cultured dermal sheet showing a DDC (*black arrow*) and a T-cell (*white arrow*) that emigrated from the tissue. Note the numerous collagen and elastin fibers of the dermis displayed in the background. **d** Population of cells that crawled-out of the human dermis after 2 days of culture. DDCs can be recognized by their dendritic morphology

junctions in the stratum granulosum to reach the LCs. Recent observations indicate that upon activation, LCs can elongate their dendrites beyond the tight junction barrier and sample antigens in the region between the most distal region of the stratum granulosum and proximal region of the cornified layer, a space that can be considered as an air–liquid interface (Kubo et al. 2009). While performing this astonishing action, LCs have to penetrate tight junction contacts between keratinocytes and to form new tight junctions between themselves and keratinocytes in order to maintain tight junction integrity. Internalized antigens co-localize with Langerin and Birbeck granules at the tip of the penetrated dendrites (Kubo et al. 2009). The elongated dendrites of LCs that reach out into the cornified layer may even have direct contact with the microbiome of the skin. In this respect it should be noted that LCs do not express TLR2, TLR4, and TLR5 on their cell surface and, as a consequence, have limited responsiveness to extracellular bacteria in terms of up-regulation of co-stimulatory molecules and production of inflammatory cytokines (van der Aar et al. 2007). The ability of LCs to stretch their dendrites beyond the surface barrier system resembles the feature of lamina propria DCs in the intestinal mucosa that are able to elongate their dendrites directly into gut lumen to sample bacteria (Rescigno et al. 2001).

Analysis of skin-draining lymphatic vessels revealed that LCs exit continuously from the epidermis under steady-state conditions at a low rate and that local inflammation markedly upregulates their emigration (Brand et al. 1999). Apparently there is a constant turnover of LCs even in the absence of inflammatory signals (Jakob et al. 2001). The LC population is maintained by local radio-resistant precursors under steady-state conditions (at least in mice), but LCs are replaced by circulating precursors during major inflammatory skin conditions (Merad et al. 2002). TNF-α and IL-1β are crucial signals to activate and amplify emigration of LCs (Cumberbatch et al. 1997), among others by inducing down-regulation of E-cadherin expression, which enables LCs to dissociate from surrounding keratinocytes (Jakob et al. 2001).

Migration of LCs in vitro and their subsequent differentiation into typical veiled cells of the afferent lymph set the paradigm for all migratory myeloid DCs, as was first discovered in mice (Schuler and Steinman 1985) and later confirmed in man (Romani et al. 1989; Teunissen et al. 1990). Although the contribution of LCs to immune responses in vivo has recently been questioned in murine models (reviewed by Romani et al. 2010), the derivation of Langerin^{+} DCs in vitro with potent cytotoxic T lymphocyte-priming capacity (Fig. 3b) continues to fuel interest in these cells as agents of immunotherapy (Mohamadzadeh et al. 2001; Ratzinger et al. 2004; Klechevsky et al. 2008; Anguille et al. 2009) reviewed by Ueno et al. (2010).

5.2 Dermal DCs

Electron microscopic and immunohistochemical studies first recognized the presence of DDCs, described variously as indeterminate cells (Murphy et al. 1983) or dermal dendrocytes (Cerio et al. 1989), but isolation and characterization of these cells were not properly achieved until 1993 (Nestle et al. 1993; Meunier et al. 1993; Lenz et al. 1993). From these early studies, primarily using spontaneously migrating cells (Fig. 3c, d), it was apparent that DDCs comprised two subsets of CD1a^{+} and CD14^{+} cells (Table 1). Most investigators suggested that they were distinct to LCs by virtue of their lower or absent CD1a expression and later, lack of Langerin. Although the alternative view that dermal CD1a^{+} DCs were simply migrating LCs that had down-regulated these markers generated confusion for a number of years, the expression of LC-restricted molecules such as E-cadherin (CD324) and EpCAM (CD326) has aided this distinction (Lukas et al. 1996; Angel et al. 2006, 2007a, b; Nagao et al. 2009). In flow cytometry and in situ studies, a small population approximately 1–2% of DDCs retain high expression of CD1a and Langerin and are presumed to represent migrating LCs.

Table 1 Phenotype of LCs, DDC subsets and macrophages in normal human skin

CD number	Alias	LC	CD1a⁺ DDC	CD14⁺ DDC	Macrophage
CD1a		+	+	–	–
CD1b		–	+	–	nd
CD1c	BDCA-1	+	+	+	–
CD1d		–	+	–	nd
CD11a	LFA-1, integrin alpha-L	–	+	+	+
CD11b	C3bi R, integrin alpha-M	–	+	+	+
CD11c	Integrin alpha-X	+	+	+	–
CD14		–	–	+	+
CD18	β-chain of CD11a, b and c	+	+	+	+
CD32	FcγR II	+	+	+	+
CD36		–	–	–/+	+
CD40		+	+	+	nd
CD45	Common leukocyte antigen	+	+	+	+
CD54	ICAM-1	+	+	+	–
CD68		–	+	+	+
CD80	B7-1, CD28 ligand 1	+	+	+	nd
CD83		+	+	–	–
CD86	B7-2, CD28 ligand 2	+	+	+	nd
CD141	BDCA-3	–	–	+	nd
CD197	CCR7	+	+	–/+	–
CD163	Hemoglobin scavenger receptor	–	–	–/+	+
CD205	DEC-205	+	+	+	–
CD206	Macrophage mannose receptor	–	+	+	+
CD207	Langerin	+	–	–	–
CD208	DC-LAMP	+	+	–	–
CD209	DC-SIGN	–	+	+	+
CD303	BDCA-2	–	–	–	–
CD304	BDCA-4, neuropilin	–	–	+	–
CD324	E-cadherin	+	–	–	–
–	DCIR, CLEC4A	+	+	+	nd
–	FXIIIa (clotting factor)	–	+	+	+

This table is compiled from various studies as indicated in the text of this review. *Arbitrary units*: – absent, + present, *nd* not determined

Analogues of CD1a$^+$ and CD14$^+$ DCs have been generated in vitro from CD34$^+$ stem cells using GM-CSF and TNF-α (Klechevsky et al. 2008; Caux et al. 1997) and from monocytes, using GM-CSF, IL-4 and TGF-β (Geissmann et al. 1998; Gogolak et al. 2007). The universal assumption is that CD1a$^+$ DCs made in this way are 'Langerhans cell-like' although the use of TGF-β gives much higher CD1a, Langerin, EpCAM and E-cadherin expression than TNF-α (Allam et al. 2003; Haniffa and Collin, unpublished). TNF-α added secondarily to monocyte-derived Langerin$^+$ cells further increases Langerin expression, although by itself is unable to generate Langerin$^+$ cells from monocytes (Geissmann et al. 2002). It is therefore possible that cells derived with TGF-β have a closer relationship with

LCs than those derived with TNF-α alone, although both are referred to as 'Langerhans cell-like' (Bechetoille et al. 2006).

At the time Langerin (CD207) was discovered (Valladeau et al. 1999), just before the millennium change, it was believed that this C-type lectin is unique to LCs and that antibodies against Langerin can be used to identify LCs. The small numbers of Langerin$^+$ cells that can be observed in the dermis were assumed to be epidermal LCs in transit to the lymph nodes. In 2007 however, three independent groups (Bursch et al. 2007; Ginhoux et al. 2007; Poulin et al. 2007) demonstrated that part of the Langerin$^+$ cells in the dermis in mice represent a novel population of DCs that are unrelated to LCs and they were simply called "dermal Langerin$^+$ DCs". These dermal Langerin$^+$ DCs represent the minority of the DDC pool, reaching 10–20% of total dermal Langerin$^+$ cells and 10% of total DDCs (Ginhoux et al. 2007; Poulin et al. 2007). In contrast, only very few Langerin$^+$ DCs are present in human dermis, as assessed by immunohistochemistry or flow cytometry (Ebner et al. 2004; Furio et al. 2005). In mice the dermal Langerin$^+$ DCs can be discriminated from Langerin$^+$ LCs and the dermal Langerin$^-$ DCs by the expression of CD103 (Bursch et al. 2007), but in humans CD103 is not a positive marker that clearly delineates this minor population from the other DC subsets. Recent studies in mice suggest that the CD207$^+$CD103$^+$ DDC is the most important DC subset to cross-present viral antigens or self antigens regardless of the presence of LCs (Bedoui et al. 2009; Henri et al. 2010). The high-sophisticated experimental methodologies used in mice to proof the existence of dermal Langerin$^+$ DCs are not feasible in humans. The search for the human equivalent of the murine dermal Langerin$^+$ DCs is still topic of investigation and to date it is not clear whether the human dermal Langerin$^+$ DCs really exists. Microarray analysis of the global mRNA transcription profile of highly purified mouse dermal Langerin$^+$ DCs may yield specific markers that are useful to detect this cell type in humans.

5.3 *Dermal Macrophages*

The distinction between DDCs and macrophages in humans has only recently been made clear through careful immunohistological studies (Ochoa et al. 2008; Zaba et al. 2007) and flow cytometry of collagenase-digested cells (Haniffa et al. 2009). Essentially, the problem of identifying the different lineages arose when two populations of migratory DCs, defined by CD14 and CD1a, were mapped to the dermis by in situ staining, without regard for a large population of dermal macrophages, which shared a number of markers with CD14$^+$ DDCs (Table 1). The most troublesome was FXIIIa, the histological marker of 'dermal dendrocytes', an ill-defined population of leukocytes with dendritic morphology (Cerio et al. 1989). When DDCs were first isolated by migration, FXIIIa was demonstrated by flow cytometry, particularly in the CD14$^+$ DCs (Klechevsky et al. 2008; Nestle et al. 1993) and these were surmised to represent the cells observed in situ. However, Zaba et al. (2007) clearly showed that FXIIIa was principally expressed by $CD163^+$ macrophages, as had been previously argued (Torocsik et al. 2005). These cells do not migrate, but can be released by collagenase digestion. The solution to identifying them by flow cytometry was revealed to be massive autofluorescence created by melanin ingestion (Haniffa et al. 2009). A further surprise emerged that macrophages were also the target of CD209 (DC-SIGN) staining in human dermis (Ochoa et al. 2008). Although sessile, non-proliferating and very slowly replaced by bone marrow-derived cells after hematopoietic stem cell transplantation, isolated dermal macrophages secrete inflammatory cytokines and are capable of stimulating memory T cells (Haniffa et al. 2009).

5.4 DC Subsets in Inflamed Skin

Under inflammatory or pathological conditions (infection, UVB-exposure, injury, skin diseases such as psoriasis, atopic dermatitis, lichen planus, etc.) the number, composition, and maturation status of the skin DC population changes dramatically. The skin-resident DC subsets may acquire an activated more mature phenotype, as shown by the expression of CD80, CD83, CD86, and lysosomal marker DC-LAMP (CD208). In addition, the amount of DCs will increase as cohorts of newly recruited (presumably blood-derived) distinct inflammatory DC subsets will infiltrate depending on the level of inflammation and type of condition. Inflammatory DCs are also expected to infiltrate the skin upon ID administration of a vaccine as the injection and vaccine will provoke local inflammation. So in this context it is relevant to discuss some of the DC subsets that are recruited in injured or diseased skin.

5.4.1 Plasmacytoid DCs

PDCs are a rare population of circulating cells that are present in the blood stream and secondary lymphoid organs under steady-state conditions. PDCs (named that way because of their plasma cell-like morphology) have a key role in the defense to viral infections through their ability to produce huge amounts of type I IFNs (IFN-α/β) in response to viral recognition (Siegal et al. 1999; Cella et al. 1999), and in addition, PDCs also link innate and adaptive immunity by controlling the function of myeloid DCs, T cells, B cells, and NK cells (Gilliet et al. 2008). Human PDCs express MHC class II^{low}, CD4, CD36, CD68, $CD123^{high}$ (IL-3 receptor α), and BDCA-4 (CD304), but lack the common lineage markers CD3, CD19, CD11b and CD11c, CD14, and CD33 (Liu 2005), whereas BDCA-2 (CD303) and ILT7 (CD85g) are specific markers for PDCs (Dzionek et al. 2001; Cao et al. 2006). Following viral stimulation immature PDCs differentiate into mature PDCs that promote the development of antigen-specific IFN-γ and IL-10-producing CD4 cells. The capacity of human PDCs to prime naive $CD4^+$ T cells to produce IFN-γ is dependent on type I IFNs and independent of IL-12, which is not expressed by PDCs but rather a typical product of activated myeloid DCs (Liu 2005). Unlike human PDCs, their counterparts in mice do express CD11c and have the capacity to produce both IFN-α and IL-12 (Asselin-Paturel et al. 2001; Boonstra et al. 2003). IFNs promote myeloid DCs to produce IL-12, IL-15, IL-18, and IL-23 (thereby favoring Th1 development) and also increase the ability of myeloid DCs to cross-present antigens to CD8 T cells (Santini et al. 2000; Le Bon et al. 2003). Human PDCs themselves also have the capacity to cross-present viral antigens to CD8 T cells (Di Pucchio et al. 2008). In addition, PDCs can prime naive $CD4^+$ T cells to differentiate into IL-10-producing regulatory T cells (Tr1 subset) (Kuwana et al. 2001).

The robust production of IFN-α/β by PDCs is linked to their unique expression of TLR7 and TLR9, which sense viral nucleic acids (single-stranded RNA and DNA, respectively) within the endosomes (Gilliet et al. 2008). In human peripheral blood, PDCs selectively express TLR7 and TLR9, but not other TLRs, whereas in contrast, myeloid DCs express TLR1 through TLR6 and TLR8 (Jarrossay et al. 2001). Of note, myeloid DCs in mice do express TLR9 and respond to TLR9 triggering (Boonstra et al. 2003). Host-derived (self) nucleic acids do not activate PDCs. However, the human antimicrobial peptide LL37 can form a complex with self-RNA and self-DNA and thereby convert these otherwise inert nucleic acids into potent agonists for TLR7 and TLR9 (Lande et al. 2007; Ganguly et al. 2009). LL37 is absent in healthy skin, but skin injury induces transient LL37 expression in keratinocytes (Dorschner et al. 2001) as well as the release of self-RNA and self-DNA from damaged cells. PDCs rapidly infiltrate skin wounds and can be triggered by the injury-induced LL37/self-nucleic acid complexes to produce type I IFNs, a process that appears to be critical for the induction of early inflammatory responses and re-epithelization of injured skin (Gregorio et al. 2010).

Synthetic oligodeoxynucleotides (ODNs) containing repeating sequences of cytosine phosphoguanosine (CpG) dinucleotides—based on bacterial unmethylated CpG dinucleotide motifs—are well-known ligands for TLR9 and potent stimulators of PDCs to produce type I IFNs. However it is important to note that some CpG-containing ODNs do not stimulate type I IFN production. CpG-containing ODNs are classified into three main groups: A-type strongly stimulates IFN-α secretion by PDCs and cytokine production by NK cells; B-type stimulates PDCs to produce IL-6 and TNF-α (but not IFN-α) and B cells to proliferate and produce antibodies; C-type combines the immune effects of A- and B-types (Gilliet et al. 2008; Vollmer et al. 2004). CpG-containing ODNs are currently being evaluated as an adjuvant to vaccines in several clinical trials (Mbow et al. 2010), including trials in which the adjuvant is administered by ID injection (Molenkamp et al. 2007).

PDCs are absent in normal human skin (Zaba et al. 2007; Wollenberg et al. 2002a), but their presence in skin is quite common under pathologic conditions such as injury, infection, some inflammatory skin diseases, cancer, and autoimmunity (Farkas et al. 2001; Wollenberg et al. 2002a; de Vries et al. 2006; Gerlini et al. 2006; Vermi et al. 2003; Bangert et al. 2003). Remarkably, atopic dermatitis lesions lack PDCs which may clarify the susceptibility of atopic dermatitis patients to viral infections (Wollenberg et al. 2002a). Human PDCs selectively express chemokine receptor CMKLR1, which guides the cells to its attractant chemerin (Zabel et al. 2005). Inactive precursor chemerin is constitutively produced by dermal endothelial cells and fibroblasts and is cleaved into the active peptide by serine proteases released during blood coagulation that can happen upon skin damage (Zabel et al. 2005). In line with the abundant presence of PDCs in lesional skin, increased chemerin expression has been reported in psoriasis (Albanesi et al. 2009), lupus erythematosus (Vermi et al. 2005), and lichen planus (Parolini et al. 2007). Chemokine receptors CXCR3 and CXCR4 are both expressed by human PDCs and also involved in the tissue-infiltration. Intriguingly, PDCs do not respond efficiently to CXCR3-ligands CXCL9, CXCL10, and CXCL11 despite high expression of CXCR3, but presence of the CXCR3-ligands dramatically increase the responsiveness to CXCR4-ligand CXCL12, suggesting that the inflammation-induced CXCR3-ligands regulate the responsiveness of PDCs to CXCL12, which is constitutively expressed by dermal endothelial cells (Vanbervliet et al. 2003). In addition, human PDCs also express the skin-homing receptor CLA (Bangert et al. 2003; Vanbervliet et al. 2003). Injury in the dermis due to vaccine administration may also elicit bioactive chemerin and induce expression of CXCR3-ligands causing rapid PDC recruitment. This assumption is supported by recent findings that skin injury induces an early and short-lived infiltration of PDCs that release type I IFNs (Gregorio et al. 2010).

5.4.2 IDECs

In addition to the classical LCs (CD1a^{high}, Langerin^{+}, Birbeck granule^{+}, CD11b^{-}, CD36^{-}), inflamed epidermis contains a second distinct DC subset (CD1a^{low}, Langerin^{-}, Birbeck granule^{-}, CD11b^{+}, CD36^{+}) called inflammatory dendritic epidermal cell or in short IDEC (Wollenberg et al. 1996, 2002a; Gros et al. 2009). The influx of IDECs seems to be driven by the expression of chemokine receptors CCR5 and CCR6 (Gros et al. 2009). The IDECs constitute a diverse (dependent on the pathologic condition) though substantial percentage of the entire CD1a^{+} cell population and varies from 50% in allergic contact dermatitis to 66% in atopic dermatitis (Wollenberg et al. 1999). While under diverse inflamed conditions both epidermal DC subsets show upregulated expression of FcγRII (CD32), the expressions of the high-affinity IgE receptor FcεRI, and co-stimulatory molecules CD80 and CD86 were more pronounced on IDECs (Wollenberg et al. 1996; Schuller et al. 2001). IDECs with activated FcεRI (via binding and cross-linking of IgE) have been shown to drive naive T-cell development into IFN-γ-producing T cells by release of IL-12 and IL-18 (Novak et al. 2004). A cardinal role in the pathogenesis of atopic dermatitis has been assumed for the IDECs because of their high expression of FcεRI that enable the highly efficient uptake and presentation of IgE-bound allergens, and notably, these cells disappear after successful topical treatment of the skin (Wollenberg et al. 2001; Bieber et al. 2010). In contrast to

LCs, IDECs express the mannose receptor CD206 that is important for the uptake of bacteria- and fungi-derived mannosylated antigens (Wollenberg et al. 2002b). The $CD1a^{-}CD1c^{-}CD11b^{+}CD11c^{+}CD36^{+}Fc\gamma RII^{+}$ antigen-presenting cells that infiltrate the epidermis after exposure to high-dose ultraviolet B radiation (Meunier et al. 1995) bear close phenotypic resemblance to IDECs.

5.4.3 SlanDCs

$CD16^{+}CD14^{-}$ slanDCs lack the skin-homing receptor CLA, which is a carbohydrate modification of P-selectin glycoprotein ligand-1 (PSGL-1) (Fuhlbrigge et al. 1997). Instead, slanDCs express the cell type-specific slan epitope (6-sulfo LacNAc), as an alternative carbohydrate modification of PSGL-1 and as a consequence they fail to bind P- and E-selectin (Schakel et al. 2002). To enter areas of inflammation, slanDCs can take advantage of their receptors for the chemotaxins C3a and C5a, which are known to mediate rapid recruitment of cells into inflamed tissue (Schakel et al. 2002). SlanDCs are present in the skin lesions of psoriasis and chronic atopic dermatitis (Schakel et al. 2006; Gschwandtner et al. 2011). Upon stimulation with LPS, slanDCs produce TNF-α in large amount, far more than other types of blood DCs (Schakel et al. 2002). In addition, LPS-triggered slanDCs can quickly produce high levels of IL-12, a feature which is inhibited in blood through the interaction of CD47 on erythrocytes and the corresponding ligand SIRPα on slanDC. This inhibitory mechanism is released when slanDCs leave the bloodstream and infiltrate inflamed tissue (Schakel et al. 2006). SlanDCs can efficiently induce neoantigen-specific $CD4^{+}$ T cells and tumor-reactive $CD8^{+}$ T cells (Schakel et al. 1998, 2002). Furthermore, LPS-activated slanDCs efficiently enhance IFN-γ secretion by NK cells and NK cell-mediated tumor-directed cytotoxicity, whereas in return NK cells strongly enhance the secretion of IL-12, thereby improving slanDC-mediated generation of $CD4^{+}$ Th1 cells (Wehner et al. 2009). Activated neutrophils directly interact with and potentiate the function of both slanDCs and NK cells, and moreover, colocalization of neutrophils, NK cells, and slanDCs, as well as of IL-12 and IFNγ, in inflamed tissues of for instance psoriasis is strongly indicative of direct reciprocal interactions and positive amplification loops (Costantini et al. 2011). It was recently demonstrated that the slan epitope can be used for targeting antigens to slanDCs and that antigens bound to the slan epitope can be taken up by slanDCs, processed and presented to T cells (Bippes et al. 2011). A multivalent anti-slanDC modular scaffold system has been developed for specific delivery of antigens to slanDCs and may be useful for human vaccines (Bippes et al. 2011).

5.4.4 Tip-DCs

Tip-DCs were originally described in mice as a distinct $CD11c^{+}CD14^{-}$ DC subset that appears during *L. monocytogenes* infection and is essential for the clearance of primary bacterial infection. These DCs have high levels of co-stimulatory molecules and MHC class II, efficiently prime naive T cells, and express enormous amounts of TNF-α and inducible nitric oxide synthase (iNOS), hence their name TNF-α and iNOS-producing DCs or in short Tip-DCs (Serbina et al. 2003). In humans, the presence of Tip-DCs was shown in the papillary dermis and dermoepidermal junction of psoriatic lesional skin (Lowes et al. 2005). In addition to high expression of TNF-α and iNOS, the infiltrated Tip-DCs also express IL-12, IL-20, and IL-23 and can be discriminated from the resident CD11c^{+} DCs by the lack of CD1c and the expression of TRAIL (Zaba et al. 2009a, 2010). Both resident CD11c^{+}CD1c^{+} DDCs and CD11c^{+}CD1c^{-} Tip-DCs can polarize T cells to become Th1 or Th17 cells, but only Tip-DCs can induce a population of activated T cells that simultaneously coproduce IFN-γ and IL-17 (Zaba et al. 2009b). Human Tip-DCs are distinct from LCs and IDECs as they lack Langerin and CD1a expression, and in addition, they lack FXIIIa, which was previously used to identify DDCs but more recently shown to be a marker of dermal macrophages (Lowes et al. 2005). It is not clear how Tip-DCs and slanDCs are related to each others as both have many characteristics in common. Perhaps CD16 is a good marker to distinguish these cells from each other. SlanDCs are CD16^{+} and already exist in blood whereas Tip-DCs are described as being differentiated from mouse Ly6C^{hi}CCR2^{+} monocytes that correspond to the human classical CD14^{+}CD16^{-} monocyte subset (Serbina et al. 2003). In connection to this, CD8^{+} T cells can be recruited rapidly into the skin (Akiba et al. 2002) contributing to the rapid development of human monocytes into Tip-DCs that express high levels of TNF-α and iNOS (Chong et al. 2011).

6 Relationship Between DC Subsets

6.1 Ontogeny of Human DCs

Extensive modeling in the mouse has recently established not only the cellular identity of committed DC progenitors, but also the control of DC differentiation by a number of transcription factors and growth factor receptor pathways (reviewed by Merad and Manz (2009) and Geissmann et al. (2010)). The homologues of monocyte/DC precursor cells, common DC precursors, and circulating precursors for classical DCs are not known in humans. Overall, the large array of data generated with monocyte-derived DCs has not hastened acceptance of a dedicated human DC precursor. Although the prevailing view is that monocytes give rise to inflammatory DCs that are not equivalent to the authentic DC lineage, few human studies have made the comparison between monocyte-derived DCs and primary blood or tissue DCs (van der Aar et al. 2007; Osugi et al. 2002; Peiser et al. 2004; Burster et al. 2005; Schnurr et al. 2005). In addition there are no compartments of human mononuclear cells that could contain an undiscovered circulating DC precursor. The most likely candidate for the circulating precursor of the classical DC is the CD1c^{+} blood DC itself (which perhaps tellingly, has no counterpart in mouse). The CD34^{+} progenitor cells might also give rise to tissue DCs although its potential is not restricted to DCs. Both cells are $FLT3^+$ and MHC class II^+, whereas murine precursors for classical DCs are MHC class II^-. Investigators looking for human precursors for classical DCs in the MHC class II^- multi-$lineage^-$ compartment of human blood will find mainly $CD123^+$ basophils, although there are also scattered $CD34^+$ cells that might have DC progenitor capacity (Bigley and Collin, unpublished).

The two principal subsets of DDCs identified by CD14 and CD1a have evident similarities with monocytes and $CD1c^+$ blood DCs, respectively. This includes parallel expression of macrophage colony-stimulating factor receptor (MCSFR), CD163, CD209 in the $CD14^+$ subset and FLT3, CD1c, and CD83 in the $CD1a^+$ subset. Monocytes and $CD14^+$ DCs are not proliferating in contrast to $CD1c^+$ blood DCs and $CD1a^+$ DDCs (Haniffa et al. 2009; Bigley and Collin, unpublished). Adoptive transfer into immunodeficient mice may be able to test these relationships.

LCs in humans are clearly able to proliferate in situ (Czernielewski et al. 1985; Czernielewski and Demarchez 1987) but whether this is sufficient for lifelong homeostasis is currently unknown. MHC-matched transplantation in the absence of graft versus host disease results in high levels of donor LC engraftment, although admittedly this is slower than for DDC subsets and a small number of recipient LCs survive long-term (Haniffa et al. 2009; Collin et al. 2006). Donor LC survival for a number of years after limb transplantation has been described (Kanitakis et al. 2004). Dermatitis increases the rate of LC proliferation (Chorro et al. 2009) and given the ease with which monocytes can be induced to express Langerin, they remain good precursor candidates following severe inflammation (Geissmann et al. 1998). In addition, it has also been suggested that LCs may develop from dermal-resident $CD14^+$ cells (Larregina et al. 2001), and according to another study, the hair follicle may be a critical reservoir of LCs that re-populate epidermis depleted of LCs by a single high-dose of ultraviolet B (Gilliam et al. 1998). The observation that patients with autosomal recessive deficiency of transcription factor IRF8 lack $CD1a^+$ and $CD14^+$ DDCs, but concurrently have a normal density of LCs, is indicative for the improbability that LCs develop directly from DDCs or, alternatively, underlines the potential for local selfrenewal of LCs (Hambleton et al. 2011).

6.2 *Functional Specialization of Cutaneous DCs in Humans*

Several studies have attempted to compare the function of LCs and different DDC subsets from human skin. These comparisons relied not only upon skin-derived DCs but also on in vitro equivalents derived from $CD34^+$ stem cells or $CD14^+$ peripheral blood monocytes. The $CD14^+$ DCs are more phagocytic, more adherent and express lower CD80, CD86, CD83, and CCR7 than the $CD1a^+$ DCs (Angel et al. 2006, 2007a; Haniffa et al. 2009; de Gruijl et al. 2006). The T-cell-stimulatory capacity of $CD14^+$ DDCs is much lower than the other DC subsets in the skin (Morelli et al. 2005). A specific role for $CD14^+$ cells in instructing IL-21-producing Tfh cells has been recently demonstrated (Klechevsky et al. 2008, 2009; Schmitt et al. 2009). This induction of human Tfh is dependent on IL-12 and transcription factor STAT4, in contrast to murine Tfh that are developing in an IL-6 and STAT3-dependent fashion (Schmitt et al. 2009). $CD1a^+$ DCs derived from $CD34^+$ cells are more potent stimulators of naive T cells, have higher cross-presenting capacity and also preferentially induce the differentiation of $CD4^+$ T cells secreting Th2 cell cytokines (Klechevsky et al. 2008; Cao et al. 2007; Duraisingham et al. 2009). One study showed that LCs migrated from skin possess a higher capacity than migrated $CD1c^+CD14^-$ DDCs to stimulate allogeneic naive $CD4^+$ T-cell proliferation and to promote the development of both Th1 and Th2 cells (Furio et al. 2010), whereas in another study (using non-purified cells) the stimulatory capacities of LCs and DDCs are comparable (Pena-Cruz et al. 2010). Nevertheless, both studies demonstrated that migrated mature LCs and DDCs have high upregulated expression of PD-L1 and PD-L2 (both involved in negative regulation of T-cell activation and induction of peripheral tolerance) and that blockade of PD-L1 and/or PD-L2 markedly enhanced T-cell activation.

DDCs have a broad TLR expression profile (TLR1 through TLR8), whereas LCs have a selective impaired expression of bacteria-sensing TLR2, TLR4 and TLR5. As a consequence LCs weakly respond to Gram-positive and Gram-negative bacteria, but their responsiveness to viruses is comparable to DDCs (van der Aar et al. 2007). The TLR profiles of monocyte-derived LCs and authentic LCs closely match (van der Aar et al. 2007), but the TLR pattern of $CD34^+$ stem cell-derived LC-like cells is dissimilar (Renn et al. 2006; Duraisingham et al. 2010), and therefore, the validity of $CD34^+$ stem cell-derived LC-like cells as a model of LCs may be questioned. LCs show deficiency in processing and MHC-II-restricted presentation of bacterial antigens and as a consequence, poorly restimulate antibacterial memory $CD4^+$ T cells and inefficiently induce bacteria-specific effector $CD4^+$ T cells from naive T cells, but rather initiate the development of regulatory $Foxp3^+CD4^+$ T cells (AMG van der Aar, EC de Jong, and MBM Teunissen, unpublished). These features of human LCs render the epidermis as a site of tolerance for the commensal bacteria of the skin, whereas the DDCs ensure immunity against bacteria that have penetrated into the dermis. Despite their inferior capacity to raise antibacterial immunity, LCs appear to be superior to DDCs for the initiation of antiviral immunity, as they efficiently stimulate naive $CD8^+$ T cells to differentiate into effector cells that express IFN-γ, TNF-α, granzyme B, and high cytotoxic activity (van der Aar et al. 2011a). This superiority of LCs is causally related to viral-induced high levels of CD70 expression, but not to IL-12 production. The high potential of LCs to activate $CD8^+$ T cells has also been reported in a recent study in which a comparison was made between LCs versus $CD14^+$ DDCs (Klechevsky et al. 2009). Vitamin D3 has immunosuppressive potential which may be exerted via modulation of DC function and leading to the induction of regulatory T cells. Remarkably, vitamin D3-exposed LCs generated $CD25^{hi}CD127^{lo}Foxp3^+$ T cells (matching the features of classical inducible regulatory T cells), whereas vitamin D3-exposed DDCs favored the development of regulatory T cells that were $Foxp3^-$ and expressing

IL-10 (corresponding to the subtype Tr1) (van der Aar et al. 2011b). In addition, the LC-derived TGF-β and DDC-derived IL-10 appeared to the key factors in the induction of Foxp3$^+$ regulatory T cells and IL-10$^+$ Tr1 cells, respectively.

LCs, migrated from cultured skin, have been shown to be the main skin DC subset capable of inducing Th17 responses dependent on the combined effects of IL-15 and IL-6 (Mathers et al. 2009). DDCs cannot synthesize IL-15 and are unable to bias Th17 responses, unless the cultures are supplemented with IL-15 and IL-6 (Mathers et al. 2009). In contrast however, in another study it is demonstrated that CD11c$^+$CD1c$^+$ DDCs are able to polarize T cells to become Th17 cells (Zaba et al. 2009b). Of note, purified CD207$^+$ LCs and CD11c$^+$CD1c$^+$DDCs can induce IL-22-producing CD4$^+$ and CD8$^+$ T cells from allogeneic peripheral blood T cells (Fujita et al. 2009). The LCs are more powerful inducers of IL-22-producing T cells than DDCs and this holds also true for monocyte-derived LCs versus monocyte-derived DCs. Surprisingly, the majority of the IL-22-producing T cells induced by LCs and DDCs lacked the expression of IL-17, IFN-γ, and IL-4 (Fujita et al. 2009).

It is very hard to compare the published data on functional analysis of human LCs and DDC subsets because there is considerable variation in the origin of the cells and the isolation methods used to obtain the distinct DC subsets. To name some of the differences: the DC subsets are either derived from skin or derived from CD14$^+$ monocytes or CD34$^+$ stem cells; the skin-derived DCs are either freshly isolated via enzymatic digestion of skin or have spontaneously crawled out the skin during in vitro culture for 1–3 days (e.g. DCs mature progressively during culture whereas CD1a expression decreases); the crawl-out DCs are derived from cultured full skin (epidermis and dermis not separated) or from epidermis and dermis that have been separated first and then cultured; the tests are performed with crude cell suspensions or the LCs and DDC subsets are purified; the purification is done by either positive or negative selection using different selection markers (for example CD1a, CD1c, or CD207 to isolate LCs); the purification is performed with either fluorescence- or magnetic-based cell-separation technologies, such as FACS, MACS, or EasySep. All these basic differences certainly lead to major differences in maturation status and functional behavior of the DCs. So, the question whether LCs and DDCs have functional specialization in certain immune responses against bacteria, viruses, fungi, or tumors still remains controversial.

7 Intradermal Vaccination and Skin DCs

7.1 Which Skin DC Subset is Important?

Functional specialization of DC subsets has been shown in mice (Ginhoux et al. 2010), but definitive evidence for similar functional specialization in man has not been provided yet, as explained in the previous section for LCs and DDC subsets

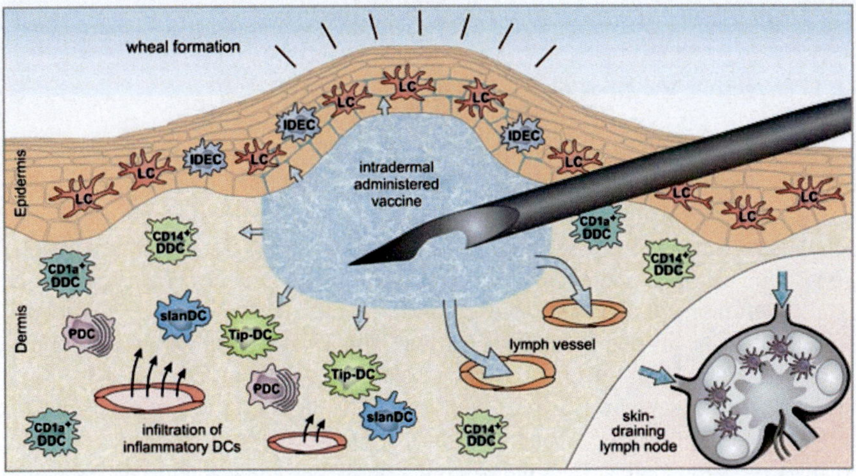

Fig. 4 Intradermal vaccination and relevant skin DC subsets. Intradermal administered vaccine can be captured by steady-state cutaneous DCs (namely LCs, CD1a$^+$ DDCs and CD14$^+$ DDCs) or by recruited inflammatory DCs (such as IDECs, slanDCs, Tip-DCs, and PDCs) and transported to the paracortical areas in the skin-draining lymph node where these DCs give rise to CD4$^+$ and CD8$^+$ effector T-cells and immunoglobulin-producing B cells for long-term protective immunity. The vaccine can also drain via the lymph vessels to the local lymph node, captured by DC subsets that reside in the lymph node, and presented to lymphocytes in a skin DC-independent fashion. A detailed description of the different DC subsets is provided in Sects. 4 and 5

that reside in normal human skin. Furthermore, ID-delivered vaccines give an impulse for inflammation, but it is not clear which of the aforementioned inflammatory DC types will be recruited into the injected skin site and participate in the process of immunization. Moreover, upon ID administration the vaccine rapidly diffuses into the surrounding tissue and is drained via the lymph vessels reaching the skin-draining lymph nodes thus directly affecting the DC subsets that reside in the lymph node. It is unknown for how long and how much of the vaccine will remain in the skin. The viscosity of the injected substance or the size of particle-based vaccines (e.g. nanoparticles, liposomes) will largely determine the time that the vaccine is stuck in the skin. In addition, the particle size can determine which DC subset is targeted and influence the Th1/Th2 cytokine balance, antibody responses, and cross-presentation (Combadiere and Mahe 2008). The physical, biochemical, and immunomodulating properties of the vaccine and adjuvant may affect the migration, phenotype, function of the skin DC subsets in different ways. So, the question as to which skin DC subset is most relevant for ID vaccination cannot simply be answered and is tightly related to the nature of the vaccine and the aim of the vaccination (for example, immunization versus tolerization). Finally, it cannot be excluded that more than one DC subset is required for optimal vaccination outcome (Fig. 4).

7.2 Improvement of Intradermal Vaccination

7.2.1 Targeting Vaccines to DC Subsets

Targeting of antigens to DCs facilitates antigen uptake and thereby enhances $CD4^+$ and $CD8^+$ T-cell responses. Targeting vaccine antigens to DCs can be achieved in various ways, for example by coupling antigens to antibodies that are specific for DCs or a certain DC subset (generally antibodies against C-type lectins) or are specific for surface molecules that are highly expressed by (activated) DCs (e.g. CD40-targeted vaccine), see companion reviews by Romani et al. and Oosterhoff et al. in this volume of Current Topics in Microbiology and Immunology (Romani et al. 2011; Oosterhoff et al. 2011). Lectin DEC-205 has been tested in multiple studies in mice and appears to be an attractive candidate for antigen targeting to DCs. All human skin DC subsets express this lectin. Flacher et al. demonstrated that ID-administered fluorescent-labeled anti-DEC-205 and anti-Langerin antibodies in murine or human skin are efficiently captured by LCs, but not DDCs, within minutes after ID injection and that targeted DCs carry the antibodies when leaving the skin (Flacher et al. 2010). Apparently, even large immunoglobulins (150 kDa) can easily diffuse from the dermis through the basement membrane into the epidermis and gain access to LCs. This result also proves that LCs are not by-passed when an immunizing antigen is administered in the dermis. The targeting antibody persists on LCs for several days, implying that targeted LCs can be exploited throughout an extended period (Flacher et al. 2010). LCs are able to present antigen to T cells when the antigen is coupled to anti-DEC-205, but not when the antigen is coupled to anti-Langerin (Flacher et al. 2010). Interestingly, targeting antigens to DCs through DEC-205 in the absence of DC activation results in tolerance induction, but if the antigen-targeting is performed with concurrent DC activation generation of immunity will occur instead (Bonifaz et al. 2004; Kretschmer et al. 2005). A similar feature has been found when antigens are targeted to CLEC9A: antigen linked to anti-CLEC9A promotes the development of antigen-specific $CD4^+Foxp3^+$ regulatory T cells in the steady state but co-administration of adjuvants prevents tolerance induction and promotes immunity (Joffre et al. 2010).

A recent study shows that targeting antigens to human DCs through DCIR-(CLEC4A) enhanced antigen-specific $CD8^+$ T-cell-immunity by all human DC subsets including in vitro-generated DCs, skin-derived LCs, and blood myeloid DCs and PDCs, which is quite remarkable as DCIR contains an immunoreceptor tyrosine-based inhibitory motif (Klechevsky et al. 2010). DCIR triggering inhibits TLR9-induced IFN-α production by PDCs while leaving up-regulation of co-stimulatory molecule expression unaffected (Meyer-Wentrup et al. 2008). Targeting PDCs through BDCA-2 may be tricky, as BDCA-2-induced signaling in PDCs diminishes the ability of activated PDCs to process and present antigens to T cells (Jahn et al. 2010). Other C-type lectins such as CLEC9A and CLEC12 are additional interesting candidates for targeting, but the expression of these lectins on skin DCs has not yet been investigated (Caminschi et al. 2009). Instead of linking antibodies to soluble antigens or vectors, antibodies can also be used to decorate antigenic particles, but in this case the particle size is crucial (Cruz et al. 2010). Alternatively, vaccine targeting to DCs, in particular to the lectin receptors of these cells, can also be achieved by glycan modification of the antigen (Singh et al. 2009).

7.2.2 Harnessing and Fine-Tuning DC Function with Adjuvants

Vaccine adjuvants are used to improve the potency of the immune response, enhance immunological memory and reduce the number of doses. Different classes of compounds display adjuvant activity in preclinical models; among them, bacterial products, mineral salts, emulsions, nanoparticles, nucleic acids, small molecules, saponins, and liposomes. However, very few have been licensed for human use as the vast majority have an unacceptable safety profile (Mbow et al. 2010; Tritto et al. 2009). Mineral salts aluminium oxyhydroxide and aluminum hydroxyphosphate (commonly referred to as alum) are still the most widely used adjuvants in vaccines and known to promote type 2 immune responses and enhance antibody production. Despite many decades of use, very little is known about the mechanism of action of alum. One proposed mechanism includes the formation of a depot from which the antigen is slowly released. Another explanation is that alum directly triggers the NLRP3 inflammasome, which leads to the production of the pro-inflammatory cytokines IL-1β, IL-18, and IL-33 (Eisenbarth et al. 2008; Hornung et al. 2008). Alternatively, due to its cytotoxicity alum causes cell death in the injection site with subsequent release of uric acid, which also activates the NLRP3 inflammasome, and in addition, attracts monocytes that differentiate into inflammatory DCs (Kool et al. 2008). Similarly to alum, the oil-in-water emulsion adjuvant MF59 increases recruitment of immune cells into the injection site, enhance monocyte differentiation into DCs, augment Ag uptake, and facilitate migration of DCs into tissue-draining lymph nodes to prime adaptive immune responses (Seubert et al. 2008; Mosca et al. 2008). It can be questioned whether these kind of adjuvants are suitable for ID vaccines, as they provoke visible inflammation in the skin for several days which may not be cosmetically acceptable.

The classical adjuvants are based on empirical knowledge, but the new generation of adjuvants is rationally designed, for example TLR9-ligand CpG and TLR4-ligand MPL have been engineered and demonstrated to be useful adjuvants. However, it is not certain whether these two adjuvants will be optimal adjuvants for ID vaccination, as DDCs lack TLR9 and LCs lack both TLR4 and TLR9. It may be that other TLR ligands are more suitable as adjuvants for immunization via the skin, for example the TLR7 agonist imiquimod, which is already licensed for topical use and potentiates immune responses in the skin. To enhance efficiency, combining TLR stimuli may be one strategy as has recently be shown in immunization experiments in mice: triggering both TLR4 and TLR7 by MPL and imiquimod causing a synergistic increase in antigen-specific, neutralizing antibodies (Kasturi et al. 2011). Application of certain adjuvants can also be used to manipulate DCs to induce distinct $CD4^{+}$ T-cell responses: the TLR3 agonist poly I:C induces strong IL-12-independent Th1 responses, whereas the Dectin-1 agonist curdlan primes for Th17 cell development (Joffre et al. 2010). It is increasingly clear that DC functions are strongly influenced by crosstalk with neighboring cells like keratinocytes that are a rich source of immunomodulatory cytokines. Vaccination via the skin offers the possibility to manipulate keratinocytes to secrete a certain cytokine (profile) that instruct DCs to promote the required type of T-cell response, for example keratinocytes can be induced to produce the cytokine TSLP which instruct DCs to promote Th2 cell development (Bogiatzi et al. 2007; Liu et al. 2007). Of course it is also possible to co-administer the desired cytokine as an adjuvant.

Local cell death and inflammation at the vaccination site occurs with the classical adjuvant alum, but this collateral damage is limited by targeting PAMP-based adjuvants to DCs. It is not clear to what extent the alum-induced triggering of the NLRP3 inflammasome contributes to the success of the immunization. It may very well be that activation of this inflammasome is an important aspect of the mechanism of action of the adjuvant alum. If so, it may be worth to include inflammasome-targeting adjuvants in vaccines.

8 Concluding Remarks and Perspectives

There are two successful and widely practiced ID vaccination strategies: (1) ID rabies vaccination has been shown to be 100% effective as pre- and post-exposure prophylaxis against human rabies encephalitis (Warrell 2011). (2) BCG vaccine; WHO recommends the ID route for the administration of the BCG vaccine against tuberculosis (World Health Organization 2004). It is clear that ID immunization is effective in humans, but the acceptance for this vaccination route is slow. Dose-sparing is one of the benefits of using ID delivery by reducing the costs of purchase, distribution and storage of vaccines, and by increasing vaccine availability in times of pandemics when vaccines may be scarce. In clinical trials it has been demonstrated that ID administration of a reduced dose of standard influenza vaccine elicited immunogenicity that was at least equal to intramuscular full dose administration (Kenney et al. 2004; Kunzi et al. 2009) and similarly, ID administration of yellow fever vaccine at a reduced dose induced protective immunity similar to conventional subcutaneous vaccination (Roukens et al. 2008). Keeping in mind that the vaccines used in these clinical trials were not specially designed for ID use but show comparable efficiency even at reduced dosages, this underlines the great potential for the skin as a vaccination site and suggests that the efficacy of ID vaccination can be further improved.

To take optimal advantage of the ID route of vaccine administration, vaccinologists should rationally design the antigen, adjuvant(s) and formulate for this purpose. The information in this review about the human skin-associated immune system and the immunobiology of the skin DC subsets may encourage vaccine engineers to create highly effective ID vaccines. The antigen should ideally target the resident and/or recruited skin DCs and via the addition of one or more adjuvants the DC-specific functions can be exploited to generate the required type of T-cell response. Of course there are more aspects that need to be improved to make ID vaccination feasible, such as the development of special devices to make the administration reliable and easy, and last but not least, the administration of the vaccine must be as painless as possible, the induration and local inflammation must be limited and scar formation negligible. The ultimate aim will be the development of excellent ID vaccines, each specifically designed to induce protective immunity against a particular pathogen, and superior to the current classical vaccines.

References

Akiba H, Kehren J, Ducluzeau MT, Krasteva M, Horand F, Kaiserlian D, Kaneko F, Nicolas JF (2002) Skin inflammation during contact hypersensitivity is mediated by early recruitment of CD8+ T cytotoxic 1 cells inducing keratinocyte apoptosis. J Immunol 168:3079–3087

Albanesi C, Scarponi C, Giustizieri ML, Girolomoni G (2005) Keratinocytes in inflammatory skin diseases. Curr Drug Targets Inflamm Allergy 4:329–334

Albanesi C, Scarponi C, Pallotta S, Daniele R, Bosisio D, Madonna S, Fortugno P, Gonzalvo-Feo S, Franssen JD, Parmentier M, De PO, Girolomoni G, Sozzani S (2009) Chemerin expression marks early psoriatic skin lesions and correlates with plasmacytoid dendritic cell recruitment. J Exp Med 206:249–258

Alcami A, Damon I, Evans D, Huggins JW, Hughes C, Jahrling PB, McFadden G, Meyer H, Moss B, Shchelkunov S, Stavskiy E, Tikunova N (2010) Scientific review of variola virus research, 1999–2010. http://www.who.int/csr/resources/publications/WHO_HSE_GAR_BDP_2010_3/en

Allam JP, Geiger E, Kraft S, Bieber T (2003) Limited reliability of E-cadherin as a specific marker for in vitro-generated Langerhans cells. Arch Dermatol Res 295:263–268

Angel CE, George E, Brooks AE, Ostrovsky LL, Brown TL, Dunbar PR (2006) Cutting edge: CD1a+ antigen-presenting cells in human dermis respond rapidly to CCR7 ligands. J Immunol 176:5730–5734

Angel CE, Lala A, Chen CJ, Edgar SG, Ostrovsky LL, Dunbar PR (2007a) CD14+ antigen-presenting cells in human dermis are less mature than their CD1a+ counterparts. Int Immunol 19:1271–1279

Angel CE, George E, Ostrovsky LL, Dunbar PR (2007b) Comprehensive analysis of MHC-II expression in healthy human skin. Immunol Cell Biol 85:363–369

Angel CE, Chen CJ, Horlacher OC, Winkler S, John T, Browning J, MacGregor D, Cebon J, Dunbar PR (2009) Distinctive localization of antigen-presenting cells in human lymph nodes. Blood 113:1257–1267

Anguille S, Smits EL, Cools N, Goossens H, Berneman ZN, Van Tendeloo VF (2009) Short-term cultured, interleukin-15 differentiated dendritic cells have potent immunostimulatory properties. J Transl Med 7:109

Ansel KM, Lee DU, Rao A (2003) An epigenetic view of helper T cell differentiation. Nat Immunol 4:616–623

Asselin-Paturel C, Boonstra A, Dalod M, Durand I, Yessaad N, Dezutter-Dambuyant C, Vicari A, O'Garra A, Biron C, Briere F, Trinchieri G (2001) Mouse type I IFN-producing cells are immature APCs with plasmacytoid morphology. Nat Immunol 2:1144–1150

Bachem A, Guttler S, Hartung E, Ebstein F, Schaefer M, Tannert A, Salama A, Movassaghi K, Opitz C, Mages HW, Henn V, Kloetzel PM, Gurka S, Kroczek RA (2010) Superior antigen cross-presentation and XCR1 expression define human CD11c+CD141+ cells as homologues of mouse CD8+ dendritic cells. J Exp Med 207:1273–1281

Badiee A, Davies N, McDonald K, Radford K, Michiue H, Hart D, Kato M (2007) Enhanced delivery of immunoliposomes to human dendritic cells by targeting the multilectin receptor DEC-205. Vaccine 25:4757–4766

Banchereau J, Steinman RM (1998) Dendritic cells and the control of immunity. Nature 392:245–252

Bangert C, Friedl J, Stary G, Stingl G, Kopp T (2003) Immunopathologic features of allergic contact dermatitis in humans: participation of plasmacytoid dendritic cells in the pathogenesis of the disease? J Invest Dermatol 121:1409–1418

Barbalat R, Ewald SE, Mouchess ML, Barton GM (2011) Nucleic acid recognition by the innate immune system. Annu Rev Immunol 29:185–214

Bauer J, Bahmer FA, Worl J, Neuhuber W, Schuler G, Fartasch M (2001) A strikingly constant ratio exists between Langerhans cells and other epidermal cells in human skin. A stereologic study using the optical disector method and the confocal laser scanning microscope. J Invest Dermatol 116:313–318

Bechetoille N, Andre V, Valladeau J, Perrier E, Dezutter-Dambuyant C (2006) Mixed Langerhans cell and interstitial/dermal dendritic cell subsets emanating from monocytes in Th2-mediated inflammatory conditions respond differently to proinflammatory stimuli. J Leukoc Biol 80:45–58

Bedoui S, Whitney PG, Waithman J, Eidsmo L, Wakim L, Caminschi I, Allan RS, Wojtasiak M, Shortman K, Carbone FR, Brooks AG, Heath WR (2009) Cross-presentation of viral and self antigens by skin-derived CD103+ dendritic cells. Nat Immunol 10:488–495

Bendelac A, Savage PB, Teyton L (2007) The biology of NKT cells. Annu Rev Immunol 25:297–336

Bieber T, Novak N, Herrman N, Koch S (2010) Role of Dendritic Cells in Atopic Dermatitis: An Update. Clin Rev Allergy Immunol. doi:10.1007/s12016-010-8224-0

Bippes CC, Feldmann A, Stamova S, Cartellieri M, Schwarzer A, Wehner R, Schmitz M, Rieber EP, Zhao S, Schakel K, Temme A, Scofield RH, Kurien BT, Bartsch H, Bachmann M (2011) A novel modular antigen delivery system for immuno targeting of human 6-sulfo LacNAc-positive blood dendritic cells (SlanDCs). PLoS One 6:e16315

Birbeck MS, Breathnach AS, Everall JD (1961) An electron microscope study of basal melanocytes and high-level clear cells (Langerhans cells) in vitiligo. J Invest Dermatol 37:51–64

Blanco P, Palucka AK, Pascual V, Banchereau J (2008) Dendritic cells and cytokines in human inflammatory and autoimmune diseases. Cytokine Growth Factor Rev 19:41–52

Bogiatzi SI, Fernandez I, Bichet JC, Marloie-Provost MA, Volpe E, Sastre X, Soumelis V (2007) Cutting edge: proinflammatory and Th2 cytokines synergize to induce thymic stromal lymphopoietin production by human skin keratinocytes. J Immunol 178:3373–3377

Bonifaz LC, Bonnyay DP, Charalambous A, Darguste DI, Fujii S, Soares H, Brimnes MK, Moltedo B, Moran TM, Steinman RM (2004) In vivo targeting of antigens to maturing dendritic cells via the DEC-205 receptor improves T cell vaccination. J Exp Med 199:815–824

Boonstra A, Asselin-Paturel C, Gilliet M, Crain C, Trinchieri G, Liu YJ, O'Garra A (2003) Flexibility of mouse classical and plasmacytoid-derived dendritic cells in directing T helper type 1 and 2 cell development: dependency on antigen dose and differential toll-like receptor ligation. J Exp Med 197:101–109

Bos JD, Kapsenberg ML (1986) The skin immune system: its cellular constituents and their interactions. Immunol Today 7:235–240

Bos JD, Meinardi MM (2000) The 500 Da rule for the skin penetration of chemical compounds and drugs. Exp Dermatol 9:165–169

Brand CU, Hunger RE, Yawalkar N, Gerber HA, Schaffner T, Braathen LR (1999) Characterization of human skin-derived CD1a-positive lymph cells. Arch Dermatol Res 291:65–72

Brandner JM, Kief S, Grund C, Rendl M, Houdek P, Kuhn C, Tschachler E, Franke WW, Moll I (2002) Organization and formation of the tight junction system in human epidermis and cultured keratinocytes. Eur J Cell Biol 81:253–263

Burgdorf S, Kurts C (2008) Endocytosis mechanisms and the cell biology of antigen presentation. Curr Opin Immunol 20:89–95

Burgdorf S, Kautz A, Bohnert V, Knolle PA, Kurts C (2007) Distinct pathways of antigen uptake and intracellular routing in CD4 and CD8 T cell activation. Science 316:612–616

Burgdorf S, Scholz C, Kautz A, Tampe R, Kurts C (2008) Spatial and mechanistic separation of cross-presentation and endogenous antigen presentation. Nat Immunol 9:558–566

Bursch LS, Wang L, Igyarto B, Kissenpfennig A, Malissen B, Kaplan DH, Hogquist KA (2007) Identification of a novel population of Langerin+ dendritic cells. J Exp Med 204:3147–3156

Burster T, Beck A, Tolosa E, Schnorrer P, Weissert R, Reich M, Kraus M, Kalbacher H, Haring HU, Weber E, Overkleeft H, Driessen C (2005) Differential processing of autoantigens in lysosomes from human monocyte-derived and peripheral blood dendritic cells. J Immunol 175:5940–5949

Burton RF (2008) Estimating body surface area from mass and height: theory and the formula of Du Bois and Du Bois. Ann Hum Biol 35:170–184

Caminschi I, Lahoud MH, Shortman K (2009) Enhancing immune responses by targeting antigen to DC. Eur J Immunol 39:931–938

Campbell DJ, Koch MA (2011) Phenotypical and functional specialization of FOXP3+ regulatory T cells. Nat Rev Immunol 11:119–130

Campbell DJ, Kim CH, Butcher EC (2003) Chemokines in the systemic organization of immunity. Immunol Rev 195:58–71

Cao W, Rosen DB, Ito T, Bover L, Bao M, Watanabe G, Yao Z, Zhang L, Lanier LL, Liu YJ (2006) Plasmacytoid dendritic cell-specific receptor ILT7-Fc epsilonRI gamma inhibits toll-like receptor-induced interferon production. J Exp Med 203:1399–1405

Cao T, Ueno H, Glaser C, Fay JW, Palucka AK, Banchereau J (2007) Both Langerhans cells and interstitial DC cross-present melanoma antigens and efficiently activate antigen-specific CTL. Eur J Immunol 37:2657–2667

Caux C, Massacrier C, Vanbervliet B, Dubois B, Durand I, Cella M, Lanzavecchia A, Banchereau J (1997) CD34+ hematopoietic progenitors from human cord blood differentiate along two independent dendritic cell pathways in response to granulocyte-macrophage colony-stimulating factor plus tumor necrosis factor alpha: II. Functional analysis. Blood 90:1458–1470

Cella M, Sallusto F, Lanzavecchia A (1997) Origin, maturation and antigen presenting function of dendritic cells. Curr Opin Immunol 9:10–16

Cella M, Jarrossay D, Facchetti F, Alebardi O, Nakajima H, Lanzavecchia A, Colonna M (1999) Plasmacytoid monocytes migrate to inflamed lymph nodes and produce large amounts of type I interferon. Nat Med 5:919–923

Cerio R, Griffiths CE, Cooper KD, Nickoloff BJ, Headington JT (1989) Characterization of factor XIIIa positive dermal dendritic cells in normal and inflamed skin. Br J Dermatol 121:421–431

Chen GY, Nunez G (2010) Sterile inflammation: sensing and reacting to damage. Nat Rev Immunol 10:826–837

Chong SZ, Wong KL, Lin G, Yang CM, Wong SC, Angeli V, Macary PA, Kemeny DM (2011) Human CD8(+) T cells drive Th1 responses through the differentiation of TNF/iNOS-producing dendritic cells. Eur J Immunol 41:1639–1651

Chorro L, Sarde A, Li M, Woollard KJ, Chambon P, Malissen B, Kissenpfennig A, Barbaroux JB, Groves R, Geissmann F (2009) Langerhans cell (LC) proliferation mediates neonatal development, homeostasis, and inflammation-associated expansion of the epidermal LC network. J Exp Med 206:3089–3100

Clark RA, Chong B, Mirchandani N, Brinster NK, Yamanaka K, Dowgiert RK, Kupper TS (2006) The vast majority of CLA+ T cells are resident in normal skin. J Immunol 176:4431–4439

Clayton E, Doupe DP, Klein AM, Winton DJ, Simons BD, Jones PH (2007) A single type of progenitor cell maintains normal epidermis. Nature 446:185–189

Cohen NR, Garg S, Brenner MB (2009) Antigen presentation by CD1 Lipids, T Cells, and NKT cells in microbial immunity. Adv Immunol 102:1–94

Collin MP, Hart DN, Jackson GH, Cook G, Cavet J, Mackinnon S, Middleton PG, Dickinson AM (2006) The fate of human Langerhans cells in hematopoietic stem cell transplantation. J Exp Med 203:27–33

Combadiere B, Mahe B (2008) Particle-based vaccines for transcutaneous vaccination. Comp Immunol Microbiol Infect Dis 31:293–315

Costantini C, Calzetti F, Perbellini O, Micheletti A, Scarponi C, Lonardi S, Pelletier M, Schakel K, Pizzolo G, Facchetti F, Vermi W, Albanesi C, Cassatella MA (2011) Human neutrophils interact with both 6-sulfo LacNAc+ DC and NK cells to amplify NK-derived IFN{gamma}: role of CD18, ICAM-1, and ICAM-3. Blood 117:1677–1686

Cox K, North M, Burke M, Singhal H, Renton S, Aqel N, Islam S, Knight SC (2005) Plasmacytoid dendritic cells (PDC) are the major DC subset innately producing cytokines in human lymph nodes. J Leukoc Biol 78:1142–1152

Crotty S (2011) Follicular helper CD4 T cells (TFH). Annu Rev Immunol 29:621–663

Crozat K, Guiton R, Contreras V, Feuillet V, Dutertre CA, Ventre E, Vu Manh TP, Baranek T, Storset AK, Marvel J, Boudinot P, Hosmalin A, Schwartz-Cornil I, Dalod M (2010a) The XC chemokine receptor 1 is a conserved selective marker of mammalian cells homologous to mouse CD8alpha+ dendritic cells. J Exp Med 207:1283–1292

Crozat K, Guiton R, Guilliams M, Henri S, Baranek T, Schwartz-Cornil I, Malissen B, Dalod M (2010b) Comparative genomics as a tool to reveal functional equivalences between human and mouse dendritic cell subsets. Immunol Rev 234:177–198

Cruz LJ, Tacken PJ, Fokkink R, Joosten B, Stuart MC, Albericio F, Torensma R, Figdor CG (2010) Targeted PLGA nano- but not microparticles specifically deliver antigen to human dendritic cells via DC-SIGN in vitro. J Control Release 144:118–126

Cumberbatch M, Dearman RJ, Kimber I (1997) Langerhans cells require signals from both tumour necrosis factor-alpha and interleukin-1 beta for migration. Immunology 92:388–395

Czernielewski JM, Demarchez M (1987) Further evidence for the self-reproducing capacity of Langerhans cells in human skin. J Invest Dermatol 88:17–20

Czernielewski J, Vaigot P, Prunieras M (1985) Epidermal Langerhans cells–a cycling cell population. J Invest Dermatol 84:424–426

de Boer OJ, van der Loos CM, Teeling P, van der Wal AC, Teunissen MBM (2007) Immunohistochemical analysis of regulatory T cell markers FOXP3 and GITR on CD4+CD25+ T cells in normal skin and inflammatory dermatoses. J Histochem Cytochem 55:891–898

de Gruijl TD, Sombroek CC, Lougheed SM, Oosterhoff D, Buter J, van den Eertwegh AJ, Scheper RJ, Pinedo HM (2006) A postmigrational switch among skin-derived dendritic cells to a macrophage-like phenotype is predetermined by the intracutaneous cytokine balance. J Immunol 176:7232–7242

de Jong A, Pena-Cruz V, Cheng TY, Clark RA, Van Rhijn I, Moody DB (2010) CD1a-autoreactive T cells are a normal component of the human alphabeta T cell repertoire. Nat Immunol 11:1102–1109

de Vries HJ, van Marle J, Teunissen MBM, Picavet D, Zorgdrager F, Bos JD, Weel J, Cornelissen M (2006) Lichen planus is associated with human herpesvirus type 7 replication and infiltration of plasmacytoid dendritic cells. Br J Dermatol 154:361–364

Degli-Esposti MA, Smyth MJ (2005) Close encounters of different kinds: dendritic cells and NK cells take centre stage. Nat Rev Immunol 5:112–124

Del Prete GF, De Carli M, Mastromauro C, Biagiotti R, Macchia D, Falagiani P, Ricci M, Romagnani S (1991) Purified protein derivative of Mycobacterium tuberculosis and excretory-secretory antigen(s) of Toxocara canis expand in vitro human T cells with stable and opposite (type 1 T helper or type 2 T helper) profile of cytokine production. J Clin Invest 88:346–350

Di Pucchio T, Chatterjee B, Smed-Sorensen A, Clayton S, Palazzo A, Montes M, Xue Y, Mellman I, Banchereau J, Connolly JE (2008) Direct proteasome-independent cross-presentation of viral antigen by plasmacytoid dendritic cells on major histocompatibility complex class I. Nat Immunol 9:551–557

Dillon SM, Robertson KB, Pan SC, Mawhinney S, Meditz AL, Folkvord JM, Connick E, McCarter MD, Wilson CC (2008) Plasmacytoid and myeloid dendritic cells with a partial activation phenotype accumulate in lymphoid tissue during asymptomatic chronic HIV-1 infection. J Acquir Immune Defic Syndr 48:1–12

Dorschner RA, Pestonjamasp VK, Tamakuwala S, Ohtake T, Rudisill J, Nizet V, Agerberth B, Gudmundsson GH, Gallo RL (2001) Cutaneous injury induces the release of cathelicidin anti-microbial peptides active against group A Streptococcus. J Invest Dermatol 117:91–97

Duhen T, Geiger R, Jarrossay D, Lanzavecchia A, Sallusto F (2009) Production of interleukin 22 but not interleukin 17 by a subset of human skin-homing memory T cells. Nat Immunol 10:857–863

Duraisingham SS, Hornig J, Gotch F, Patterson S (2009) TLR-stimulated CD34 stem cell-derived human skin-like and monocyte-derived dendritic cells fail to induce Th17 polarization of naive T cells but do stimulate Th1 and Th17 memory responses. J Immunol 183:2242–2251

Duraisingham SS, Hornig J, Gotch F, Patterson S (2010) CD34-derived human Langerhans cells stimulate a T helper type 2 response independently of extracellular-signal-regulated kinase phosphorylation. Immunology 131:210–219

Dzionek A, Fuchs A, Schmidt P, Cremer S, Zysk M, Miltenyi S, Buck DW, Schmitz J (2000) BDCA-2, BDCA-3, and BDCA-4: three markers for distinct subsets of dendritic cells in human peripheral blood. J Immunol 165:6037–6046

Dzionek A, Sohma Y, Nagafune J, Cella M, Colonna M, Facchetti F, Gunther G, Johnston I, Lanzavecchia A, Nagasaka T, Okada T, Vermi W, Winkels G, Yamamoto T, Zysk M, Yamaguchi Y, Schmitz J (2001) BDCA-2, a novel plasmacytoid dendritic cell-specific type II C-type lectin, mediates antigen capture and is a potent inhibitor of interferon alpha/beta induction. J Exp Med 194:1823–1834

Ebner S, Ehammer Z, Holzmann S, Schwingshackl P, Forstner M, Stoitzner P, Huemer GM, Fritsch P, Romani N (2004) Expression of C-type lectin receptors by subsets of dendritic cells in human skin. Int Immunol 16:877–887

Eisenbarth SC, Colegio OR, O'Connor W, Sutterwala FS, Flavell RA (2008) Crucial role for the Nalp3 inflammasome in the immunostimulatory properties of aluminium adjuvants. Nature 453:1122–1126

Engering A, Geijtenbeek TB, van Kooyk Y (2002) Immune escape through C-type lectins on dendritic cells. Trends Immunol 23:480–485

Engering A, van Vliet SJ, Hebeda K, Jackson DG, Prevo R, Singh SK, Geijtenbeek TB, van Krieken H, van Kooyk Y (2004) Dynamic populations of dendritic cell-specific ICAM-3 grabbing nonintegrin-positive immature dendritic cells and liver/lymph node-specific ICAM-3 grabbing nonintegrin-positive endothelial cells in the outer zones of the paracortex of human lymph nodes. Am J Pathol 164:1587–1595

Eto H, Suga H, Matsumoto D, Inoue K, Aoi N, Kato H, Araki J, Yoshimura K (2009) Characterization of structure and cellular components of aspirated and excised adipose tissue. Plast Reconstr Surg 124:1087–1097

Eyler JM (2003) Smallpox in history: the birth, death, and impact of a dread disease. J Lab Clin Med 142:216–220

Faith A, Peek E, McDonald J, Urry Z, Richards DF, Tan C, Santis G, Hawrylowicz C (2007) Plasmacytoid dendritic cells from human lung cancer draining lymph nodes induce Tc1 responses. Am J Respir Cell Mol Biol 36:360–367

Farkas L, Beiske K, Lund-Johansen F, Brandtzaeg P, Jahnsen FL (2001) Plasmacytoid dendritic cells (natural interferon- alpha/beta-producing cells) accumulate in cutaneous lupus erythematosus lesions. Am J Pathol 159:237–243

Flacher V, Tripp CH, Stoitzner P, Haid B, Ebner S, Del FB, Koch F, Park CG, Steinman RM, Idoyaga J, Romani N (2010) Epidermal Langerhans cells rapidly capture and present antigens from C-type lectin-targeting antibodies deposited in the dermis. J Invest Dermatol 130:755–762

Foster CA, Yokozeki H, Rappersberger K, Koning F, Volc-Platzer B, Rieger A, Coligan JE, Wolff K, Stingl G (1990) Human epidermal T cells predominantly belong to the lineage expressing alpha/beta T cell receptor. J Exp Med 171:997–1013

Fuchs E, Raghavan S (2002) Getting under the skin of epidermal morphogenesis. Nat Rev Genet 3:199–209

Fuhlbrigge RC, Kieffer JD, Armerding D, Kupper TS (1997) Cutaneous lymphocyte antigen is a specialized form of PSGL-1 expressed on skin-homing T cells. Nature 389:978–981

Fujii S, Shimizu K, Hemmi H, Steinman RM (2007) Innate Valpha14(+) natural killer T cells mature dendritic cells, leading to strong adaptive immunity. Immunol Rev 220:183–198

Fujita H, Nograles KE, Kikuchi T, Gonzalez J, Carucci JA, Krueger JG (2009) Human Langerhans cells induce distinct IL-22-producing CD4+ T cells lacking IL-17 production. Proc Natl Acad Sci USA 106:21795–21800

Furio L, Berthier-Vergnes O, Ducarre B, Schmitt D, Peguet-Navarro J (2005) UVA radiation impairs phenotypic and functional maturation of human dermal dendritic cells. J Invest Dermatol 125:1032–1038

Furio L, Briotet I, Journeaux A, Billard H, Peguet-Navarro J (2010) Human langerhans cells are more efficient than CD14(-)CD1c(+) dermal dendritic cells at priming naive CD4(+) T cells. J Invest Dermatol 130:1345–1354

Ganguly D, Chamilos G, Lande R, Gregorio J, Meller S, Facchinetti V, Homey B, Barrat FJ, Zal T, Gilliet M (2009) Self-RNA-antimicrobial peptide complexes activate human dendritic cells through TLR7 and TLR8. J Exp Med 206:1983–1994

Geijtenbeek TB, Gringhuis SI (2009) Signalling through C-type lectin receptors: shaping immune responses. Nat Rev Immunol 9:465–479

Geijtenbeek TB, van Vliet SJ, Engering A, ‘t Hart BA, van Kooyk Y (2004) Self- and nonself-recognition by C-type lectins on dendritic cells. Annu Rev Immunol 22:33–54

Geissmann F, Prost C, Monnet JP, Dy M, Brousse N, Hermine O (1998) Transforming growth factor beta1, in the presence of granulocyte/macrophage colony-stimulating factor and interleukin 4, induces differentiation of human peripheral blood monocytes into dendritic Langerhans cells. J Exp Med 187:961–966

Geissmann F, Dieu-Nosjean MC, Dezutter C, Valladeau J, Kayal S, Leborgne M, Brousse N, Saeland S, Davoust J (2002) Accumulation of immature Langerhans cells in human lymph nodes draining chronically inflamed skin. J Exp Med 196:417–430

Geissmann F, Jung S, Littman DR (2003) Blood monocytes consist of two principal subsets with distinct migratory properties. Immunity 19:71–82

Geissmann F, Manz MG, Jung S, Sieweke MH, Merad M, Ley K (2010) Development of monocytes, macrophages, and dendritic cells. Science 327:656–661

Gerlini G, Hefti HP, Kleinhans M, Nickoloff BJ, Burg G, Nestle FO (2001) Cd1d is expressed on dermal dendritic cells and monocyte-derived dendritic cells. J Invest Dermatol 117:576–582

Gerlini G, Mariotti G, Bianchi B, Pimpinelli N (2006) Massive recruitment of type I interferon producing plasmacytoid dendritic cells in varicella skin lesions. J Invest Dermatol 126:507–509

Gilliam AC, Kremer IB, Yoshida Y, Stevens SR, Tootell E, Teunissen MBM, Hammerberg C, Cooper KD (1998) The human hair follicle: a reservoir of CD40+ B7-deficient Langerhans cells that repopulate epidermis after UVB exposure. J Invest Dermatol 110:422–427

Gilliet M, Cao W, Liu YJ (2008) Plasmacytoid dendritic cells: sensing nucleic acids in viral infection and autoimmune diseases. Nat Rev Immunol 8:594–606

Ginhoux F, Collin MP, Bogunovic M, Abel M, Leboeuf M, Helft J, Ochando J, Kissenpfennig A, Malissen B, Grisotto M, Snoeck H, Randolph G, Merad M (2007) Blood-derived dermal langerin+ dendritic cells survey the skin in the steady state. J Exp Med 204:3133–3146

Ginhoux F, Ng LG, Merad M (2010) Understanding the murine cutaneous dendritic cell network to improve intradermal vaccination strategies. Curr Top Microbiol Immunol 351:1–24

Glaser R, Navid F, Schuller W, Jantschitsch C, Harder J, Schroder JM, Schwarz A, Schwarz T (2009) UV-B radiation induces the expression of antimicrobial peptides in human keratinocytes in vitro and in vivo. J Allergy Clin Immunol 123:1117–1123

Gogolak P, Rethi B, Szatmari I, Lanyi A, Dezso B, Nagy L, Rajnavolgyi E (2007) Differentiation of CD1a- and CD1a+ monocyte-derived dendritic cells is biased by lipid environment and PPARgamma. Blood 109:643–652

Gordon S, Taylor PR (2005) Monocyte and macrophage heterogeneity. Nat Rev Immunol 5:953–964

Gregorio J, Meller S, Conrad C, Di Nardo A, Homey B, Lauerma A, Arai N, Gallo RL, Digiovanni J, Gilliet M (2010) Plasmacytoid dendritic cells sense skin injury and promote wound healing through type I interferons. J Exp Med 207:2921–2930

Gros E, Bussmann C, Bieber T, Forster I, Novak N (2009) Expression of chemokines and chemokine receptors in lesional and nonlesional upper skin of patients with atopic dermatitis. J Allergy Clin Immunol 124:753–760

Gschwandtner M, Schakel K, Werfel T, Gutzmer R (2011) Histamine H(4) receptor activation on human slan-dendritic cells down-regulates their pro-inflammatory capacity. Immunology 132:49–56

Guermonprez P, Saveanu L, Kleijmeer M, Davoust J, van Endert P, Amigorena S (2003) ER-phagosome fusion defines an MHC class I cross-presentation compartment in dendritic cells. Nature 425:397–402

Hambleton S, Salem S, Bustamante J, Bigley V, Boisson-Dupuis S, Azevedo J, Fortin A, Haniffa M, Ceron-Gutierrez L, Bacon CM, Menon G, Trouillet C, McDonald D, Carey P, Ginhoux F, Alsina L, Zumwalt TJ, Kong XF, Kumararatne D, Butler K, Hubeau M, Feinberg J, Al-Muhsen S, Cant A, Abel L, Chaussabel D, Doffinger R, Talesnik E, Grumach A, Duarte A, Abarca K, Moraes-Vasconcelos D, Burk D, Berghuis A, Geissmann F, Collin M, Casanova JL, Gros P (2011) IRF8 mutations and human dendritic-cell immunodeficiency. N Engl J Med 365:127–138

Haniffa M, Ginhoux F, Wang XN, Bigley V, Abel M, Dimmick I, Bullock S, Grisotto M, Booth T, Taub P, Hilkens C, Merad M, Collin M (2009) Differential rates of replacement of human dermal dendritic cells and macrophages during hematopoietic stem cell transplantation. J Exp Med 206:371–385

Hansen TH, Bouvier M (2009) MHC class I antigen presentation: learning from viral evasion strategies. Nat Rev Immunol 9:503–513

Harrington LE, Hatton RD, Mangan PR, Turner H, Murphy TL, Murphy KM, Weaver CT (2005) Interleukin 17-producing CD4+ effector T cells develop via a lineage distinct from the T helper type 1 and 2 lineages. Nat Immunol 6:1123–1132

Henri S, Poulin LF, Tamoutounour S, Ardouin L, Guilliams M, de Bovis B, Devilard E, Viret C, Azukizawa H, Kissenpfennig A, Malissen B (2010) CD207+ CD103+ dermal dendritic cells cross-present keratinocyte-derived antigens irrespective of the presence of Langerhans cells. J Exp Med 207:189–206

Hochrein H, Shortman K, Vremec D, Scott B, Hertzog P, O'Keeffe M (2001) Differential production of IL-12, IFN-alpha, and IFN-gamma by mouse dendritic cell subsets. J Immunol 166:5448–5455

Homey B, Alenius H, Muller A, Soto H, Bowman EP, Yuan W, McEvoy L, Lauerma AI, Assmann T, Bunemann E, Lehto M, Wolff H, Yen D, Marxhausen H, To W, Sedgwick J, Ruzicka T, Lehmann P, Zlotnik A (2002) CCL27-CCR10 interactions regulate T cell-mediated skin inflammation. Nat Med 8:157–165

Hornung V, Bauernfeind F, Halle A, Samstad EO, Kono H, Rock KL, Fitzgerald KA, Latz E (2008) Silica crystals and aluminum salts activate the NALP3 inflammasome through phagosomal destabilization. Nat Immunol 9:847–856

Huysamen C, Willment JA, Dennehy KM, Brown GD (2008) CLEC9A is a novel activation C-type lectin-like receptor expressed on BDCA3+ dendritic cells and a subset of monocytes. J Biol Chem 283:16693–16701

Ingersoll MA, Spanbroek R, Lottaz C, Gautier EL, Frankenberger M, Hoffmann R, Lang R, Haniffa M, Collin M, Tacke F, Habenicht AJ, Ziegler-Heitbrock L, Randolph GJ (2010)

Comparison of gene expression profiles between human and mouse monocyte subsets. Blood 115:e10–e19

Ito M, Liu Y, Yang Z, Nguyen J, Liang F, Morris RJ, Cotsarelis G (2005) Stem cells in the hair follicle bulge contribute to wound repair but not to homeostasis of the epidermis. Nat Med 11:1351–1354

Jahn PS, Zanker KS, Schmitz J, Dzionek A (2010) BDCA-2 signaling inhibits TLR-9-agonist-induced plasmacytoid dendritic cell activation and antigen presentation. Cell Immunol 265:15–22

Jakob T, Ring J, Udey MC (2001) Multistep navigation of Langerhans/dendritic cells in and out of the skin. J Allergy Clin Immunol 108:688–696

Jarrossay D, Napolitani G, Colonna M, Sallusto F, Lanzavecchia A (2001) Specialization and complementarity in microbial molecule recognition by human myeloid and plasmacytoid dendritic cells. Eur J Immunol 31:3388–3393

Joffre OP, Sancho D, Zelenay S, Keller AM, Reis e Sousa C (2010) Efficient and versatile manipulation of the peripheral CD4+ T-cell compartment by antigen targeting to DNGR-1/CLEC9A. Eur J Immunol 40:1255–1265

Jongbloed SL, Kassianos AJ, McDonald KJ, Clark GJ, Ju X, Angel CE, Chen CJ, Dunbar PR, Wadley RB, Jeet V, Vulink AJ, Hart DN, Radford KJ (2010) Human CD141+ (BDCA-3)+ dendritic cells (DCs) represent a unique myeloid DC subset that cross-presents necrotic cell antigens. J Exp Med 207:1247–1260

Kalinski P, Hilkens CM, Wierenga EA, Kapsenberg ML (1999) T-cell priming by type-1 and type-2 polarized dendritic cells: the concept of a third signal. Immunol Today 20:561–567

Kanitakis J (2002) Anatomy, histology and immunohistochemistry of normal human skin. Eur J Dermatol 12:390–399

Kanitakis J, Petruzzo P, Dubernard JM (2004) Turnover of epidermal Langerhans' cells. N Engl J Med 351:2661–2662

Kapsenberg ML (2003) Dendritic-cell control of pathogen-driven T-cell polarization. Nat Rev Immunol 3:984–993

Kasturi SP, Skountzou I, Albrecht RA, Koutsonanos D, Hua T, Nakaya HI, Ravindran R, Stewart S, Alam M, Kwissa M, Villinger F, Murthy N, Steel J, Jacob J, Hogan RJ, Garcia-Sastre A, Compans R, Pulendran B (2011) Programming the magnitude and persistence of antibody responses with innate immunity. Nature 470:543–547

Kato M, Khan S, d'Aniello E, McDonald KJ, Hart DN (2007) The novel endocytic and phagocytic C-Type lectin receptor DCL-1/CD302 on macrophages is colocalized with F-actin, suggesting a role in cell adhesion and migration. J Immunol 179:6052–6063

Kawai T, Akira S (2010) The role of pattern-recognition receptors in innate immunity: update on Toll-like receptors. Nat Immunol 11:373–384

Kawai T, Akira S (2011) Toll-like receptors and their crosstalk with other innate receptors in infection and immunity. Immunity 34:637–650

Keller M, Ruegg A, Werner S, Beer HD (2008) Active caspase-1 is a regulator of unconventional protein secretion. Cell 132:818–831

Kenney RT, Frech SA, Muenz LR, Villar CP, Glenn GM (2004) Dose sparing with intradermal injection of influenza vaccine. N Engl J Med 351:2295–2301

Kim YC, Jarrahian C, Zehrung D, Mitragotri S, Prausnitz MR (2011) Delivery systems for intradermal vaccination. Curr Top Microbiol Immunol 351:77–112

King C, Tangye SG, Mackay CR (2008) T follicular helper (TFH) cells in normal and dysregulated immune responses. Annu Rev Immunol 26:741–766

Klechevsky E, Morita R, Liu M, Cao Y, Coquery S, Thompson-Snipes L, Briere F, Chaussabel D, Zurawski G, Palucka AK, Reiter Y, Banchereau J, Ueno H (2008) Functional specializations of human epidermal Langerhans cells and CD14+ dermal dendritic cells. Immunity 29:497–510

Klechevsky E, Liu M, Morita R, Banchereau R, Thompson-Snipes L, Palucka AK, Ueno H, Banchereau J (2009) Understanding human myeloid dendritic cell subsets for the rational design of novel vaccines. Hum Immunol 70:281–288

Klechevsky E, Flamar AL, Cao Y, Blanck JP, Liu M, O'Bar A, Agouna-Deciat O, Klucar P, Thompson-Snipes L, Zurawski S, Reiter Y, Palucka AK, Zurawski G, Banchereau J (2010) Cross-priming $CD8^{+}$ T cells by targeting antigens to human dendritic cells through DCIR. Blood 116:1685–1697

Kool M, Soullie T, van Nimwegen M, Willart MA, Muskens F, Jung S, Hoogsteden HC, Hammad H, Lambrecht BN (2008) Alum adjuvant boosts adaptive immunity by inducing uric acid and activating inflammatory dendritic cells. J Exp Med 205:869–882

Kretschmer K, Apostolou I, Hawiger D, Khazaie K, Nussenzweig MC, von Boehmer H (2005) Inducing and expanding regulatory T cell populations by foreign antigen. Nat Immunol 6:1219–1227

Kubo A, Nagao K, Yokouchi M, Sasaki H, Amagai M (2009) External antigen uptake by Langerhans cells with reorganization of epidermal tight junction barriers. J Exp Med 206:2937–2946

Kunzi V, Klap JM, Seiberling MK, Herzog C, Hartmann K, Kursteiner O, Kompier R, Grimaldi R, Goudsmit J (2009) Immunogenicity and safety of low dose virosomal adjuvanted influenza vaccine administered intradermally compared to intramuscular full dose administration. Vaccine 27:3561–3567

Kupper TS, Fuhlbrigge RC (2004) Immune surveillance in the skin: mechanisms and clinical consequences. Nat Rev Immunol 4:211–222

Kuwana M, Kaburaki J, Wright TM, Kawakami Y, Ikeda Y (2001) Induction of antigen-specific human CD4(+) T cell anergy by peripheral blood DC2 precursors. Eur J Immunol 31:2547–2557

Lahoud MH, Proietto AI, Ahmet F, Kitsoulis S, Eidsmo L, Wu L, Sathe P, Pietersz S, Chang HW, Walker ID, Maraskovsky E, Braley H, Lew AM, Wright MD, Heath WR, Shortman K, Caminschi I (2009) The C-type lectin Clec12A present on mouse and human dendritic cells can serve as a target for antigen delivery and enhancement of antibody responses. J Immunol 182:7587–7594

Lai Y, Gallo RL (2009) AMPed up immunity: how antimicrobial peptides have multiple roles in immune defense. Trends Immunol 30:131–141

Lakadamyali M, Rust MJ, Zhuang X (2006) Ligands for clathrin-mediated endocytosis are differentially sorted into distinct populations of early endosomes. Cell 124:997–1009

Lande R, Gregorio J, Facchinetti V, Chatterjee B, Wang YH, Homey B, Cao W, Wang YH, Su B, Nestle FO, Zal T, Mellman I, Schroder JM, Liu YJ, Gilliet M (2007) Plasmacytoid dendritic cells sense self-DNA coupled with antimicrobial peptide. Nature 449:564–569

Langerhans P (1868) Ueber die Nerven der menschlichen Haut. Virchows Arch Pathol Anat 44:325–337

Lanzavecchia A, Sallusto F (2001) The instructive role of dendritic cells on T cell responses: lineages, plasticity and kinetics. Curr Opin Immunol 13:291–298

Larregina AT, Morelli AE, Spencer LA, Logar AJ, Watkins SC, Thomson AW, Falo LD Jr (2001) Dermal-resident CD14+ cells differentiate into Langerhans cells. Nat Immunol 2:1151–1158

Le Bon A, Etchart N, Rossmann C, Ashton M, Hou S, Gewert D, Borrow P, Tough DF (2003) Cross-priming of CD8+ T cells stimulated by virus-induced type I interferon. Nat Immunol 4:1009–1015

Lenz A, Heine M, Schuler G, Romani N (1993) Human and murine dermis contain dendritic cells. Isolation by means of a novel method and phenotypical and functional characterization. J Clin Invest 92:2587–2596

Lin ML, Zhan Y, Villadangos JA, Lew AM (2008) The cell biology of cross-presentation and the role of dendritic cell subsets. Immunol Cell Biol 86:353–362

Lindstedt M, Lundberg K, Borrebaeck CA (2005) Gene family clustering identifies functionally associated subsets of human in vivo blood and tonsillar dendritic cells. J Immunol 175:4839–4846

Liu YJ (2005) IPC: professional type 1 interferon-producing cells and plasmacytoid dendritic cell precursors. Annu Rev Immunol 23:275–306

Liu YJ, Soumelis V, Watanabe N, Ito T, Wang YH, de Waal Malefyt R, Omori M, Zhou B, Ziegler SF (2007) TSLP: an epithelial cell cytokine that regulates T cell differentiation by conditioning dendritic cell maturation. Annu Rev Immunol 25:193–219

Lowes MA, Chamian F, Abello MV, Fuentes-Duculan J, Lin SL, Nussbaum R, Novitskaya I, Carbonaro H, Cardinale I, Kikuchi T, Gilleaudeau P, Sullivan-Whalen M, Wittkowski KM, Papp K, Garovoy M, Dummer W, Steinman RM, Krueger JG (2005) Increase in TNF-alpha and inducible nitric oxide synthase-expressing dendritic cells in psoriasis and reduction with efalizumab (anti-CD11a). Proc Natl Acad Sci U S A 102:19057–19062

Lukas M, Stossel H, Hefel L, Imamura S, Fritsch P, Sepp NT, Schuler G, Romani N (1996) Human cutaneous dendritic cells migrate through dermal lymphatic vessels in a skin organ culture model. J Invest Dermatol 106:1293–1299

Luther SA, Tang HL, Hyman PL, Farr AG, Cyster JG (2000) Coexpression of the chemokines ELC and SLC by T zone stromal cells and deletion of the ELC gene in the plt/plt mouse. Proc Natl Acad Sci U S A 97:12694–12699

MacDonald KP, Munster DJ, Clark GJ, Dzionek A, Schmitz J, Hart DN (2002) Characterization of human blood dendritic cell subsets. Blood 100:4512–4520

Manfredi AA, Capobianco A, Bianchi ME, Rovere-Querini P (2009) Regulation of dendritic- and T-cell fate by injury-associated endogenous signals. Crit Rev Immunol 29:69–86

Mantoux C (1910) L'intradermo-réaction a la tuberculine et son interprétation clinique. La Presse Médicale 2:10–15

Martinon F, Tschopp J (2005) NLRs join TLRs as innate sensors of pathogens. Trends Immunol 26:447–454

Martinon F, Mayor A, Tschopp J (2009) The inflammasomes: guardians of the body. Annu Rev Immunol 27:229–265

Mathers AR, Janelsins BM, Rubin JP, Tkacheva OA, Shufesky WJ, Watkins SC, Morelli AE, Larregina AT (2009) Differential capability of human cutaneous dendritic cell subsets to initiate Th17 responses. J Immunol 182:921–933

Matzinger P (2007) Friendly and dangerous signals: is the tissue in control? Nat Immunol 8:11–13

Matzinger P, Kamala T (2011) Tissue-based class control: the other side of tolerance. Nat Rev Immunol 11:221–230

Mbow ML, De Gregorio E, Valiante NM, Rappuoli R (2010) New adjuvants for human vaccines. Curr Opin Immunol 22:411–416

McClain DJ, Harrison S, Yeager CL, Cruz J, Ennis FA, Gibbs P, Wright MS, Summers PL, Arthur JD, Graham JA (1997) Immunologic responses to vaccinia vaccines administered by different parenteral routes. J Infect Dis 175:756–763

McGeachy MJ, Cua DJ (2008) Th17 cell differentiation: the long and winding road. Immunity 28:445–453

McIlroy D, Troadec C, Grassi F, Samri A, Barrou B, Autran B, Debre P, Feuillard J, Hosmalin A (2001) Investigation of human spleen dendritic cell phenotype and distribution reveals evidence of in vivo activation in a subset of organ donors. Blood 97:3470–3477

Medzhitov R, Janeway CA Jr (1997) Innate immunity: the virtues of a nonclonal system of recognition. Cell 91:295–298

Merad M, Manz MG (2009) Dendritic cell homeostasis. Blood 113:3418–3427

Merad M, Manz MG, Karsunky H, Wagers A, Peters W, Charo I, Weissman IL, Cyster JG, Engleman EG (2002) Langerhans cells renew in the skin throughout life under steady-state conditions. Nat Immunol 3:1135–1141

Meunier L, Gonzalez-Ramos A, Cooper KD (1993) Heterogeneous populations of class II MHC+ cells in human dermal cell suspensions. Identification of a small subset responsible for potent dermal antigen-presenting cell activity with features analogous to Langerhans cells. J Immunol 151:4067–4080

Meunier L, Bata-Csorgo Z, Cooper KD (1995) In human dermis, ultraviolet radiation induces expansion of a CD36+ CD11b+ CD1- macrophage subset by infiltration and proliferation;

CD1+ Langerhans-like dendritic antigen-presenting cells are concomitantly depleted. J Invest Dermatol 105:782–788
Meyer-Wentrup F, Benitez-Ribas D, Tacken PJ, Punt CJ, Figdor CG, de Vries IJ, Adema GJ (2008) Targeting DCIR on human plasmacytoid dendritic cells results in antigen presentation and inhibits IFN-alpha production. Blood 111:4245–4253
Mittag D, Proietto AI, Loudovaris T, Mannering SI, Vremec D, Shortman K, Wu L, Harrison LC (2011) Human dendritic cell subsets from spleen and blood are similar in phenotype and function but modified by donor health status. J Immunol 186:6207–6217
Mohamadzadeh M, Berard F, Essert G, Chalouni C, Pulendran B, Davoust J, Bridges G, Palucka AK, Banchereau J (2001) Interleukin 15 skews monocyte differentiation into dendritic cells with features of Langerhans cells. J Exp Med 194:1013–1020
Molenkamp BG, van Leeuwen PA, Meijer S, Sluijter BJ, Wijnands PG, Baars A, van den Eertwegh AJ, Scheper RJ, de Gruijl TD (2007) Intradermal CpG-B activates both plasmacytoid and myeloid dendritic cells in the sentinel lymph node of melanoma patients. Clin Cancer Res 13:2961–2969
Moody DB, Porcelli SA (2003) Intracellular pathways of CD1 antigen presentation. Nat Rev Immunol 3:11–22
Morelli AE, Rubin JP, Erdos G, Tkacheva OA, Mathers AR, Zahorchak AF, Thomson AW, Falo LD Jr, Larregina AT (2005) CD4+ T cell responses elicited by different subsets of human skin migratory dendritic cells. J Immunol 175:7905–7915
Mosca F, Tritto E, Muzzi A, Monaci E, Bagnoli F, Iavarone C, O'Hagan D, Rappuoli R, De GE (2008) Molecular and cellular signatures of human vaccine adjuvants. Proc Natl Acad Sci USA 105:10501–10506
Mosmann TR, Coffman RL (1989) TH1 and TH2 cells: different patterns of lymphokine secretion lead to different functional properties. Annu Rev Immunol 7:145–173
Murphy GF, Bhan AK, Harrist TJ, Mihm MC Jr (1983) In situ identification of T6-positive cells in normal human dermis by immunoelectron microscopy. Br J Dermatol 108:423–431
Nagao K, Ginhoux F, Leitner WW, Motegi S, Bennett CL, Clausen BE, Merad M, Udey MC (2009) Murine epidermal Langerhans cells and langerin-expressing dermal dendritic cells are unrelated and exhibit distinct functions. Proc Natl Acad Sci U S A 106:3312–3317
Nestle FO, Zheng XG, Thompson CB, Turka LA, Nickoloff BJ (1993) Characterization of dermal dendritic cells obtained from normal human skin reveals phenotypic and functionally distinctive subsets. J Immunol 151:6535–6545
Nestle FO, Di MP, Qin JZ, Nickoloff BJ (2009) Skin immune sentinels in health and disease. Nat Rev Immunol 9:679–691
Nishikawa Y, Sato H, Oka T, Yoshino T, Takahashi K (2009) Immunohistochemical discrimination of plasmacytoid dendritic cells from myeloid dendritic cells in human pathological tissues. J Clin Exp Hematop 49:23–31
Novak N, Valenta R, Bohle B, Laffer S, Haberstok J, Kraft S, Bieber T (2004) FcepsilonRI engagement of Langerhans cell-like dendritic cells and inflammatory dendritic epidermal cell-like dendritic cells induces chemotactic signals and different T-cell phenotypes in vitro. J Allergy Clin Immunol 113:949–957
Ochoa MT, Loncaric A, Krutzik SR, Becker TC, Modlin RL (2008) "Dermal dendritic cells" comprise two distinct populations: CD1+ dendritic cells and CD209+ macrophages. J Invest Dermatol 128:2225–2231
Oosterhoff D, Sluijter BJ, Hangalapura BN, de Gruijl TD (2011) The dermis as a portal for dendritic cell-targeted immunotherapy of cutaneous melanoma. Curr Top Microbiol Immunol 351:181–220
Osugi Y, Vuckovic S, Hart DN (2002) Myeloid blood CD11c(+) dendritic cells and monocyte-derived dendritic cells differ in their ability to stimulate T lymphocytes. Blood 100: 2858–2866
Oura J, Tamura Y, Kamiguchi K, Kutomi G, Sahara H, Torigoe T, Himi T, Sato N (2011) Extracellular heat shock protein 90 plays a role in translocating chaperoned antigen from endosome to proteasome for generating antigenic peptide to be cross-presented by dendritic cells. Int Immunol 23:223–237

Pack M, Trumpfheller C, Thomas D, Park CG, Granelli-Piperno A, Munz C, Steinman RM (2008) DEC-205/CD205+ dendritic cells are abundant in the white pulp of the human spleen, including the border region between the red and white pulp. Immunology 123:438–446

Palm NW, Medzhitov R (2009) Pattern recognition receptors and control of adaptive immunity. Immunol Rev 227:221–233

Parolini S, Santoro A, Marcenaro E, Luini W, Massardi L, Facchetti F, Communi D, Parmentier M, Majorana A, Sironi M, Tabellini G, Moretta A, Sozzani S (2007) The role of chemerin in the colocalization of NK and dendritic cell subsets into inflamed tissues. Blood 109:3625–3632

Passlick B, Flieger D, Ziegler-Heitbrock HW (1989) Identification and characterization of a novel monocyte subpopulation in human peripheral blood. Blood 74:2527–2534

Peiser M, Wanner R, Kolde G (2004) Human epidermal Langerhans cells differ from monocyte-derived Langerhans cells in CD80 expression and in secretion of IL-12 after CD40 cross-linking. J Leukoc Biol 76:616–622

Pena-Cruz V, McDonough SM, Diaz-Griffero F, Crum CP, Carrasco RD, Freeman GJ (2010) PD-1 on immature and PD-1 ligands on migratory human Langerhans cells regulate antigen-presenting cell activity. J Invest Dermatol 130:2222–2230

Piccioli D, Tavarini S, Borgogni E, Steri V, Nuti S, Sammicheli C, Bardelli M, Montagna D, Locatelli F, Wack A (2007) Functional specialization of human circulating CD16 and CD1c myeloid dendritic-cell subsets. Blood 109:5371–5379

Poulin LF, Henri S, de Bovis B, Devilard E, Kissenpfennig A, Malissen B (2007) The dermis contains langerin+ dendritic cells that develop and function independently of epidermal Langerhans cells. J Exp Med 204:3119–3131

Poulin LF, Salio M, Griessinger E, Anjos-Afonso F, Craciun L, Chen JL, Keller AM, Joffre O, Zelenay S, Nye E, Le Moine A, Faure F, Donckier V, Sancho D, Cerundolo V, Bonnet D, Reis e Sousa C (2010) Characterization of human DNGR-1+ BDCA3+ leukocytes as putative equivalents of mouse CD8alpha+ dendritic cells. J Exp Med 207:1261–1271

Proksch E, Brandner JM, Jensen JM (2008) The skin: an indispensable barrier. Exp Dermatol 17:1063–1072

Ratzinger G, Baggers J, de Cos MA, Yuan J, Dao T, Reagan JL, Munz C, Heller G, Young JW (2004) Mature human Langerhans cells derived from CD34+ hematopoietic progenitors stimulate greater cytolytic T lymphocyte activity in the absence of bioactive IL-12p70, by either single peptide presentation or cross-priming, than do dermal-interstitial or monocyte-derived dendritic cells. J Immunol 173:2780–2791

Reiner SL, Sallusto F, Lanzavecchia A (2007) Division of labor with a workforce of one: challenges in specifying effector and memory T cell fate. Science 317:622–625

Renn CN, Sanchez DJ, Ochoa MT, Legaspi AJ, Oh CK, Liu PT, Krutzik SR, Sieling PA, Cheng G, Modlin RL (2006) TLR activation of Langerhans cell-like dendritic cells triggers an antiviral immune response. J Immunol 177:298–305

Rescigno M, Urbano M, Valzasina B, Francolini M, Rotta G, Bonasio R, Granucci F, Kraehenbuhl JP, Ricciardi-Castagnoli P (2001) Dendritic cells express tight junction proteins and penetrate gut epithelial monolayers to sample bacteria. Nat Immunol 2:361–367

Robbins SH, Walzer T, Dembele D, Thibault C, Defays A, Bessou G, Xu H, Vivier E, Sellars M, Pierre P, Sharp FR, Chan S, Kastner P, Dalod M (2008) Novel insights into the relationships between dendritic cell subsets in human and mouse revealed by genome-wide expression profiling. Genome Biol 9:R17

Romagnani S, Maggi E, Liotta F, Cosmi L, Annunziato F (2009) Properties and origin of human Th17 cells. Mol Immunol 47:3–7

Romani N, Lenz A, Glassel H, Stossel H, Stanzl U, Majdic O, Fritsch P, Schuler G (1989) Cultured human Langerhans cells resemble lymphoid dendritic cells in phenotype and function. J Invest Dermatol 93:600–609

Romani N, Clausen BE, Stoitzner P (2010) Langerhans cells and more: langerin-expressing dendritic cell subsets in the skin. Immunol Rev 234:120–141

Romani N, Flacher V, Tripp CH, Sparber F, Ebner S, Stoitzner P (2011) Targeting skin dendritic cells to improve intradermal vaccination. Curr Top Microbiol Immunol 351:113–138

Roukens AH, Vossen AC, Bredenbeek PJ, van Dissel JT, Visser LG (2008) Intradermally administered yellow fever vaccine at reduced dose induces a protective immune response: a randomized controlled non-inferiority trial. PLoS One 3:e1993

Rubartelli A, Lotze MT (2007) Inside, outside, upside down: damage-associated molecular-pattern molecules (DAMPs) and redox. Trends Immunol 28:429–436

Sacks D, Sher A (2002) Evasion of innate immunity by parasitic protozoa. Nat Immunol 3:1041–1047

Sakaguchi S, Miyara M, Costantino CM, Hafler DA (2010) FOXP3+ regulatory T cells in the human immune system. Nat Rev Immunol 10:490–500

Sakuraba A, Sato T, Kamada N, Kitazume M, Sugita A, Hibi T (2009) Th1/Th17 immune response is induced by mesenteric lymph node dendritic cells in Crohn's disease. Gastroenterology 137:1736–1745

Sallusto F, Lanzavecchia A (2009) Heterogeneity of CD4+ memory T cells: functional modules for tailored immunity. Eur J Immunol 39:2076–2082

Sallusto F, Schaerli P, Loetscher P, Schaniel C, Lenig D, Mackay CR, Qin S, Lanzavecchia A (1998) Rapid and coordinated switch in chemokine receptor expression during dendritic cell maturation. Eur J Immunol 28:2760–2769

Sallusto F, Geginat J, Lanzavecchia A (2004) Central memory and effector memory T cell subsets: function, generation, and maintenance. Annu Rev Immunol 22:745–763

Santini SM, Lapenta C, Logozzi M, Parlato S, Spada M, Di Pucchio T, Belardelli F (2000) Type I interferon as a powerful adjuvant for monocyte-derived dendritic cell development and activity in vitro and in Hu-PBL-SCID mice. J Exp Med 191:1777–1788

Savina A, Jancic C, Hugues S, Guermonprez P, Vargas P, Moura IC, Lennon-Dumenil AM, Seabra MC, Raposo G, Amigorena S (2006) NOX2 controls phagosomal pH to regulate antigen processing during crosspresentation by dendritic cells. Cell 126:205–218

Schakel K, Mayer E, Federle C, Schmitz M, Riethmuller G, Rieber EP (1998) A novel dendritic cell population in human blood: one-step immunomagnetic isolation by a specific mAb (M-DC8) and in vitro priming of cytotoxic T lymphocytes. Eur J Immunol 28:4084–4093

Schakel K, Kannagi R, Kniep B, Goto Y, Mitsuoka C, Zwirner J, Soruri A, von Kietzell M, Rieber E (2002) 6-Sulfo LacNAc, a novel carbohydrate modification of PSGL-1, defines an inflammatory type of human dendritic cells. Immunity 17:289–301

Schakel K, von Kietzell M, Hansel A, Ebling A, Schulze L, Haase M, Semmler C, Sarfati M, Barclay AN, Randolph GJ, Meurer M, Rieber EP (2006) Human 6-sulfo LacNAc-expressing dendritic cells are principal producers of early interleukin-12 and are controlled by erythrocytes. Immunity 24:767–777

Schmitt N, Morita R, Bourdery L, Bentebibel SE, Zurawski SM, Banchereau J, Ueno H (2009) Human dendritic cells induce the differentiation of interleukin-21-producing T follicular helper-like cells through interleukin-12. Immunity 31:158–169

Schnurr M, Chen Q, Shin A, Chen W, Toy T, Jenderek C, Green S, Miloradovic L, Drane D, Davis ID, Villadangos J, Shortman K, Maraskovsky E, Cebon J (2005) Tumor antigen processing and presentation depend critically on dendritic cell type and the mode of antigen delivery. Blood 105:2465–2472

Schon MP, Zollner TM, Boehncke WH (2003) The molecular basis of lymphocyte recruitment to the skin: clues for pathogenesis and selective therapies of inflammatory disorders. J Invest Dermatol 121:951–962

Schuler G, Steinman RM (1985) Murine epidermal Langerhans cells mature into potent immunostimulatory dendritic cells in vitro. J Exp Med 161:526–546

Schuller E, Teichmann B, Haberstok J, Moderer M, Bieber T, Wollenberg A (2001) In situ expression of the costimulatory molecules CD80 and CD86 on langerhans cells and inflammatory dendritic epidermal cells (IDEC) in atopic dermatitis. Arch Dermatol Res 293:448–454

Segre JA (2006) Epidermal barrier formation and recovery in skin disorders. J Clin Invest 116:1150–1158

Serbina NV, Salazar-Mather TP, Biron CA, Kuziel WA, Pamer EG (2003) TNF/iNOS-producing dendritic cells mediate innate immune defense against bacterial infection. Immunity 19:59–70
Seubert A, Monaci E, Pizza M, O'Hagan DT, Wack A (2008) The adjuvants aluminum hydroxide and MF59 induce monocyte and granulocyte chemoattractants and enhance monocyte differentiation toward dendritic cells. J Immunol 180:5402–5412
Shortman K, Heath WR (2010) The CD8+ dendritic cell subset. Immunol Rev 234:18–31
Siedlar M, Frankenberger M, Ziegler-Heitbrock LH, Belge KU (2000) The M-DC8-positive leukocytes are a subpopulation of the CD14+ CD16+ monocytes. Immunobiology 202:11–17
Siegal FP, Kadowaki N, Shodell M, Fitzgerald-Bocarsly PA, Shah K, Ho S, Antonenko S, Liu YJ (1999) The nature of the principal type 1 interferon-producing cells in human blood. Science 284:1835–1837
Sigmundsdottir H, Pan J, Debes GF, Alt C, Habtezion A, Soler D, Butcher EC (2007) DCs metabolize sunlight-induced vitamin D3 to 'program' T cell attraction to the epidermal chemokine CCL27. Nat Immunol 8:285–293
Singh SK, Stephani J, Schaefer M, Kalay H, Garcia-Vallejo JJ, den Haan J, Saeland E, Sparwasser T, van Kooyk Y (2009) Targeting glycan modified OVA to murine DC-SIGN transgenic dendritic cells enhances MHC class I and II presentation. Mol Immunol 47:164–174
Singh SK, Streng-Ouwehand I, Litjens M, Kalay H, Burgdorf S, Saeland E, Kurts C, Unger WW, van Kooyk Y (2011) Design of neo-glycoconjugates that target the mannose receptor and enhance TLR-independent cross-presentation and Th1 polarization. Eur J Immunol 41:916–925
Sonnenberg GF, Fouser LA, Artis D (2011) Border patrol: regulation of immunity, inflammation and tissue homeostasis at barrier surfaces by IL-22. Nat Immunol 12:383–390
Steinman RM, Banchereau J (2007) Taking dendritic cells into medicine. Nature 449:419–426
Steinman RM, Cohn ZA (1973) Identification of a novel cell type in peripheral lymphoid organs of mice. I. Morphology, quantitation, tissue distribution. J Exp Med 137:1142–1162
Steinman RM, Cohn ZA (1974) Identification of a novel cell type in peripheral lymphoid organs of mice. II. Functional properties in vitro. J Exp Med 139:380–397
Stingl G, Wolff-Schreiner EC, Pichler WJ, Gschnait F, Knapp W, Wolff K (1977) Epidermal Langerhans cells bear Fc and C3 receptors. Nature 268:245–246
Stingl G, Tamaki K, Katz SI (1980) Origin and function of epidermal Langerhans cells. Immunol Rev 53:149–174
Stockinger B, Bourgeois C, Kassiotis G (2006) CD4+ memory T cells: functional differentiation and homeostasis. Immunol Rev 211:39–48
Streilein JW (1983) Skin-associated lymphoid tissues (SALT): origins and functions. J Invest Dermatol 80(Suppl):12s–16s
Summers KL, Hock BD, McKenzie JL, Hart DN (2001) Phenotypic characterization of five dendritic cell subsets in human tonsils. Am J Pathol 159:285–295
Takahashi K, Asagoe K, Zaishun J, Yanai H, Yoshino T, Hayashi K, Akagi T (1998) Heterogeneity of dendritic cells in human superficial lymph node: in vitro maturation of immature dendritic cells into mature or activated interdigitating reticulum cells. Am J Pathol 153:745–755
Takeuchi O, Akira S (2010) Pattern recognition receptors and inflammation. Cell 140:805–820
Tanis W, Mancham S, Binda R, Janssen HL, Bezemer G, IJzermans JN, Tilanus HW, Laman JD, de Wit H, Drexhage HA, Schalm SW, Kwekkeboom J (2004) Human hepatic lymph nodes contain normal numbers of mature myeloid dendritic cells but few plasmacytoid dendritic cells. Clin Immunol 110:81–88
Teunissen MBM (2005) Langerhans cells and other skin dendritic cells. In: Bos JD (ed) Skin immune system - Cutaneous immunology and clinical immunodermatology, 3rd edn. CRC Press, Boca Raton
Teunissen MBM, Wormmeester J, Krieg SR, Peters PJ, Vogels IM, Kapsenberg ML, Bos JD (1990) Human epidermal Langerhans cells undergo profound morphologic and phenotypical changes during in vitro culture. J Invest Dermatol 94:166–173

Torocsik D, Bardos H, Nagy L, Adany R (2005) Identification of factor XIII-A as a marker of alternative macrophage activation. Cell Mol Life Sci 62:2132–2139

Trifari S, Kaplan CD, Tran EH, Crellin NK, Spits H (2009) Identification of a human helper T cell population that has abundant production of interleukin 22 and is distinct from T(H)-17, T(H)1 and T(H)2 cells. Nat Immunol 10:864–871

Tritto E, Mosca F, De Gregorio E (2009) Mechanism of action of licensed vaccine adjuvants. Vaccine 27:3331–3334

Trombetta ES, Mellman I (2005) Cell biology of antigen processing in vitro and in vivo. Annu Rev Immunol 23:975–1028

Udey MC (1997) Cadherins and langerhans cell immunobiology. Clin Exp Immunol 107(Suppl 1):6–8

Ueno H, Schmitt N, Klechevsky E, Pedroza-Gonzalez A, Matsui T, Zurawski G, Oh S, Fay J, Pascual V, Banchereau J, Palucka K (2010) Harnessing human dendritic cell subsets for medicine. Immunol Rev 234:199–212

Underhill DM (2007) Collaboration between the innate immune receptors dectin-1, TLRs, and Nods. Immunol Rev 219:75–87

Valladeau J, Saeland S (2005) Cutaneous dendritic cells. Semin Immunol 17:273–283

Valladeau J, Duvert-Frances V, Pin JJ, Dezutter-Dambuyant C, Vincent C, Massacrier C, Vincent J, Yoneda K, Banchereau J, Caux C, Davoust J, Saeland S (1999) The monoclonal antibody DCGM4 recognizes Langerin, a protein specific of Langerhans cells, and is rapidly internalized from the cell surface. Eur J Immunol 29:2695–2704

Valladeau J, Ravel O, Dezutter-Dambuyant C, Moore K, Kleijmeer M, Liu Y, Duvert-Frances V, Vincent C, Schmitt D, Davoust J, Caux C, Lebecque S, Saeland S (2000) Langerin, a novel C-type lectin specific to langerhans cells, is an endocytic receptor that induces the formation of birbeck granules. Immunity 12:71–81

van der Aar AM, Sylva-Steenland RM, Bos JD, Kapsenberg ML, de Jong EC, Teunissen MBM (2007) Loss of TLR2, TLR4, and TLR5 on Langerhans cells abolishes bacterial recognition. J Immunol 178:1986–1990

van der Aar AM, de Groot R, Sanchez-Hernandez M, Taanman EW, van Lier RA, Teunissen MBM, de Jong EC, Kapsenberg ML (2011a) Virus selectively primes human Langerhans cells for CD70 expression promoting CD8+ T cell responses. J Immunol in press

van der Aar AM, Sibiryak DS, Bakdash G, van Capel TM, van der Kleij HP, Opstelten DJ, Teunissen MBM, Kapsenberg ML, de Jong EC (2011b) Vitamin D3 targets epidermal and dermal dendritic cells for induction of distinct regulatory T cells. J Allergy Clin Immunol 127:1532–1540

Vanbervliet B, Bendriss-Vermare N, Massacrier C, Homey B, de Bouteiller O, Briere F, Trinchieri G, Caux C (2003) The inducible CXCR3 ligands control plasmacytoid dendritic cell responsiveness to the constitutive chemokine stromal cell-derived factor 1 (SDF-1)/CXCL12. J Exp Med 198:823–830

Velasquez-Lopera MM, Correa LA, Garcia LF (2008) Human spleen contains different subsets of dendritic cells and regulatory T lymphocytes. Clin Exp Immunol 154:107–114

Vermi W, Bonecchi R, Facchetti F, Bianchi D, Sozzani S, Festa S, Berenzi A, Cella M, Colonna M (2003) Recruitment of immature plasmacytoid dendritic cells (plasmacytoid monocytes) and myeloid dendritic cells in primary cutaneous melanomas. J Pathol 200:255–268

Vermi W, Riboldi E, Wittamer V, Gentili F, Luini W, Marrelli S, Vecchi A, Franssen JD, Communi D, Massardi L, Sironi M, Mantovani A, Parmentier M, Facchetti F, Sozzani S (2005) Role of ChemR23 in directing the migration of myeloid and plasmacytoid dendritic cells to lymphoid organs and inflamed skin. J Exp Med 201:509–515

Volc-Platzer B, Stingl G, Wolff K, Hinterberg W, Schnedl W (1984) Cytogenetic identification of allogeneic epidermal Langerhans cells in a bone-marrow-graft recipient. N Engl J Med 310:1123–1124

Vollmer J, Weeratna R, Payette P, Jurk M, Schetter C, Laucht M, Wader T, Tluk S, Liu M, Davis HL, Krieg AM (2004) Characterization of three CpG oligodeoxynucleotide classes with distinct immunostimulatory activities. Eur J Immunol 34:251–262

Warrell MJ (2011) Intradermal rabies vaccination: the evolution and future of pre- and post-exposure prophylaxis. Curr Top Microbiol Immunol 351:139–157

Wehner R, Lobel B, Bornhauser M, Schakel K, Cartellieri M, Bachmann M, Rieber EP, Schmitz M (2009) Reciprocal activating interaction between 6-sulfo LacNAc+ dendritic cells and NK cells. Int J Cancer 124:358–366

Wollenberg A, Kraft S, Hanau D, Bieber T (1996) Immunomorphological and ultrastructural characterization of Langerhans cells and a novel, inflammatory dendritic epidermal cell (IDEC) population in lesional skin of atopic eczema. J Invest Dermatol 106:446–453

Wollenberg A, Wen S, Bieber T (1999) Phenotyping of epidermal dendritic cells: clinical applications of a flow cytometric micromethod. Cytometry 37:147–155

Wollenberg A, Sharma S, von Bubnoff D, Geiger E, Haberstok J, Bieber T (2001) Topical tacrolimus (FK506) leads to profound phenotypic and functional alterations of epidermal antigen-presenting dendritic cells in atopic dermatitis. J Allergy Clin Immunol 107:519–525

Wollenberg A, Wagner M, Gunther S, Towarowski A, Tuma E, Moderer M, Rothenfusser S, Wetzel S, Endres S, Hartmann G (2002a) Plasmacytoid dendritic cells: a new cutaneous dendritic cell subset with distinct role in inflammatory skin diseases. J Invest Dermatol 119:1096–1102

Wollenberg A, Mommaas M, Oppel T, Schottdorf EM, Gunther S, Moderer M (2002b) Expression and function of the mannose receptor CD206 on epidermal dendritic cells in inflammatory skin diseases. J Invest Dermatol 118:327–334

World Health Organization (2004) BCG vaccination—WHO position paper. Weekly epidemiological record 79:27–38

Zaba LC, Fuentes-Duculan J, Steinman RM, Krueger JG, Lowes MA (2007) Normal human dermis contains distinct populations of CD11c+BDCA-1+ dendritic cells and CD163+FXIIIA+ macrophages. J Clin Invest 117:2517–2525

Zaba LC, Krueger JG, Lowes MA (2009a) Resident and "inflammatory" dendritic cells in human skin. J Invest Dermatol 129:302–308

Zaba LC, Fuentes-Duculan J, Eungdamrong NJ, Abello MV, Novitskaya I, Pierson KC, Gonzalez J, Krueger JG, Lowes MA (2009b) Psoriasis is characterized by accumulation of immunostimulatory and Th1/Th17 cell-polarizing myeloid dendritic cells. J Invest Dermatol 129:79–88

Zaba LC, Fuentes-Duculan J, Eungdamrong NJ, Johnson-Huang LM, Nograles KE, White TR, Pierson KC, Lentini T, Suarez-Farinas M, Lowes MA, Krueger JG (2010) Identification of TNF-related apoptosis-inducing ligand and other molecules that distinguish inflammatory from resident dendritic cells in patients with psoriasis. J Allergy Clin Immunol 125:1261–1268

Zabel BA, Silverio AM, Butcher EC (2005) Chemokine-like receptor 1 expression and chemerin-directed chemotaxis distinguish plasmacytoid from myeloid dendritic cells in human blood. J Immunol 174:244–251

Delivery Systems for Intradermal Vaccination

Y. C. Kim, C. Jarrahian, D. Zehrung, S. Mitragotri and M. R. Prausnitz

Abstract Intradermal (ID) vaccination can offer improved immunity and simpler logistics of delivery, but its use in medicine is limited by the need for simple, reliable methods of ID delivery. ID injection by the Mantoux technique requires special training and may not reliably target skin, but is nonetheless used currently for BCG and rabies vaccination. Scarification using a bifurcated needle was extensively used for smallpox eradication, but provides variable and inefficient delivery into the skin. Recently, ID vaccination has been simplified by introduction of a simple-to-use hollow microneedle that has been approved for ID injection of influenza vaccine in Europe. Various designs of hollow microneedles have been studied preclinically and in humans. Vaccines can also be injected into skin using needle-free devices, such as jet injection, which is receiving renewed clinical attention for ID vaccination. Projectile delivery using powder and gold particles (i.e., gene gun) have also been used clinically for ID vaccination. Building off the scarification approach, a number of preclinical studies have examined solid microneedle patches for use with vaccine coated onto metal microneedles, encapsulated within dissolving microneedles or added topically to skin after

Y. C. Kim · M. R. Prausnitz (✉)
School of Chemical and Biomolecular Engineering, Georgia Institute of Technology, Atlanta, GA 30332, USA
e-mail: prausnitz@gatech.edu

Y. C. Kim
Department of Microbiology and Immunology, Emory University School of Medicine, Atlanta, GA 30322, USA

C. Jarrahian · D. Zehrung
PATH, Seattle, WA 98121, USA

S. Mitragotri
Department of Chemical Engineering, University of California Santa Barbara, Santa Barbara, CA 93106, USA

Current Topics in Microbiology and Immunology (2012) 351: 77–112
DOI: 10.1007/82_2011_123

Published Online: 7 April 2011

microneedle pretreatment, as well as adapting tattoo guns for ID vaccination. Finally, technologies designed to increase skin permeability in combination with a vaccine patch have been studied through the use of skin abrasion, ultrasound, electroporation, chemical enhancers, and thermal ablation. The prospects for bringing ID vaccination into more widespread clinical practice are encouraging, given the large number of technologies for ID delivery under development.

Contents

1 Introduction

1.1 Immunologic Motivation for Intradermal Delivery

The skin contains high concentrations of antigen-presenting cells, and is thus a site capable of inducing potent immune responses. The skin is composed of multiple layers, each with characteristic resident and transient immune cell subsets. Outermost is the thin layer of the epidermis (0.05–0.2 mm), which is primarily made up of epithelial cells as well as Langerhans cells, melanocytes, and Merkel cells. Beneath the epidermis, the dermis is a thicker layer (1.5–3 mm) consisting of a network of collagen fibers. Cells of the adaptive and innate system reside in or circulate through the dermis, including macrophages, mast cells, Langerhans cells, and dermal dendritic cells. Antigen-presenting cells in the skin perform an essential role in processing incoming antigens, resulting in immune system activation or immune tolerance of self or harmless antigens (Nicolas and Guy 2008). For these reasons, it is possible that delivery of vaccines to the epidermis or dermis may result in superior immune responses compared to other anatomical sites (Glenn and Kenney 2006; Lambert and Laurent 2008; Nicolas and Guy 2008). Alternatively, an equivalent immune response could be stimulated by delivery of a smaller quantity of vaccine antigen to the skin. Either of these mechanisms could be beneficial for developing vaccines against new disease targets, improving immune responses in hard-to-treat groups, or lowering the cost of vaccine antigens, and may be particularly valuable for improving access to vaccines in low-resource settings.

While a substantial number of clinical studies evaluating intradermal (ID) delivery of vaccines have been performed, the majority of studies have not been designed to evaluate whether ID delivery is immunologically superior to other routes. In most cases, to simplify administration, a reduced dose (10 or 20%) delivered ID was compared to the full dose delivered either subcutaneously (SC) or intramuscularly (IM). Only a few studies have compared delivery of the same dose of vaccine ID and SC/IM. Further research will be needed to establish whether the potential for dose-sparing is unique to ID delivery (PATH 2009). However, some ID delivery devices in development offer additional desirable features such as needle-free delivery or improved ease of administration, which may be drivers for further adoption of ID vaccine delivery even if there is no net immunologic benefit.

1.2 Current Intradermal Vaccines

1.2.1 Smallpox

Vaccines for smallpox have been delivered to the skin dating back to Edward Jenner's first experiments in 1796 demonstrating that exposure to cowpox could protect against smallpox infection. A variety of scarification techniques and devices have been used to allow virus introduction, including knives, needles, scalpels, and rotary lancets. During the global smallpox eradication campaign, both multi-dose nozzle jet injectors and bifurcated needles were used for ID vaccinia virus inoculation (Henderson et al. 2008).

1.2.2 BCG

Bacille Calmette-Guérin (BCG) vaccine for tuberculosis is globally the most widely delivered ID vaccine. ID injection by needle and syringe is the most commonly used method, but in some areas BCG is also delivered to the skin using a multipuncture device. New versions of BCG are under development in an effort to improve immune protection, and are also delivered ID (Hoft et al. 2008).

1.2.3 Rabies

Rabies vaccines are conventionally delivered IM, but due to the high cost of cell-culture-derived vaccines and the pressing need for affordable vaccination regimens in endemic regions, ID delivery has been extensively studied. Both post-exposure prophylaxis and pre-exposure prophylaxis ID regimens induce protective titers, and WHO has recommended ID delivery of reduced doses of rabies vaccines since 1991 (WHO 2005; 2007). Given equivalent doses of antigen, delivery to the dermis appears to be either superior or equivalent to IM/SC (Bernard et al. 1982; Bernard et al. 1987; Fishbein et al. 1987; Phanuphak et al. 1990). A detailed review on ID rabies vaccination can be found elsewhere in this special volume on ID immunization (Warrell 2011).

1.3 Clinical Studies on other Intradermal Vaccines

1.3.1 Influenza

Multiple studies of reduced-dose delivery of influenza vaccines have been conducted, providing some of the most informative clinical data on the potential for dose-sparing through ID delivery. One study found that ID delivery of 6 μg HA per influenza strain was comparably immunogenic as the standard IM dose of 15 μg HA per strain (Belshe et al. 2004). A later comparison of 3, 6, and 9 μg delivered both ID and IM found equivalent responses for the two delivery routes for each dose (Belshe et al. 2007). Trials have also been conducted with influenza using novel microneedle devices to aid accurate ID delivery, as discussed in Sect. 3.2.

1.3.2 Hepatitis B

ID delivery of reduced doses of hepatitis B vaccine has been evaluated in healthy infant, child, and adult populations as well as in immuno-compromised patient groups. Meta-analyses have concluded that seroconversion rates are lower than full-dose IM delivery, although responses are higher in children and females (Chen and Gluud 2005; Sangare et al. 2009). When the same dose of hepatitis B antigen has been delivered ID and IM, immune responses were equivalent for both routes (Ayoola 1984; Milne et al. 1986; Heijtink et al. 1989; Coberly et al. 1994; Rahman et al. 2000).

1.3.3 Hepatitis A

Hepatitis A vaccines have also been proposed as a possible target for reduced-dose ID delivery. Two studies found that reduced doses delivered ID produced comparable immune responses to IM delivery, while a third indicated that the ID route was inferior (Brindle et al. 1994; Carlsson et al. 1996; Pancharoen et al. 2005). Local reactogenicity was observed for alum-adjuvanted formulations.

1.3.4 Polio

In a few countries, ID was originally the standard route of delivery for inactivated poliovirus vaccine, but injection depth was later shifted to IM (Weniger and Papania 2008). Studies have found that ID delivery of reduced doses is capable of inducing seroconversion, which may help make this vaccine more affordable for use in developing countries (Samuel et al. 1991; Samuel et al. 1992; Nirmal et al. 1998). More recently, the WHO Global Polio Eradication Initiative has worked to determine the potential for this mode of delivery to be used in post-eradication settings after phase-out of oral polio vaccine.

1.3.5 Measles

Several studies have been conducted evaluating ID delivery of measles vaccine, with mixed results (Burland 1969; Kok et al. 1983; Whittle et al. 1984; de Moraes et al. 1994). However, the vaccine dose and method used to deliver the vaccine varied, and it is possible that trials using older generation delivery technology did not deliver vaccine reliably to the dermis (PATH 2009). Transcutaneous immunization of measles vaccine on a coated patch has also been attempted. Although a salivary sIgA response was observed, the key marker of immunity, an increase in neutralizing serum IgG, was not detected (Etchart et al. 2007).

1.3.6 Yellow Fever

Studies were conducted delivering the 17D attenuated yellow fever virus vaccine by scarification, but this delivery mode was abandoned as efficacy was low. More recently, a clinical trial compared full dose SC delivery of a 17D vaccine to 1/5 dose delivered ID by Mantoux injection, which found equivalent seroprotection between the two routes (Roukens et al. 2008). A more extensive description on ID vaccination against yellow fever is provided elsewhere in this special volume on ID immunization (Roukens et al. 2011).

1.3.7 Others

A number of other vaccines have been considered for ID delivery. Research has shown that a reduced ID dose of vaccines for diphtheria-tetanus-pertussis, tetanus toxoid, and tick-borne encephalitis can generate a comparable immune response to the standard dose and way of injection (Stanfield et al. 1972; Zoulek et al. 1984; Zoulek et al. 1986; Dimache et al. 1990). ID delivery is also under investigation for a number of vaccines in development, including vaccines for tuberculosis, enterotoxigenic *E. coli*, and pandemic influenza, as well as DNA vaccines.

1.4 Difficulties to Make Intradermal Delivery More Widespread

The traditional methods used for ID delivery of vaccines have limitations which may hinder adoption of ID delivery. Bifurcated needles and multipuncture devices have been used successfully for delivery of smallpox and BCG vaccines, but do not deliver reproducible quantities of vaccine antigen to the dermis and are therefore unlikely to be appropriate delivery devices for new vaccines (Lambert and Laurent 2008). The Mantoux method of inserting a needle at a shallow angle into the skin can also be inconsistent, and requires additional training and skill to perform correctly (Flynn et al. 1994). The perceived difficulty of performing an ID injection using this method may prevent development of vaccines for ID delivery. New generations of devices, such as those discussed in the rest of this article, may improve the reliability of ID delivery and enable adoption of the ID route for more vaccines.

2 Injecting into the Skin

Most vaccines are administered IM or SC using a hypodermic needle. To achieve ID vaccination, conventional hypodermic needles can be used by employing the Mantoux technique to inject into the skin. Simpler and more reliable ID injection is being pursued through adaptations of hypodermic needle technology, as well as novel hollow microneedle devices produced by microfabrication (Prausnitz et al. 2009).

2.1 Hypodermic Needles: Mantoux Intradermal Injection

The Mantoux technique is an ID injection method characterized by a needle inserted at a 5–15 degree angle, approximately 1 mm deep into the dermis, to

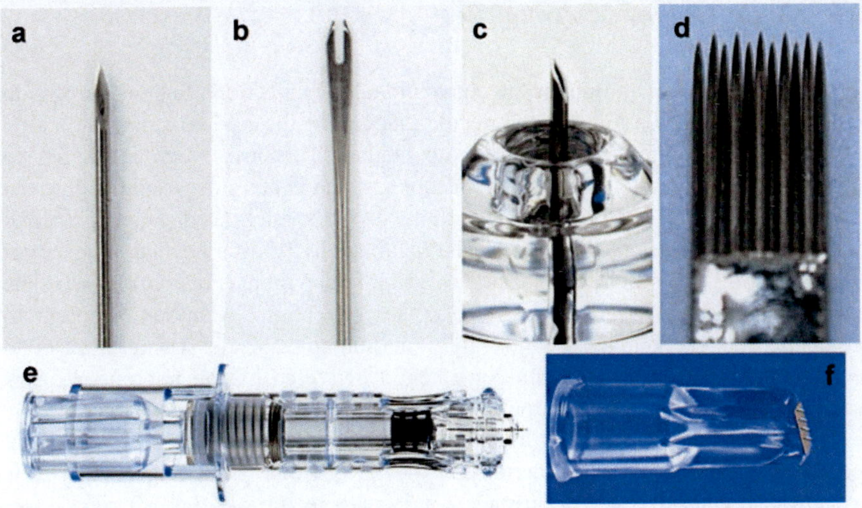

Fig. 1 Needles used for ID vaccination. **a** 32 gauge hypodermic needle with ID bevel used for Mantoux technique injections. **b** Bifurcated needles used for smallpox vaccination by scarification. **c** Hollow microneedle developed for reliable ID injection, currently used for ID influenza vaccination (Courtesy of BD). **d** Mag-11 tattoo needle. **e** Microneedle injection system, consisting of a single-use syringe coupled to a microneedle shown in part **c** (Courtesy of BD). **f** Microneedle injection system containing of a row of four microneedles (Courtesy of NanoPass Technologies)

inject a vaccine or drug (Fig. 1a). This method was developed by Charles Mantoux in the early 20th century, and it has been used to identify tuberculosis infection by the ID injection of tuberculin (Mantoux 1909). However, this technique requires training and is often considered an inconsistent delivery method, thus preventing vaccine makers or medical practitioners from using ID injection as a common immunization method (Lambert and Laurent 2008). Also, age or elasticity-related skin conditions have a significant effect on adequate placement of the needle in the dermis for the traditional ID injection technique (Dean et al. 2005; Laurent et al. 2007), thus leading to inadequate vaccination. Other disadvantages of Mantoux technique injection include inaccurately delivered dosage of vaccine, vaccine wastage in dead space of the needle, and variable injection success when using different gauge needles (Flynn et al. 1994). Moreover, success rate of ID injection by untrained personnel was found to be 80–90% (Howard et al. 1997). In an effort to reduce training requirements and to improve the reliability of the Mantoux injection technique, an intradermal adapter is under development by PATH (Seattle, WA, USA), a nonprofit, international health agency that develops and advances health technologies for low resource settings, and SID Technologies. This device fits over a conventional hypodermic needle and syringe and limits the angle and depth of penetration of the needle into the skin in order to facilitate delivery to the dermis.

2.2 Single Hollow Microneedles

To overcome these limitations of conventional ID injection, Becton–Dickinson (BD) has developed a micro-sized needle that can be inserted into skin vertically, unlike the angled injection of the Mantoux method. This novel microneedle device has been studied in animals and human subjects, and is currently used in approved influenza vaccines (INTANZA® and IDflu®). BD's microneedle device (called Soluvia™) uses a 30 gauge microneedle that extends 1.5 mm beyond an insertion depth-limiting tip, which is connected to a prefilled syringe (Figs. 1c and 1e). The microneedle system was evaluated versus the conventional Mantoux technique to compare delivery efficiency and safety in human subjects. Using ultrasound echography analysis, the distribution of fluid delivered by the microneedle was seen to be larger than the Mantoux injection control. In addition, the microneedle system had a high ID administration success rate (95%) and, in a study of patient compliance and safety, the microneedle device showed promising results. This system also caused fewer occurrences of injuries to the papillary dermis, lesser pain than Mantoux injection and was administered easily by untrained personnel (Laurent et al. 2007).

2.2.1 Preclinical Studies

An earlier prototype of the BD microneedle using a 1 mm, 34 gauge needle has been tested in rats for delivery of influenza vaccines which showed dose sparing effects compared to an IM control. ID microneedle administration of a low dose (0.01 μg) of inactivated virus vaccine induced similar serum antibody response as IM injection of a dose 100 times larger (1 μg). Additionally, using microneedles for ID immunization with split-viron vaccine (seasonal H1N1 strain) showed approximately ten-fold dose-sparing compared to IM immunization. In the same study, ID immunization using plasmid DNA vaccine encoding the hemagglutinin protein of influenza A virus showed similar dose-sparing effects after multiple immunizations (Alarcon et al. 2007). The BD microneedle was also used to deliver a live attenuated vaccine against Japanese encephalitis (ChimeriVax™–JE) in non-human primates. In this study, ID microneedle injection was compared to SC injection and transcutaneous microabrasion (see Sect. 6.1). The microneedle ID injection provided the best and most consistent immune responses (i.e., neutralizing antibodies) of the three types of immunizations (Dean et al. 2005).

A further study compared anthrax vaccine delivery using ID microneedle immunization, IM injection, intranasal delivery, and epidermal delivery by microabrasion (Mikszta et al. 2005) into mice (10 μg dose) and rabbits (50 μg dose). Microneedle ID vaccination showed slightly better response in the murine model than the other routes used, while all treatments in the rabbit had similar responses. A follow-up ID immunization was performed to compare ID injection with IM injection over a range of doses in a rabbit model: 10, 0.2, and 0.08 μg of anthrax vaccine (Mikszta et al. 2006). After prime immunization, ID injection showed significantly higher immunogenicity than IM injection when using 10 and 0.2 μg dosages. Interestingly, ID injection with 0.2 μg showed a statistically equivalent response to IM administration of the 10 μg dose. After administration of a booster immunization, this dose-sparing phenomenon continued. Furthermore, an aerosol lethal challenge with anthrax spores showed that a 10 μg ID injection completely protected the immunized rabbits, whereas IM injection of the same dose protected only 71% of the rabbits.

2.2.2 Clinical Trials

An early prototype of the BD microneedle system was first tested in a clinical study examining influenza vaccine delivery in healthy adults (18–60 yrs) and elderly adults (>60 yrs) (Belshe et al. 2004). In this study, 6 μg of hemagglutinin was delivered by ID injection and compared to a full dose (15 μg) delivered by IM immunization. It was found that in younger participants, ID immunization was not significantly different from immunization by IM, as shown by geometric mean hemagglutination inhibition (HAI) titers. However, ID administration showed lower HAI titers than IM in elderly patients. Further evaluation of ID microneedle vaccination against influenza was performed in clinical studies of healthy adults (18–57 yrs) (Leroux-Roels et al. 2008; Beran et al. 2009) and elderly persons (>60 yrs) (Holland et al. 2008; Arnou et al. 2009). For healthy adults, 9 μg of hemagglutinin (H1, H3, and B strains) was delivered by ID injection and was compared to a 15 μg IM immunization. This study confirmed previous results that reduced-dose ID injection was equally immunogenic as full-dose IM injection (Leroux-Roels et al. 2008).

In a Phase II clinical trial, the effects of lower dose ID immunization was investigated using 3, 6, and 9 μg of hemagglutinin (ID) and 15 μg of hemagglutinin (IM). ID immunization using 3 and 6 μg of hemagglutinin induced inferior immune response as shown by HAI titer, but a dose of 9 μg showed comparable response compared to full-dose (15 μg) IM vaccination (Beran et al. 2009). For elderly subjects (>60 years old), a booster vaccine (15 μg) was administered due to the inferior immune system generally found in the elderly compared to younger adults (Goodwin et al. 2006). Therefore, 15 μg of hemagglutinin was administered twice by either ID or IM routes in elderly subjects. In this phase II clinical trial, ID immunization showed significantly better immune response as determined by post-immunization GMT (geometric mean titer), seroprotection (% participants with HAI titers ≥40), GMTR (geometric mean ratio of post-immunization titer to pre-immunization titer), and rate of seroconversion (post-immunization titer in participants with a pre-immunization titer <10). Therefore, ID microneedle vaccination provided superior immunogenicity in a high priority population for protection from influenza due to high vulnerability (Holland et al. 2008). These findings were further confirmed in a phase III clinical trial for elderly persons (>60 years old), where ID immunization showed superior seroprotection, GMTR, and rate of seroconversion compared to IM after prime immunization.

After administration of two booster immunizations, ID immunization induced consistently higher seroprotection rates than IM immunization (Arnou et al. 2009).

As a final note, ID immunization caused more local inflammatory-like reactions than IM immunization. It is possible that because ID delivery occurs in the skin, inflammatory or immunologic reactions are more easily visible than those that may occur after IM immunization, which presents the antigen deep into the muscle layer where an inflammatory reaction would not be visible to the eye (Belshe et al. 2004; Holland et al. 2008; Arnou et al. 2009; Beran et al. 2009; Van Damme et al. 2009).

2.3 Arrays of Hollow Microneedles

Hollow microneedles have also been developed as multi-needle arrays, which have involved shorter needles (<<1 mm) produced by novel microfabrication techniques, including laser micromachining (Davis et al. 2005), silicon-based MEMS technique using deep reactive-ion etching (Gardeniers et al. 2003; Roxhed et al. 2007), integrated lithographic molding technique (Luttge et al. 2007), deep X-ray photolithography (Perennes et al. 2006), photolithography with micromolding technique (Wang et al. 2009), drawing lithography with viscoelastic polymer (Lee et al. 2010) and others. In addition, glass hollow microneedles have been fabricated by drawn glass micropipette techniques (Wang et al. 2006). A recently developed hollow microneedle array (MicronJet from NanoPass Technologies) was used in a human clinical trial involving healthy adults (Van Damme et al. 2009). This device consists of a row of four hollow silicon microneedles that are 450 μm in length (Fig. 1f). In this study, ID injection with the array using 20 and 40% of the IM dose (15 μg) induced similar immune response as measured by GMT increase, seroconversion rate, and seroprotection rate.

3 Shooting into the Skin

ID delivery can also be achieved via jet injection or particle injection routes, which are needle-free methods of vaccine and drug delivery. There have been decades of clinical experience with jet injection, and more recent studies are being conducted with newer innovations in this technology.

3.1 Jet Injector

Needle-free jet injectors create a fine stream of pressurized liquid that penetrates the skin. The depth of delivery—ID, SC, or IM—is largely determined by design variables such as the injection stream coherence, quality, and pressure; orifice size, skin and tissue thickness, and the angle of the injection relative to the skin (Schramm-Baxter and Mitragotri 2004; Weniger and Papania 2008). Vaccines that have been shown to achieve immunity when administered via jet injection to conventional depths (i.e., ID, SC, or IM, depending on the vaccine) include typhoid, cholera, BCG, tetanus-diphtheria for adults, whole cell diphtheria-tetanus-pertussis (DTP), measles, meningococcal A and C, smallpox, yellow fever, hepatitis A, hepatitis B, influenza, plague, polio, and tetanus (Weniger and Papania 2008).

3.1.1 History

Historically, multi-use nozzle jet injector (MUNJI) devices with reusable nozzles were used successfully worldwide in the latter half of the 20th century to deliver countless millions, or by some estimates billions of doses of vaccines to both adults and children over the course of several decades (Weniger and Papania 2008). In response to the risks of disease transmission due to cross contamination from reuse of injection devices, a new generation of jet injector designs were developed starting in the late 1980s to address this safety concern. These new jet injectors utilize a sterile, disposable cartridge or syringe for each patient injection and a reusable hand-piece that relies on a power source, such as a manually powered spring or gas canister. A number of disposable-syringe jet injectors (DSJIs) have been developed and approved by national regulatory authorities for a variety of applications and uses, including vaccine delivery. Some of these are low-cost, manually powered DSJI technologies, developed specifically for application to developing countries' immunization requirements and needs, which include design features to prevent reuse ('auto-disable') of the needle-free syringes. DSJIs in clinical development for ID delivery include the Biojector® 2000 and Zetajet® (Bioject), and PharmaJet® (PharmaJet Inc.).

There is a long history of ID delivery via the jet injector route through the use of modified syringe orifice nozzles that can either have direct contact to the skin or can involve a setback feature or 'spacer' intended to introduce a gap between the nozzle orifice and the injection site, thereby weakening the injection stream and limiting deposition to the dermal space (Weniger and Papania 2008) (Figs. 2a, b). MUNJI devices provided millions of ID smallpox doses during the implementation of the smallpox eradication program (Millar and Foege 1969; Weniger and Papania 2008). Jet injectors have also been utilized historically for ID vaccination of rabies (Bernard et al. 1982; Bernard et al. 1987), hepatitis A (Williams et al. 2000), BCG (Paul et al. 1978; Parker 1984), DTP combination vaccine (Stanfield et al. 1972), measles (Burland 1969; Kok et al. 1983), and influenza vaccine (Weniger and Papania 2008).

3.1.2 Recent Intradermal Vaccination Clinical Studies

A number of studies have been or will soon be implemented to address the application of DSJI ID delivery to vaccines of importance to global public health.

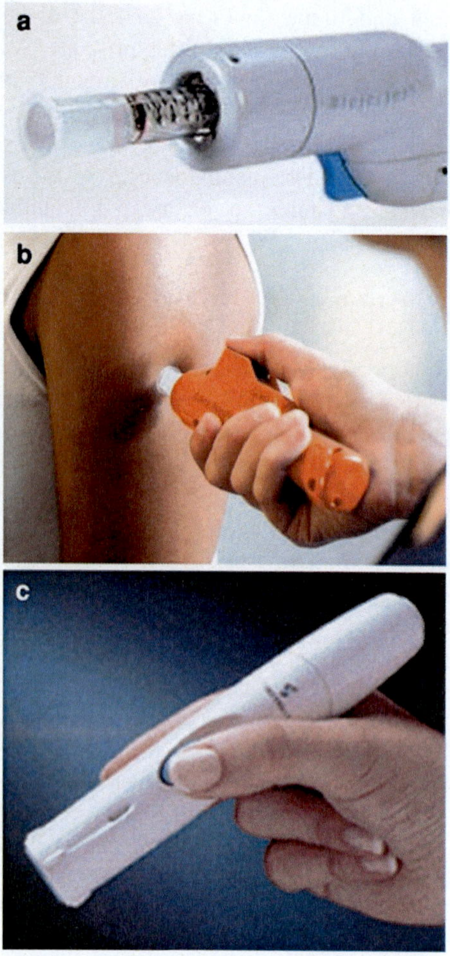

Fig. 2 Liquid jet and solid projectile injectors. **a** Jet injector (Biojector 2000) with ID spacer (white portion at end of syringe), used for investigational use only (Courtesy of BioJect). **b** Jet injector applied to the skin for injection (Courtesy of PharmaJet). **c** Epidermal powder immunization device for ID projectile injection (Courtesy of PowderMed)

For example, the US Centers for Disease Control and Prevention is leading a study on seasonal influenza vaccine delivered ID via a DSJI technology in children of 6–24 months of age. This study compares full and fractional dose IM with ID vaccination. Results-to-date indicate that injections were generally tolerable with few study-related adverse events. Initial blinded assay results demonstrate comparable immune response rates. Final study results and analysis can be found in Gomez et al. (2010).

The WHO Global Polio Eradication Initiative has worked to determine the potential for DSJI ID delivery of inactivated poliovirus vaccine (IPV) to be used in post-eradication settings after phasing out the use of oral polio vaccine. Studies have been conducted in Oman, Cuba, and India to evaluate reduced ('fractional') dose of IPV delivered with two different DSJI devices. Compared to IM, inferior seroconversion rates were found when ID doses were delivered at 6, 10, and

14 weeks of age, but non-inferior rates of protection (>95%) were seen using a later 2, 4, and 6 month schedule. When IPV was used as a booster to oral polio vaccine, inferior seroconversion rates were observed for ID compared to IM delivery (Sutter 2009; Mohammed et al. 2010; Resik et al. 2010).

DSJI technology has also been used for the delivery of DNA vaccines for malaria in young adults (Epstein et al. 2002; Wang et al. 2006) and an HIV-vaccine candidate (PATH 2009). A pilot study assessment of human papillomavirus vaccine has also recently occurred (PATH 2009). PATH is also working to implement a new study of purified Vero cell rabies vaccine for ID post-exposure prophylaxis using a DSJI technology in India. Results of this study are anticipated in 2012. Other vaccine trials of ID vaccine delivery are planned for other applications including BCG, IPV, varicella zoster virus, H1N1 and yellow fever (PATH 2009).

3.2 *Projectile Delivery*

Epidermal powder immunization (EPI) and particle-mediated epidermal delivery (PMED) utilize helium gas to deliver powdered proteins, polysaccharides, inactivated pathogens, or DNA-coated particles into the epidermis at supersonic speeds (Weniger and Papania 2008) (Fig. 2c). Companies involved in developing this technology include Powderject, PowderMed (acquired by Pfizer in 2006), and Iaculor Injection. It is not known if this device technology class is still in active development (PATH 2009). Conventional protein antigens must be specially formulated for delivery by EPI, and are spray dried into powders of suitable density and size (20–70 μm). A clinical trial has been conducted evaluating delivery of a powdered inactivated influenza vaccine by EPI injection, which found that immunogenicity was comparable to standard delivery by IM needle and syringe (Dean and Chen 2004). EPI has also shown efficacy in preclinical studies with hepatitis B and HIV vaccines (Chen et al. 2002; Osorio et al. 2003).

In PMED, gold beads 1–3 μm in diameter are coated with vaccine and delivered by needle-free jet injection into the epidermis. This approach may be particularly suited to DNA vaccines, as deposition of coated particles into the stratum corneum and epidermis may encourage DNA uptake and expression by resident antigen-presenting cells. DNA vaccines for hepatitis B delivered by PMED have induced protective antibodies (Roy et al. 2000; Roberts et al. 2005). Clinical studies have also been conducted with DNA vaccines for seasonal influenza to evaluate the feasibility of this approach. Results have been promising, but immune responses are not yet equivalent to standard vaccine delivery methods (Drape et al. 2006; Jones et al. 2009). EPI and PMED delivery of DNA vaccines for a variety of other diseases have also shown immunogenicity preclinically, including malaria, avian influenza, herpes simplex virus, HIV, non-small cell lung cancer, Eurasian encephalitic viruses, hantaviruses, SARS coronavirus, and smallpox (Weniger and Papania 2008).

4 Piercing into the Skin

For more than 200 years, various sharp instruments have been used for vaccination by creating small holes in the skin that allow vaccine to penetrate into the body (Weniger and Papania 2008). Although most vaccine administration is currently performed by hypodermic needle injection, sharp tools such as bifurcated needles have historically been used for smallpox (Frey et al. 2002) and BCG (Darmanger et al. 1977) vaccination and remain in use to this day. Over the past decade, new skin piercing technologies for ID drug transport have been developed, and include techniques such as microneedles (Prausnitz 2004) and tattooing (Bins et al. 2005). Recently these methods, especially microneedles, have shown promise for delivering vaccines to the skin, thereby enabling improved immunogenicity and simpler patient administration.

4.1 Bifurcated Needles

The bifurcated needle (Fig. 1b) was invented by Benjamin Rubin in 1961 for smallpox vaccination. It consists of two sharp prongs which hold vaccine fluid by capillary action between the two tines. The use of this device is simple and does not require trained personnel (Baxby 2002; Weniger and Papania 2008). The needles are dipped into vaccine and then punctured perpendicularly into skin repeatedly over an area of about 5 mm diameter by a process called scarification (WHO 2010). Although this method was effective for the smallpox eradication program, poorly controlled dosing, inefficient use of vaccine and needle-stick injuries were significant shortcomings that have limited the use of bifurcated needles for other vaccines.

4.2 Solid Microneedles

In addition to hollow microneedles discussed in Sect. 2, solid microneedles can be used to pierce the skin and thereby deposit vaccine in the epidermal and/or dermal space (Prausnitz et al. 2009). Techniques for vaccination using solid microneedles include the use of microneedles that penetrate the skin to make a hole through which vaccine can be transported. Vaccine formulations may be placed on the skin after microneedle penetration, coated onto microneedles or embedded within microneedles and released into the skin after insertion. Solid microneedles can be prepared as patches that can be easily applied to the skin, perhaps by self administration.

4.2.1 Coated Microneedles

Coated microneedles have been the most extensively studied technique for ID microneedle vaccination (Figs. 3a, b). Using this approach, vaccine forms a solid-state coating on the surface of solid microneedles that dissolves off within the skin upon application. Typically, this method provides a bolus delivery of a sub-milligram dose of antigen within minutes of application, which is often suitable for delivery of vaccines. An effective microneedle coating process typically involves dip-coating metal microneedles in a coating solution containing the vaccine, a surfactant to promote wetting of the microneedle surface, and a viscosity enhancer to increase coating thickness (Gill and Prausnitz 2007b; Gill and Prausnitz 2007a). Using this technique, compounds over a large range of sizes including small molecules, proteins, DNA, and virus particles have been coated onto microneedles. Novel coated microneedle designs for improved delivery have been demonstrated, such as the three-dimensional grooves-embedded microneedle (Han et al. 2009) and the pocketed microneedle (Gill and Prausnitz 2008). The first ID vaccination using coated microneedles delivered ovalbumin as a model protein antigen to

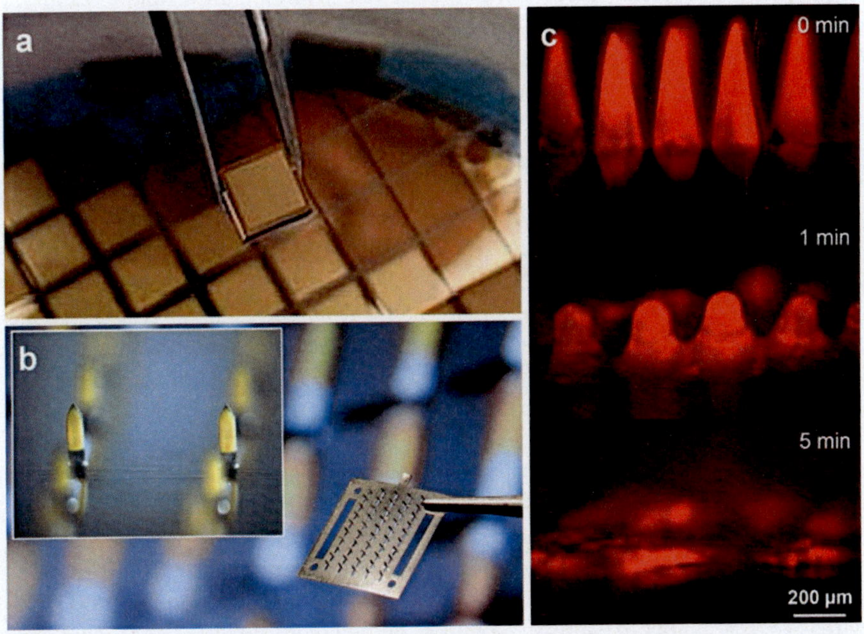

Fig. 3 Solid microneedle patches. **a** Arrays of solid silicon microneedles coated with gold. (Courtesy of University of Queensland). **b** Array of solid stainless steel microneedles coated with yellow dye. Each 12 mm by 12 mm device contains 50 microneedles measuring 700 μm tall. Inset shows magnified view of two coated microneedles (Courtesy of Georgia Institute of Technology). **c** Dissolving microneedles shown intact before insertion into skin, partially dissolved 1 min after insertion into skin and fully dissolved 5 min after insertion into skin (Reproduced from (Sullivan et al. 2010); Courtesy of Georgia Institute of Technology)

hairless guinea pigs (Matriano et al. 2002; Widera et al. 2006). In these studies, ID microneedle vaccination showed a better immune response than an equivalent SC or IM injection at low dose. The investigators also found that immune response by microneedle vaccination was dose-dependent.

Among the various vaccine candidates, influenza vaccine has received the most attention by ID immunization using small arrays of coated microneedles measuring approximately 700 μm in length (Zhu et al. 2009). Microneedles coated with 10 μg of seasonal influenza H1N1 inactivated virus vaccine induced complete protection against lethal virus infection in mice. However, subsequent studies showed that influenza vaccine lost more than 95% of its antigenicity during the coating process (Kim et al. 2010b). In order to maintain antigenicity, the disaccharide trehalose was added to the coating formulation to serve as a stabilizer. This enabled successful immunizations requiring smaller doses of vaccine (0.4 μg) as compared to immunizations with similar immune responses by conventional IM immunization (Kim et al. 2009; Kim et al. 2011). Coated microneedles also showed improved thermal stability of vaccine compared to the liquid form of vaccine (Kim et al. 2010b). More detailed studies showed that coated microneedle vaccination with inactivated influence virus vaccine induced similar antibody IgG response, HAI titer, and neutralizing activity as conventional IM immunization in mice (Kim et al. 2009; Kim et al. 2010b). To account for antigenic changes to the vaccine during the coating process, vaccine coated on microneedles was dissolved off the needles and then delivered IM by injection. In this case, vaccination using microneedles showed a better primary immune response than corresponding IM immunization using the same antigen formulation (Quan et al. 2009).

Vaccination by coated microneedles induced robust immunity to influenza after challenge in a mouse model (Kim et al. 2011). Notably, microneedle-immunized mice were shown to have undetectable levels of influenza virus titer in their lungs after challenge, unlike IM immunized mice, which had virus titers at least 100-fold higher. Additional assays for immune response from corresponding lung samples such as lung cytokine and lung IgG also consistently showed microneedle immunization to be superior to IM. As evidence for microneedle-enhanced immune system memory response, the microneedle immunized group was found to have significantly higher levels of total IgG and isotypes IgG1 and IgG2a post-challenge than pre-challenge, but antibody levels in IM immunized mice were lower post-challenge than pre-challenge (Kim et al. 2011). In addition to improved humoral immunity, coated microneedles also induced cellular recall response such as MHC II-associated $CD4^{+}$ T helper cell response (Kim et al. 2009). Finally, microneedle immunization performed using a different strain of influenza (H3N2) virus vaccine induced similar complete protection against lethal challenge (Koutsonanos et al. 2009). Studies using virus-like particle (VLP) vaccine coated on microneedles were also performed. The VLP dose was controlled using a coating formulation including antigen concentration and a number of coating dips (Kim et al. 2010a). When a 0.35 μg dose of VLP was delivered, microneedle vaccination induced a stronger immune response than IM, as measured by IgG, IgG subtype (IgG1, IgG2a, IgG2b), HAI, neutralizing activity, lung IgG, lung cytokine, and more suppression of lung virus infection. Microneedle immunization by VLP showed complete protection from a lethal viral challenge without major body weight loss, unlike IM after the same dose, which partially protected mice from lethal viral infection (40%) and caused significant body weight loss (Quan et al. 2010).

A novel approach to coated microneedles involved the use of polyphosphazene (PCPP), which served as both an effective coating excipient and an immune adjuvant (Andrianov et al. 2009). ID microneedle immunization with hepatitis B surface antigen (HBsAg) in pigs using the PCPP coating formulation was superior in inducing antigen-specific IgG compared to ID injection by hypodermic needle with or without PCPP. Another study demonstrated effective generation of cellular immune responses to a hepatitis C DNA vaccine administered to mice using coated microneedles (Gill et al. 2010). Other studies have sought to specifically target delivery to antigen-presenting Langerhans cells using extremely short (~100 μm) needles that penetrate only into the epidermis. These short needles were coated using a novel coating process involving gas-jet drying (Chen et al. 2009). In an initial study, vaccination with ovalbumin-coated needles induced similar immune response to IM immunization. In a follow-up study, microneedles coated with a low dose of hemagglutinin-based influenza vaccine generated a similar immune response as IM vaccination at a 100-times larger dose. The authors proposed that these short, densely packed microneedles could deliver more than half of the antigen directly to antigen-presenting cells such as epidermal Langerhans cells and dermal dendritic cells (Fernando et al. 2010).

Methods for long-term vaccine storage without significant immunogenicity loss, especially without refrigeration, are important for vaccination campaigns. Microneedles are coated with vaccine in the solid state, which is expected to confer thermal stability. In a stability study of microneedles coated with inactivated influenza vaccine, mice immunized with coated microneedles stored at room temperature for 1 month produced similar IgG responses to those of mice immunized by microneedles stored for 1 day. Furthermore, both groups were completely protected from lethal challenge after viral infection. In vitro assay of the microneedles, however, showed a decrease in antigenicity by about 80% (Kim et al. 2010c).

4.2.2 Dissolving Microneedles

As an improvement over coated microneedles, dissolving microneedles have been developed in order to eliminate sharp, biohazardous waste after vaccination (Fig. 3c). Unlike non-dissolving (e.g., metal) microneedles coated with a vaccine formulation, dissolving microneedles are made solely of material such as polymers or sugars that will safely dissolve in the skin after insertion, which leaves behind only the microneedle patch backing. Typically, the vaccine is incorporated into the matrix of the microneedle and is released into the skin upon microneedle dissolution. Dissolving microneedles have been made using a number of different materials, including polyvinylpyrrolidone (Sullivan et al. 2008), maltose (Kolli and Banga 2008), carboxymethylcellulose (Lee et al. 2008), polylactic and/or polyglycolic acid (Park et al. 2005; Park et al. 2006) and dextrin (Ito et al. 2006). In a recent study, dissolving microneedles were prepared by encapsulating inactivated influenza vaccine in a polyvinylpyrrolidone matrix and used to immunize mice. The vaccine was gently encapsulated without significant damage to immunogenicity and was shown to generate similar antibody and cellular immune responses compared to IM injection of the same dose and provided complete protection against lethal challenge. Compared to IM injection, dissolving microneedle vaccination resulted in more efficient lung virus clearance and enhanced cellular recall responses after challenge (Sullivan et al. 2010). TheraJect has also developed biodegradable microneedles using carboxymethylcellulose containing various biomolecules including influenza vaccine (Oh et al. 2006).

4.2.3 Pretreatment with Solid Microneedles

As a simpler, albeit probably less efficient, method, microneedles can be used to pierce the skin to make it more permeable and thereby enable entry of topically applied vaccines. This method is attractive because the micro-scale pores made by microneedle insertion are generally too small for penetration of microorganisms (Donnelly et al. 2009), yet large enough for delivery of sub-unit and possibly viral vaccines. After insertion and removal of the microneedles, vaccine can be applied using a patch or other topical formulation for slow delivery by diffusion through long-lived pores (Kalluri and Banga 2011). This approach was investigated for transcutaneous vaccination using diphtheria toxoid and influenza vaccine (Ding et al. 2009a; Ding et al. 2009b). When diphtheria toxoid was applied to microneedle-pretreated skin in combination with cholera toxin adjuvant, a similar immune response was induced compared to SC injection. However, microneedle pretreatment did not enhance immune response for influenza vaccine. This vaccination approach has also been studied in an ex vivo human skin model to investigate skin immune cell responses (Ng et al. 2009). Using a related approach, blunt-tipped microneedles were used to scrape the skin, thereby making microtroughs in the skin through which a DNA vaccine encoding HBsAg was administered (Mikszta et al. 2002). This approach generated stronger humoral and cellular immune responses than IM or ID injection.

4.3 Tattoo Vaccination

Tattoo guns use high-frequency oscillating needles to make thousands of punctures in the skin, which is conventionally used to deposit tattoo ink in the dermis, but has been adapted to deliver ID vaccines (Fig. 1d). In one study, hemagglutinin-expressing DNA vaccine was administered to pigs and derived humoral and protective immunity as shown by methods including HAI titer and improved virus clearance from nasal swabbing (Eriksson et al. 1998). To overcome the slow processing of an immune response induced by DNA vaccination, DNA tattooing was suggested for short-interval DNA vaccination (Bins et al. 2005). In this study, it was shown that short-interval ID DNA tattoo immunization generated fast and stable T cell responses to human papillomavirus and complete protection from influenza virus challenge. When compared to the IM route, DNA tattoo vaccination elicited much stronger and quicker humoral and cellular immune responses. In addition, studies indicated that even IM immunization with adjuvant was inferior to DNA tattoo immunization (Pokorna et al. 2009). To determine the effect of the tattooing process on DNA vaccine stability, the DNA topology change was evaluated, including critical factors for antigen expression and immune response (Quaak et al. 2009). It was found that the DNA tattooing tool had negligible effect on DNA structure and activity. Other vaccines including an adenoviral vector vaccine against respiratory syncytial virus (Potthoff et al. 2009) and a peptide vaccine against human papillomavirus (Pokorna et al. 2009) were administrated by ID tattooing. In the case of the adenoviral vector vaccine, tattooing showed similar performance to ID injection. Tattooing of the peptide vaccine with CpG motifs adjuvant showed better response than IM vaccination with adjuvant.

DNA tattooing was evaluated in non-human primates, which have previously shown poor DNA vaccine immunization effect, but showed remarkable enhancement of immune response by this method administering an HIV vaccine (Verstrepen et al. 2008). In order to advance this technique to human clinical trials, a human ex vivo skin model was tested, which showed that DNA concentration was the most critical factor for effective DNA vaccination by tattooing (van den Berg et al. 2009). A human clinical trial for treating melanoma is planned (Quaak et al. 2008). A comprehensive review on DNA tattooing can be found in one of the accompanying papers in this special volume on ID immunization (Oosterhuis et al. 2010).

5 Permeabilizing the Skin

Most of the ID vaccination methods described so far involve minimally invasive needle-based methods or non-invasive jet-based methods that actively deposit vaccine within the skin. Another set of approaches involve mostly non-invasive methods that increase skin permeability to enable vaccine transport into the skin in a transiently permeabilized state. The key to success using these approaches is disruption of skin's outer layer, called stratum corneum. Although the stratum corneum is only 10–20 μm thick, it provides a highly effective barrier to the permeation of xenogens, including topically applied vaccine formulations (Scheuplein and Blank 1971). A number of methods to increase skin permeability have been developed, largely for drug delivery applications, many of which have been tested for vaccination (Mitragotri 2005; Prausnitz and Langer 2008).

5.1 Abrasion

A number of studies have demonstrated that the skin barrier can be broken by abrasion. A variety of abrasion methods including rough surfaces (Frerichs et al. 2008), tape-stripping (Takigawa et al. 2001; Peachman et al. 2003; Inoue and Aramaki 2007; Vandermeulen et al. 2009), and microdermabrasion devices (Gill et al. 2009) have been shown to induce adequate removal of the stratum corneum. Repeated peeling by tape (for example, Scotch® tape) effectively removes the stratum corneum. Application of tumor epitope peptides on tape-stripped mouse skin primed tumor-specific cytotoxic T cells in the lymph nodes and the spleen, protected mice against a subsequent challenge with the corresponding tumor cells, and also suppressed the growth of established tumors (Takigawa et al. 2001). Skin abrasion using a razor and a toothbrush followed by application of adenoviral vectors has yielded promising results in humans (Van Kampen et al. 2005).

Skin abrasion using an abrasive paper is perhaps the most commonly used method of disrupting the stratum corneum for immunization. For example, abrasion with emery paper, after skin hydration, has been shown to induce adequate penetration of anthrax vaccine (Matyas et al. 2004) and influenza virus vaccine (Guebre-Xabier et al. 2003), among others. This has led to the development of a Skin Prep System (SPS) to provide a controlled method of stratum corneum disruption for transcutaneous immunization currently under development by Intercell (Frerichs et al. 2008) (Fig. 4a). This technique has been shown to be effective in humans. Specifically, the skin was prepared by use of two mild strokes with the skin preparation device containing a mild abrasive affixed to a pressure-controlled device. The device was a single-use, disposable system and was discarded immediately after use. Following skin preparation, the patch containing vaccine against traveler's diarrhea (LT patch) was applied within the marked area and worn for 6 h at each vaccination, then removed and discarded by the participant. 59 LT-patch recipients were protected against moderate-to-severe diarrhea (protective efficacy of 75%) and severe diarrhea (protective efficacy of 84%). LT-patch recipients who became ill had shorter episodes of diarrhea (0.5 vs 2.1 days) with fewer loose stools than placebo (Frech et al. 2008). In another study, a similar technique was used to boost response against influenza vaccine. In this case, prior to application, the patch area was lightly abraded with ECG-grade emery paper on skin wetted with 10% glycerol/70% alcohol to disrupt the stratum corneum. In weeks following vaccination, hemagglutination inhibition (HAI) responses in LT immunostimulatory patch recipients showed improvement over those receiving vaccine alone (Frech et al. 2005).

Microdermabrasion is a common cosmetic procedure that has been adapted to remove superficial skin layers by sandblasting and thereby enable selective removal of the stratum corneum barrier. This approach has been shown to increase skin permeability and thereby enable topical application of live attenuated vaccinia virus on microdermabraded skin to generate virus-specific antibodies in the blood (Gill et al. 2009). As mentioned in Sect. 4.2.3, a microneedle-based abrasion method has also been successfully used for vaccination.

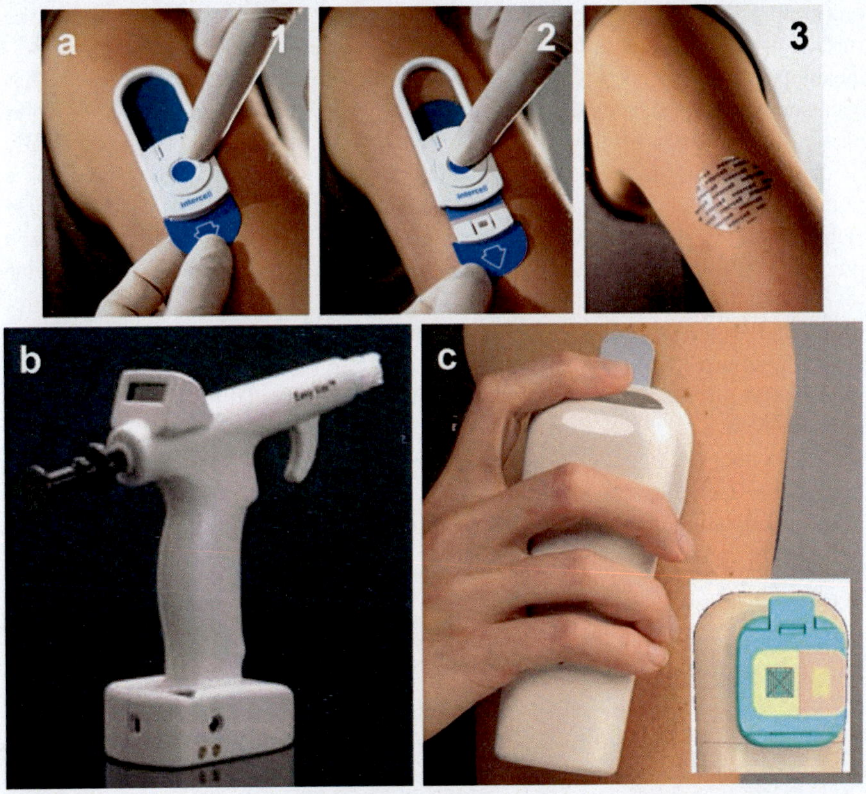

Fig. 4 Skin permeabilization methods. **a** Skin abrasion device, in which a sandpaper device is placed on the skin (1), scraped across the skin in a controlled fashion (2) and then a vaccine patch is applied to the abraded skin (3) (Courtesy of Intecell). **b** Hand-held skin electroporation device, which uses microneedles as electrodes to cause highly localized electroporation in the skin to facilitate DNA vaccine delivery into skin cells (Courtesy of Cyto Pulse Sciences). **c** Heat-based device for thermal ablation of the skin. The microheater array (*left side of inset*) is used to ablate the skin and then a vaccine patch (*right side of inset*) is applied to the ablated skin (Courtesy of Altea Therapeutics)

5.2 Ultrasound

Ultrasound, especially at low frequencies, is very effective in permeabilizing the skin (Tezel et al. 2001). It is now understood that acoustic cavitation, which is formation, pulsation, and collapse of gaseous bubbles under the oscillating pressure field of ultrasound, is the principal mediator for ultrasound-induced enhanced skin permeability. Several studies have shown that during ultrasound exposure, transient cavitation is predominantly induced in the coupling medium (the liquid present between the ultrasound transducer and the skin) and is primarily responsible for skin permeabilization (Tang et al. 2002; Tezel et al. 2002; Tezel and Mitragotri 2003). An estimated 10 bubble collapses/s/cm^2 in the form of symmetric collapses (generating shock waves) or asymmetric collapses (producing microjets) near the surface of the skin are sufficient to explain the experimentally-observed skin permeability enhancements by ultrasound-induced skin permeabilization. Ultrasound has been shown to enhance the delivery of vaccines into skin (Tezel et al. 2005). Studies performed in mice have shown that the immune response generated by ultrasonically delivered vaccine was about 10-fold greater compared with SC injection per unit dose of the vaccine that entered the skin (about 1% of the topically applied dose entered the skin) (Tezel et al. 2005). Compared to simple topical administration, ultrasound pretreatment showed increased vaccine delivery, thereby enabling sufficient vaccine to enter the skin to activate the immune response. Furthermore, application of ultrasound resulted in activation of Langerhans cells, the reasons behind which are not clear. In another study, it was shown that application of tetanus toxoid to skin pretreated with ultrasound generated anti-tetanus toxoid IgG and neutralizing antibody titers (Dahlan et al. 2009). Several parameters, including concentration of co-applied sodium dodecyl sulfate and ultrasound duty cycle, impacted the magnitude of antibody titers. The authors concluded that the main mechanism of ultrasound-assisted skin immunization involved factors in addition to enhancement of skin permeability to topically applied antigen.

5.3 *Electroporation*

Electroporation involves the application of high-voltage, short-duration electric pulses to transiently disrupt lipid barriers in the body. For vaccination, electroporation has been used to increase stratum corneum permeability and thereby enable vaccine entry into the skin. Electroporation has also been used to permeabilize cells within the skin and thereby drive, for example, DNA vaccines into epidermal and dermal cells (Fig. 4b). Electroporation has been well established as a tool for delivering molecules across the stratum corneum (Prausnitz et al. 1993) or across the cell membranes (Bilitewski et al. 2003). Many studies have focused on the use of electroporation for DNA vaccination. This is not surprising given the long history of use of electroporation for delivery of DNA into cells in vitro. However, many electroporation studies involve insertion of electrode needles into the skin. Some studies have demonstrated the use of electroporation for topical vaccine delivery (Zhao et al. 2006). In one study, electroporation has been found to stimulate the exodus of Langerhans cells from the skin, which is likely to have an adjuvant-like effect (Zhao et al. 2006). In this study, the efficacy of peptide delivery was found to be comparable to that of ID injected with Freund's complete adjuvant. Further, the peptide-specific CTL response to the vaccine delivered by electroporation was equivalent to that delivered by ID injection.

Electroporation has been shown to induce an effective immune response after delivery of DNA vaccines (Peachman et al. 2003; Foldvari et al. 2006; Medi and Singh 2008; Vandermeulen et al. 2009). For example, studies in pigs have shown the ability of electroporation to deliver HBsAg gene using a single-needle or a six-needle electrode (Babiuk et al. 2002). Studies have demonstrated that in vivo skin electroporation may be used to increase transgene expression relative to naked DNA injection (Drabick et al. 2001). Transfected cells were principally located in dermis and included adipocytes, fibroblasts, endothelial cells, and numerous mononuclear cells with dendritic processes in a porcine model. Transfected cells were also observed in lymph nodes draining electropermeabilized sites. A HBsAg-coding plasmid was used to test skin electroporation-mediated nucleic acid vaccination in a murine model. Applications for these findings include modulation of immune responses to pathogens, allergens, and tumor-associated antigens and the modification of tolerance. In another study, in vivo electroporation has shown protection against avian influenza in non-human primates (Laddy et al. 2009). A number of human clinical trials testing vaccination enhanced by electroporation are currently under way.

5.4 Chemical Enhancers

Several chemicals are known to interact with the skin and disrupt the highly ordered lipid bilayer structure in the stratum corneum. This observation led to the study of chemical agents to enhance transport across skin. More than 300 chemicals have been studied for their ability to increase skin permeability (Karande et al. 2004). Chemical permeation enhancers are relatively inexpensive and easy to formulate, they offer flexibility in their design, are simple in application and allow the freedom of self-administration to the patient. Chemical enhancers comprise a wide variety of different chemical functional groups and facilitate drug transport across the skin by a variety of complex mechanisms. They can directly exert their effect on skin structure by acting on intercellular lipids or corneocytes. Chemical enhancers can extract lipids from the skin thereby creating diffusion pathways for transdermal permeation. Alternatively, they can partition themselves into the lipid bilayers thereby disrupting the highly ordered lipid lamellae and causing their fluidization. Chemical enhancers can also significantly increase skin transport of a drug by enhancing its thermodynamic activity in the formulation (Karande et al. 2005).

Recently, chemical enhancers have been shown to possess the ability to deliver antigens and generate immune responses. This was achieved by designing formulations that possess the ability to enhance skin permeability as well as exhibit high adjuvanticity. The rational design of such multi-functional formulations from first principles requires in-depth knowledge of interactions between chemical enhancers and skin, which exist for a very limited pool of chemicals. Hence, combinatorial libraries of chemical mixtures were screened. Studies have shown that in a randomly selected population of chemical formulations, certain binary mixtures of chemicals are far more potent in permeabilizing the skin as compared to single chemicals (Karande et al. 2004). In vaccination studies, a third chemical was added with the goal of enhancing the ability to offer adjuvanticity. The lead chemical formulations were tested in mice using the model antigen ovalbumin. The formulations that exhibited high permeation and adjuvanticity potential in in vitro screening also induced high IgG titers in mice (Karande et al. 2009). In another study, penetration enhancers and immunomodulators oleic acid and retinoic acid were used to enhance transcutaneous immunization with inactivated influenza virus across tape-stripped skin (Skountzou et al. 2006). Pretreatment of mouse skin with oleic acid elicited increased levels of influenza virus-specific binding and neutralizing antibodies to levels equivalent to those induced by intranasal immunization with inactivated influenza virus. Oleic acid and retinoic acid treatments differentially affected the pattern of cytokine production upon stimulation with influenza viral antigen and provided enhanced protection.

5.5 Thermal Ablation

Thermal poration of skin has been used to deliver vaccines into skin. Microporation systems are designed to porate the skin and are being developed by a number of companies. In this method, an array of micropores is created in the skin by removal of stratum corneum by the application of focused thermal energy based on resistive heating via the contact of electrically heated small-diameter wires to the skin surface (Bramson et al. 2003) (Fig. 4c) or other methods based on radiofrequency or laser-based approaches. In this study, the microporation tip was comprised of a set of 80 μm diameter tungsten wires with control circuitry allowing for precise control of the electrical current pulses that were passed through each wire. The software user interface was designed to enable the control of various microporation parameters including micropore density, resistive element temperature, current pulse width, number of pulses, pulses pacing, and contact pressure. The temperature of the tip that was placed in contact with the skin was calibrated by an optical calibrator device. The study showed that microporation significantly increased the penetration of topically delivered vaccine. Microporation enhanced expression of luciferase upon placement of adenovirus vectors by 100–300-fold. The same procedure led to increased CTL response and increased IFN-γ secreting cells. In a related study, the same technology has been shown to deliver influenza vaccine into mouse skin. Eighty micropores were created in 1 cm^2 area and the vaccine was placed on the porated skin. This procedure generated adequate protective response in mice (Garg et al. 2007).

6 Discussion

6.1 Immunologic Advantages of Intradermal Vaccination

ID vaccination offers potential immunologic advantages to public health. The skin is known to be a site rich in antigen-presenting cells, some of which are specific to the skin, including epidermal Langerhans cells and dermal dendritic cells

(Glenn and Kenney 2006). In addition, antigen may be taken up directly by lymphatic vessels for transport to antigen-presenting cells in the lymph nodes. At a minimum, the ID route of vaccination appears to follow different pathways to immunity compared to IM or SC routes. However, there is evidence that the ID route is not only different, but is also beneficial (Glenn and Kenney 2006; Lambert and Laurent 2008; Nicolas and Guy 2008).

The possibility of dose sparing enabled by ID vaccination has been suggested by previous preclinical and clinical studies; however, the successful application of this approach has yet to be definitively confirmed for many vaccines (Glenn and Kenney 2006; Lambert and Laurent 2008; Nicolas and Guy 2008). Although the conclusions vary between different studies and different vaccines, there is an indication that dose sparing may be possible. However, it is not currently clear under what conditions the skin's unique immune environment can be harnessed for optimal effect. In addition to dose sparing, there is preclinical study evidence of other beneficial differences of ID vaccination. Studies with microneedles showed improved influenza virus clearance from the lungs and enhanced memory responses compared to IM vaccination (Kim et al. 2011). Studies with EPI showed a specific role for Langerhans cells to generate robust antibody responses (Chen et al. 2004). Studies with ultrasound-mediated vaccination suggested an adjuvant effect on the skin (Dahlan et al. 2009).

6.2 Logistical Advantages of Intradermal Vaccination

ID vaccination offers potential value to public health also in terms of possible logistical advantages. For comparison, IM and SC vaccination can only be carried out by hypodermic needle injection with few other options beside jet injection. ID vaccination opens the door to many other technologies because the skin is readily accessible at the surface of the body. As a result, ID injection may enable vaccination methods that generate no biohazardous sharp waste, can be administered by personnel with minimal training, and simplify transportation and storage logistics (Table 1).

Mantoux technique injection requires specialized training by clinical personnel. Microneedle systems and patch-based delivery (accompanied by skin permeabilization technologies) offer the promise of simplified vaccination methods that require minimal training and may permit self-vaccination by patients in certain scenarios. This not only benefits routine vaccination scenarios, but is especially important to mass vaccination campaigns associated with disease eradication programs or pandemic emergencies. In contrast, some of the novel ID delivery methods, such as projectile delivery and tattoo guns, introduce new, sophisticated devices that require additional training of clinical personnel. Assuming the injection is done properly, the Mantoux technique can administer essentially all of the vaccine into the skin. Hollow microneedles and projectile delivery can be similarly efficient. However, solid microneedles typically retain some vaccine on the device

Table 1 Capabilities of intradermal vaccination systems

ID delivery method	Ease of use[a]	Vaccine utilization[b]	Biohazardous sharp waste[c]	Technology development[d]	Vaccine reformulation[e]	Device cost[f]
Mantoux injection	++	+++	+	+++	++	+++
Single hollow microneedle	++	+++	++	++	++	++
Array of hollow microneedles	++	+++	++	++	++	++
Jet injection	+	+++	+++	+++	++	+
Powder/gene gun	+	+++	+++	++	+	+
Bifurcated needle	+++	+	+	+++	++	+++
Coated microneedles	+++	++	++	+	+	++
Dissolving microneedles	+++	++	+++	+	+	++
Pretreatment with microneedles	+++	+	++	+	+	++
Tattoo gun	+	+	+	+	++	+
Skin abrasion	+++	+	+++	++	+	+++
Ultrasound	+	+	+++	+	+	+
Electroporation	+	+	+++	+	+	+
Chemical enhancer	+++	+	+++	+	+	+++
Thermal ablation	+++	+	+++	+	+	++

[a] +++ requires little or no personnel training, ++ requires personnel training, + requires personnel training and maintenance of a dedicated device

[b] +++ almost 100% in skin, ++ >50% in skin, + <50% in skin

[c] +++ no biohazardous sharp waste, ++ microscopic biohazardous sharp waste, + macroscopic biohazardous sharp waste

[d] +++ in widespread clinical practice, ++ published vaccination data in humans, + preclinical

[e] +++ no reformulation required, ++ possible new liquid formulation required, + reformulation required to produce solid-state vaccine

[f] +++ inexpensive disposable device, ++ specialty disposable device, + reusable device. Per-injection cost of reusable devices will depend on the number of times the device can be used and the cost of any disposable components

and patch-based skin permeabilization methods are extremely inefficient, such that most vaccine typically remains on the skin surface. The efficiency of vaccine utilization will be of critical importance for new, costly vaccines, as well as in developing countries where vaccine cost can be a significant barrier to access.

Eliminating the hypodermic needle from vaccination is a major objective of public health, given that close to one million people die each year from disease transmission from contaminated needles (Miller and Pisani 1999; Kermode 2004). Microneedles are a step in the right direction, but still generate biohazardous sharp waste, with the exception of dissolving microneedles. Projectile delivery and patch-based methods eliminate needles and therefore offer an improved safety profile.

However, some ID delivery methods can cause added tissue trauma to the skin (Bremseth and Pass 2001). Most of the new methods of ID vaccination require significant technology development. While jet injection is already in widespread clinical use, many other technologies are only in the preclinical stage of development for vaccination. That being said, many of those technologies are in much later stage of development or use for non-vaccine applications, which will facilitate their adaptation to ID vaccination.

Most of the new ID vaccination technologies also require vaccine reformulation. Hollow microneedle, jet and tattoo-based methods may use standard, currently available liquid formulation, but in some cases will need to be concentrated or otherwise modified. The other methods mostly use a solid-state vaccine formulation, which offers likely advantages in terms of vaccine stability during storage, but, however, requires significant reformulation, with associated research, regulatory, and manufacturing hurdles. Finally, device cost is a significant consideration, given that a hypodermic needle and syringe are extremely inexpensive, disposable devices. Microneedle systems and some of the patch-based methods are expected to have low manufacturing cost in mass production. However, many of the other technologies require multiple device components, which may be engineered into disposable devices with added cost or reusable devices with disposable components that require an initial investment that can be amortized over many patients.

6.3 Future Outlook

ID vaccination has already made significant impact on public health as the primary means of immunization during smallpox eradication and continues to play a role in BCG and rabies vaccination in current clinical practice (Plotkin et al. 2008). However, as discussed in this article, there are many more opportunities for ID vaccination to potentially improve immunogenicity and simplify logistics of the administration of other vaccines. A number of new ID vaccination technologies have been successful in human clinical trials. ID vaccination using the BD hollow microneedle was approved in Europe in 2009 for ID administration of the Sanofi Pasteur seasonal influenza vaccine and was introduced in Australia and New Zealand during the 2010 influenza season (Holland et al. 2008; Beran et al. 2009). This microneedle device may be adapted for use to administer other vaccines as well. Jet injectors have a long history of use for vaccination and are receiving renewed attention for ID delivery of vaccines in clinical trials, especially to address developing countries' needs, through support from WHO and US Centers for Disease Control and Prevention (see Sect. 3.1.2.). Skin abrasion as a pretreatment before applying a vaccine patch is also in clinical trials for prevention of influenza and traveler's diarrhea (Frech et al. 2005; Frech et al. 2008). Projectile based delivery by EPI and PMED have been studied in a number of human clinical trials for both DNA and protein-based vaccines (Dean and Chen 2004; Jones et al. 2009), although it is unclear as to what extent this technology is under continued commercial development.

Other ID delivery devices are under advanced preclinical study. Solid coated microneedles have been the subject of numerous vaccination studies in mice and larger animals to administer influenza and other vaccines (see Sect. 5.2), and have been used in a Phase II clinical trial of a drug, parathyroid hormone (Cosman et al. 2009). Likewise, skin electroporation, in some cases in combination with microneedles, has been studied in animals for skin vaccination. As evidence for clinical feasibility, electroporation of skin for targeted delivery of chemotherapeutic agents to skin tumors is approved and used in Europe (Gehl 2008). Tattooing is of course in widespread human use, and its application to vaccination has been studied preclinically. Other methods to increase skin permeability, such as ultrasound, chemical enhancers and heat, are also in clinical use or trials for transdermal drug delivery applications (Prausnitz and Langer 2008), which compliment preclinical studies of their use for vaccination. Given the large number of technologies for ID vaccination under development, and the advanced clinical status of many of them, the future outlook for bringing ID vaccination into more widespread clinical practice appears encouraging. The optimal delivery method will depend on the specific application and other factors, such as immunologic response, logistical needs, and financial constraints.

References

Alarcon JB, Hartley AW, Harvey NG, Mikszta JA (2007) Preclinical evaluation of microneedle technology for intradermal delivery of influenza vaccines. Clin Vaccine Immunol 14:375–381

Andrianov AK, DeCollibus DP, Gillis HA, Kha HH, Marin A, Prausnitz MR, Babiuk LA, Townsend H, Mutwiri G (2009) Poly [di (carboxylatophenoxy) phosphazene] is a potent adjuvant for intradermal immunization. Proc Natl Acad Sci USA 106:18936–18941

Arnou R, Icardi G, De Decker M, Ambrozaitis A, Kazek MP, Weber F, Van Damme P (2009) Intradermal influenza vaccine for older adults: a randomized controlled multicenter phase III study. Vaccine 27:7304–7312

Ayoola EA (1984) Hepatitis B vaccine in developing countries: problems and prospects. IARC Sci Publ 63:297–305

Babiuk S, Baca-Estrada ME, Foldvari M, Storms M, Rabussay D, Widera G, Babiuk LA (2002) Electroporation improves the efficacy of DNA vaccines in large animals. Vaccine 20:3399–3408

Baxby D (2002) Smallpox vaccination techniques; from knives and forks to needles and pins. Vaccine 20:2140–2149

Belshe RB, Newman FK, Cannon J, Duane C, Treanor J, Van Hoecke C, Howe BJ, Dubin G (2004) Serum antibody responses after intradermal vaccination against influenza. New Engl J Med 351:2286–2294

Belshe RB, Newman FK, Wilkins K, Graham IL, Babusis E, Ewell M, Frey SE (2007) Comparative immunogenicity of trivalent influenza vaccine administered by intradermal or intramuscular route in healthy adults. Vaccine 25:6755–6763

Beran J, Ambrozaitis A, Laiskonis A, Mickuviene N, Bacart P, Calozet Y, Demanet E, Heijmans S, Van Belle P, Weber F, Salamand C (2009) Intradermal influenza vaccination of healthy adults using a new microinjection system: a 3-year randomised controlled safety and immunogenicity trial. BMC Med 7:13

Bernard KW, Roberts MA, Sumner J, Winkler WG, Mallonee J, Baer GM, Chaney R (1982) Human diploid cell rabies vaccine. Effectiveness of immunization with small intradermal or subcutaneous doses. JAMA 247:1138–1142

Bernard KW, Mallonee J, Wright JC, Reid FL, Makintubee S, Parker RA, Dwyer DM, Winkler WG (1987) Preexposure immunization with intradermal human diploid cell rabies vaccine. Risks and benefits of primary and booster vaccination. JAMA 257:1059–1063

Bilitewski U, Genrich M, Kadow S, Mersal G (2003) Biochemical analysis with microfluidic systems. Anal Bioanal Chem 377:556–569

Bins AD, Jorritsma A, Wolkers MC, Hung CF, Wu TC, Schumacher TNM, Haanen JBAG (2005) A rapid and potent DNA vaccination strategy defined by in vivo monitoring of antigen expression. Nat Med 11:899–904

Bramson J, Dayball K, Evelegh C, Wan YH, Page D, Smith A (2003) Enabling topical immunization via microporation: a novel method for pain-free and needle-free delivery of adenovirus-based vaccines. Gene Ther 10:251–260

Bremseth DL, Pass F (2001) Delivery of insulin by jet injection: recent observations. Diabetes Technol Ther 3:225–232

Brindle RJ, Morris CA, Berger R, Kurtz JB (1994) Inadequate response to intradermal hepatitis A vaccine. Vaccine 12:483–484

Burland WL (1969) Measles vaccination by the intradermal route. Postgrad Med J 45:323–326

Carlsson U, Brudin L, Eliasson I, Hansson BG (1996) Hepatitis A vaccination by intracutaneous low dose administration: a less expensive alternative. Scand J Infect Dis 28:435–438

Chen W, Gluud C (2005) Vaccines for preventing hepatitis B in health-care workers. Cochrane Database Syst Rev, Issue 4. Art. No.: CD000100. doi:10.1002/14651858.CD000100.pub3

Chen D, Zuleger C, Chu Q, Maa YF, Osorio J, Payne LG (2002) Epidermal powder immunization with a recombinant HIV gp120 targets Langerhans cells and induces enhanced immune responses. AIDS Res Hum Retroviruses 18:715–722

Chen D, Burger M, Chu Q, Endres R, Zuleger C, Dean H, Payne LG (2004) Epidermal powder immunization: cellular and molecular mechanisms for enhancing vaccine immunogenicity. Virus Res 103:147–153

Chen XF, Prow TW, Crichton ML, Jenkins DWK, Roberts MS, Frazer IH, Fernando GJP, Kendall MAF (2009) Dry-coated microprojection array patches for targeted delivery of immunotherapeutics to the skin. J Control Release 139:212–220

Coberly JS, Townsend T, Repke J, Fields H, Margolis H, Halsey NA (1994) Suboptimal response following intradermal hepatitis B vaccine in infants. Vaccine 12:984–987

Cosman F, Lane NE, Bolognese MA, Zanchetta JR, Garcia-Hernandez PA, Sees K, Matriano JA, Gaumer K, Daddona PE (2009) Effect of transdermal teriparatide administration on bone mineral density in postmenopausal women. J Clin Endocrinol Metab 95:151–158

Dahlan A, Alpar HO, Stickings P, Sesardic D, Murdan S (2009) Transcutaneous immunisation assisted by low-frequency ultrasound. Int J Pharm 368:123–128

Darmanger AM, Nekzad SM, Kuis M, Tendam HG (1977) BCG vaccination by bifurcated needle in a pilot vaccination program. Bull WHO 55:49–61

Davis SP, Martanto W, Allen MG, Prausnitz MR (2005) Hollow metal microneedles for insulin delivery to diabetic rats. IEEE Trans Biomed Eng 52:909–915

de Moraes JC, Leon ME, Souza VA, Pannuti C, Travisanello C, Halsey NA, de Quadros CA (1994) Intradermal administration of measles vaccines. Bull Pan Am Health Organ 28:250–255

Dean HJ, Chen D (2004) Epidermal powder immunization against influenza. Vaccine 23:681–686

Dean CH, Alarcon JB, Waterston AM, Draper K, Early R, Guirakhoo F, Monath TP, Mikszta JA (2005) Cutaneous delivery of a live, attenuated chimeric flavivirus vaccine against Japanese encephalitis (ChimeriVax)-JE) in non-human primates. Hum Vaccine 1:106–111

Dimache G, Stoean C, Durbaca S, Croitoru M, Ionescu M, Nedelcu IN, Corbu I (1990) Study of specific immune response to unadsorbed concentrated tetanus vaccine administered by intradermal route to non-immunized persons in the last ten years. Arch Roum Pathol Exp Microbiol 49:51–62

Ding Z, Van Riet E, Romeijn S, Kersten GFA, Jiskoot W, Bouwstra JA (2009a) Immune modulation by adjuvants combined with diphtheria toxoid administered topically in BALB/c mice after microneedle array pretreatment. Pharm Res 26:1635–1643

Ding Z, Verbaan FJ, Bivas-Benita M, Bungener L, Huckriede A, van den Berg DJ, Kersten G, Bouwstra JA (2009b) Microneedle arrays for the transcutaneous immunization of diphtheria and influenza in BALB/c mice. J Control Release 136:71–78

Donnelly RF, Singh TRR, Tunney MM, Morrow DIJ, McCarron PA, O'Mahony C, Woolfson AD (2009) Microneedle arrays allow lower microbial penetration than hypodermic needles in vitro. Pharm Res 26:2513–2522

Drabick JJ, Glasspool-Malone J, King A, Malone RW (2001) Cutaneous transfection and immune responses to intradermal nucleic acid vaccination are significantly enhanced by in vivo electropermeabilization. Mol Ther 3:249–255

Drape RJ, Macklin MD, Barr LJ, Jones S, Haynes JR, Dean HJ (2006) Epidermal DNA vaccine for influenza is immunogenic in humans. Vaccine 24:4475–4481

Epstein JE, Gorak EJ, Charoenvit Y, Wang R, Freydberg N, Osinowo O, Richie TL, Stoltz EL, Trespalacios F, Nerges J, Ng J, Fallarme-Majam V, Abot E, Goh L, Parker S, Kumar S, Hedstrom RC, Norman J, Stout R, Hoffman SL (2002) Safety, tolerability, and lack of antibody responses after administration of a PfCSP DNA malaria vaccine via needle or needle-free jet injection, and comparison of intramuscular and combination intramuscular/intradermal routes. Hum Gene Ther 13:1551–1560

Eriksson E, Yao F, Svensjo T, Winkler T, Slama J, Macklin MD, Andree C, McGregor M, Hinshaw V, Swain WF (1998) In vivo gene transfer to skin and wound by microseeding. J Surg Res 78:85–91

Etchart N, Hennino A, Friede M, Dahel K, Dupouy M, Goujon-Henry C, Nicolas JF, Kaiserlian D (2007) Safety and efficacy of transcutaneous vaccination using a patch with the live-attenuated measles vaccine in humans. Vaccine 25:6891–6899

Fernando GJP, Chen XF, Prow TW, Crichton ML, Fairmaid EJ, Roberts MS, Frazer IH, Brown LE, Kendall MAF (2010) Potent immunity to low doses of influenza vaccine by probabilistic guided micro-targeted skin delivery in a mouse model. PLoS One 5:e10266

Fishbein DB, Pacer RE, Holmes DF, Ley AB, Yager P, Tong TC (1987) Rabies preexposure prophylaxis with human diploid cell rabies vaccine: a dose-response study. J Infect Dis 156:50–55

Flynn PM, Shenep JL, Mao L, Crawford R, Williams BF, Williams BG (1994) Influence of needle gauge in Mantoux skin testing. Chest 106:1463–1465

Foldvari M, Babiuk S, Badea I (2006) DNA delivery for vaccination and therapeutics through the skin. Curr Drug Deliv 3:17–28

Frech SA, Kenney RT, Spyr CA, Lazar H, Viret JF, Herzog C, Gluck R, Glenn GM (2005) Improved immune responses to influenza vaccination in the elderly using an immunostimulant patch. Vaccine 23:946–950

Frech SA, Dupont HL, Bourgeois AL, McKenzie R, Belkind-Gerson J, Figueroa JF, Okhuysen PC, Guerrero NH, Martinez-Sandoval FG, Melendez-Romero JH, Jiang ZD, Asturias EJ, Halpern J, Torres OR, Hoffman AS, Villar CP, Kassem RN, Flyer DC, Andersen BH, Kazempour K, Breisch SA, Glenn GM (2008) Use of a patch containing heat-labile toxin from *Escherichia coli* against travellers' diarrhoea: a phase II, randomised, double-blind, placebo-controlled field trial. Lancet 371:2019–2025

Frerichs DM, Ellingsworth LR, Frech SA, Flyer DC, Villar CP, Yu J, Glenn GM (2008) Controlled, single-step, stratum corneum disruption as a pretreatment for immunization via a patch. Vaccine 26:2782–2787

Frey SE, Couch RB, Tacket CO, Treanor JJ, Wolff M, Newman FK, Atmar RL, Edelman R, Nolan CM, Belshe RB (2002) Clinical responses to undiluted and diluted smallpox vaccine. New Engl J Med 346:1265–1274

Gardeniers HJGE, Luttge R, Berenschot EJW, de Boer MJ, Yeshurun SY, Hefetz M, van't Oever R, van den Berg A (2003) Silicon micromachined hollow microneedles for transdermal liquid transport. J MEMS 12:855–862

Garg S, Hoelscher M, Belser JA, Wang C, Jayashankar L, Guo Z, Durland RH, Katz JM, Sambhara S (2007) Needle-free skin patch delivery of a vaccine for a potentially pandemic influenza virus provides protection against lethal challenge in mice. Clin Vaccine Immunol 14:926–928

Gehl J (2008) Electroporation for drug and gene delivery in the clinic: doctors go electric. Methods Mol Biol 423:351–359

Gill HS, Prausnitz MR (2007a) Coated microneedles for transdermal delivery. J Control Release 117:227–237

Gill HS, Prausnitz MR (2007b) Coating formulations for microneedles. Pharm Res 24:1369–1380

Gill HS, Prausnitz MR (2008) Pocketed microneedles for drug delivery to the skin. J Phys Chem Solids 69:1537–1541

Gill HS, Andrews SN, Sakthivel SK, Fedanov A, Williams IR, Garber DA, Priddy FH, Yellin S, Feinberg MB, Staprans SI, Prausnitz MR (2009) Selective removal of stratum corneum by microdermabrasion to increase skin permeability. Eur J Pharm Sci 38:95–103

Gill HS, Sõderholm J, Prausnitz MR, Sällberg M (2010) Cutaneous vaccination using microneedles coated with hepatitis C DNA vaccine. Gene Ther 17:811–814

Glenn GM, Kenney RT (2006) Mass vaccination: solutions in the skin. Curr Top Microbiol Immunol 304:247–268

Gomez V, Palomeque FS, Feris J et al. (2010) Still-blinded safety and immunogenicity data from a trial of reduced-dose, intradermal, influenza vaccination by needle-free jet injection. 13th Annual Conference on Vaccine Research, Bethesda, MD

Goodwin K, Viboud C, Simonsen L (2006) Antibody response to influenza vaccination in the elderly: a quantitative review. Vaccine 24:1159–1169

Guebre-Xabier M, Hammond SA, Epperson DE, Yu J, Ellingsworth L, Glenn GM (2003) Immunostimulant patch containing heat-labile enterotoxin from *Escherichia coli* enhances immune responses to injected influenza virus vaccine through activation of skin dendritic cells. J Virol 77:5218–5225

Han M, Kim DK, Kang SH, Yoon HR, Kim BY, Lee SS, Kim KD, Lee HG (2009) Improvement in antigen-delivery using fabrication of a grooves-embedded microneedle array. Sens Act B 137:274–280

Heijtink RA, Knol RM, Schalm SW (1989) Low-dose (2 micrograms) hepatitis B vaccination in medical students: comparable immunogenicity for intramuscular and intradermal routes. J Med Virol 27:151–154

Henderson DA, Borio BL, Grabenstein JD (2008) Smallpox and vaccinia. In: Plotkin S, Orenstein WA, Offit PA (eds) Vaccines, vol 5. Elsevier, Amsterdam, pp 773–803

Hoft DF, Blazevic A, Abate G, Hanekom WA, Kaplan G, Soler JH, Weichold F, Geiter L, Sadoff JC, Horwitz MA (2008) A new recombinant bacille Calmette-Guerin vaccine safely induces significantly enhanced tuberculosis-specific immunity in human volunteers. J Infect Dis 198:1491–1501

Holland D, Booy R, De Looze F, Eizenberg P, McDonald J, Karrasch J, McKeirnan M, Salem H, Mills G, Reid J, Weber F, Saville M (2008) Intradermal influenza vaccine administered using a new microinjection system produces superior immunogenicity in elderly adults: a randomized controlled trial. J Infect Dis 198:650–658

Howard A, Mercer P, Nataraj HC, Kang BC (1997) Bevel-down superior to bevel-up in intradermal skin testing. Ann Allergy Asthma Immunol 78:594–596

Inoue J, Aramaki Y (2007) Toll-like receptor-9 expression induced by tape-stripping triggers on effective immune response with CpG-oligodeoxynucleotides. Vaccine 25:1007–1013

Ito Y, Hagiwara E, Saeki A, Sugioka N, Takada K (2006) Feasibility of microneedles for percutaneous absorption of insulin. Eur J Pharm Sci 29:82–88

Jones S, Evans K, McElwaine-Johnn H, Sharpe M, Oxford J, Lambkin-Williams R, Mant T, Nolan A, Zambon M, Ellis J, Beadle J, Loudon PT (2009) DNA vaccination protects against an influenza challenge in a double-blind randomised placebo-controlled phase 1b clinical trial. Vaccine 27:2506–2512

Kalluri H, Banga AK (2011) Formation and closure of microchannels in skin following microporation. Pharm Res 28:82–94

Karande P, Jain A, Mitragotri S (2004) Discovery of transdermal penetration enhancers by high-throughput screening. Nat Biotechnol 22:192–197

Karande P, Jain A, Ergun K, Kispersky V, Mitragotri S (2005) Design principles of chemical penetration enhancers for transdermal drug delivery. Proc Natl Acad Sci USA 102:4688–4693

Karande P, Arora A, Pham TK, Stevens D, Wojicki A, Mitragotri S (2009) Transcutaneous immunization using common chemicals. J Control Release 138:134–140

Kermode M (2004) Unsafe injections in low-income country health settings: need for injection safety promotion to prevent the spread of blood-borne viruses. Health Promot Int 19:95–103

Kim YC, Quan FS, Yoo DG, Compans RW, Kang SM, Prausnitz MR (2009) Improved influenza vaccination in the skin using vaccine coated-microneedles. Vaccine 27:6932–6938

Kim YC, Quan FS, Compans RW, Kang SM, Prausnitz MR (2010a) Fomulation of microneedles coated with influenza virus-like particle vaccine. AAPS PharmSciTech 11:1193–1201

Kim YC, Quan FS, Yoo DG, Compans RW, Kang SM, Prausnitz MR (2010b) Enhanced memory responses to seasonal H1N1 influenza vaccination of the skin with the use of vaccine-coated microneedles. J Infect Dis 201:190–198

Kim YC, Quan FS, Compans RW, Kang SM, Prausnitz MR (2010c) Formulation and coating of microneedles with inactivated influenza virus to improve vaccine stability and immunogenicity. J Control Release 142:187–195

Kim YC, Quan FS, Compans RW, Kang SM, Prausnitz MR (2011) Stability kinetics of influenza vaccine coated onto microneedles during drying and storage. Pharm Res 28:135–144

Kok PW, Kenya PR, Ensering H (1983) Measles immunization with further attenuated heat-stable measles vaccine using five different methods of administration. Trans Roy Soc Trop Med Hyg 77:171–176

Kolli CS, Banga AK (2008) Characterization of solid maltose microneedles and their use for transdermal delivery. Pharm Res 25:104–113

Koutsonanos DG, Martin MdP, Zarnitsyn VG, Sullivan SP, Compans RW, Prausnitz MR, Skountzou I (2009) Transdermal influenza immunization with vaccine-coated microneedle arrays. PLoS One 4:e4773

Laddy DJ, Yan J, Khan AS, Andersen H, Cohn A, Greenhouse J, Lewis M, Manischewitz J, King LR, Golding H, Draghia-Akli R, Weiner DB (2009) Electroporation of synthetic DNA antigens offers protection in nonhuman primates challenged with highly pathogenic avian influenza virus. J Virol 83:4624–4630

Lambert PH, Laurent PE (2008) Intradermal vaccine delivery: will new delivery systems transform vaccine administration? Vaccine 26:3197–3208

Laurent PE, Bonnet S, Alchas P, Regolini P, Mikszta JA, Pettis R, Harvey NG (2007) Evaluation of the clinical performance of a new intradermal vaccine administration technique and associated delivery system. Vaccine 25:8833–8842

Lee JW, Park JH, Prausnitz MR (2008) Dissolving microneedles for transdermal drug delivery. Biomaterials 29:2113–2124

Lee K, Lee HC, Lee DS, Jung H (2010) Drawing lithography: three-dimensional fabrication of an ultrahigh-aspect-ratio microneedle. Adv Mat 22:483–486

Leroux-Roels I, Vets E, Freese R, Seiberling M, Weber F, Salamand C, Leroux-Roels G (2008) Seasonal influenza vaccine delivered by intradermal microinjection: a randomised controlled safety and immunogenicity trial in adults. Vaccine 26:6614–6619

Luttge R, Berenschot EJW, de Boer MJ, Altpeter DM, Vrouwe EX, van den Berg A, Elwenspoek M (2007) Integrated lithographic molding for microneedle-based devices. J MEMS 16:872–884

Mantoux C (1909) Tuberculin intradermo reactions in the treatment of tuberculosis: intradermi-tuberculisation. C R Hebd Seances Acad Sci 148:996–998

Matriano JA, Cormier M, Johnson J, Young WA, Buttery M, Nyam K, Daddona PE (2002) Macroflux® microprojection array patch technology: a new and efficient approach for intracutaneous immunization. Pharm Res 19:63–70

Matyas GR, Friedlander AM, Glenn GM, Little S, Yu J, Alving CR (2004) Needle-free skin patch vaccination method for anthrax. Infect Immun 72:1181–1183

Medi BM, Singh J (2008) Delivery of DNA into skin via electroporation. Methods Mol Biol 423:225–232

Mikszta JA, Alarcon JB, Brittingham JM, Sutter DE, Pettis RJ, Harvey NG (2002) Improved genetic immunization via micromechanical disruption of skin-barrier function and targeted epidermal delivery. Nat Med 8:415–419

Mikszta JA, Sullivan VJ, Dean C, Waterston AM, Alarcon JB, Dekker JP, Brittingham JM, Huang J, Hwang CR, Ferriter M, Jiang G, Mar K, Saikh KU, Stiles BG, Roy CJ, Ulrich RG, Harvey NG (2005) Protective immunization against inhalational anthrax: a comparison of minimally invasive delivery platforms. J Infect Dis 191:278–288

Mikszta JA, Dekker JP, Harvey NG, Dean CH, Brittingham JM, Huang J, Sullivan VJ, Dyas B, Roy CJ, Ulrich RG (2006) Microneedle-based intradermal delivery of the anthrax recombinant protective antigen vaccine. Infect Immun 74:6806–6810

Millar JD, Foege WH (1969) Status of eradication of smallpox (and control of measles) in West and Central Africa. J Infect Dis 120:725–732

Miller MA, Pisani E (1999) The cost of unsafe injections. Bull WHO 77:808–811

Milne A, Allwood GK, Pearce NE, Lucas CR, Krugman S (1986) Low dose hepatitis B vaccination in children. New Zeal Med J 99:47–49

Mitragotri S (2005) Immunization without needles. Nat Rev Immun 5:905–916

Mohammed AJ, AlAwaidy S, Bawikar S, Kurup PJ, Elamir E, Shaban MMA, Sharif SM, van der Avoort HGAM, Pallansch MA, Malankar P, Burton A, Sreevatsava M, Sutter RW (2010) Fractional doses of inactivated poliovirus vaccine in Oman. New Engl J Med 362:2351–2359

Ng KW, Pearton M, Coulman S, Anstey A, Gateley C, Morrissey A, Allender C, Birchall J (2009) Development of an ex vivo human skin model for intradermal vaccination: tissue viability and Langerhans cell behaviour. Vaccine 27:5948–5955

Nicolas JF, Guy B (2008) Intradermal, epidermal and transcutaneous vaccination: from immunology to clinical practice. Expert Rev Vaccines 7:1201–1214

Nirmal S, Cherian T, Samuel BU, Rajasingh J, Raghupathy P, John TJ (1998) Immune response of infants to fractional doses of intradermally administered inactivated poliovirus vaccine. Vaccine 16:928–931

Oh SJ, Harrison T, D'Andrea A, Kwon SY, Burkoth TL, Burke R (2006) Intradermal influenza vaccine delivery using skin-penetrating dissolvable vaccine microneedles. AAPS Annual Meeting. San Antonio, TX

Oosterhuis K, van den Berg JH, Schumacher TN, Haanen JBAG (2010) DNA vaccines and intradermal vaccination by DNA tattooing. Curr Top Microbiol Immunol 351:221–250

Osorio JE, Zuleger CL, Burger M, Chu Q, Payne LG, Chen D (2003) Immune responses to hepatitis B surface antigen following epidermal powder immunization. Immunol Cell Biol 81:52–58

Pancharoen C, Mekmullica J, Thisyakorn U, Kasempimolporn S, Wilde H, Herzog C (2005) Reduced-dose intradermal vaccination against hepatitis A with an aluminum-free vaccine is immunogenic and can lower costs. Clin Infect Dis 41:1537–1540

Park JH, Allen MG, Prausnitz MR (2005) Biodegradable polymer microneedles: fabrication, mechanics and transdermal drug delivery. J Control Release 104:51–66

Park JH, Allen MG, Prausnitz MR (2006) Polymer microneedles for controlled-release drug delivery. Pharm Res 23:1008–1019

Parker V (1984) Jet gun or syringe? A trial of alternative methods of BCG vaccination. Public Health 98:315–320

PATH (2009) Intradermal delivery of vaccines: a review of the literature and the potential for development for use in low- and middle-income countries. PATH/WHO, Ferney Voltaire, France. http://www.path.org/publications/detail.php?i=1746 14 Sept 2010.

Paul SS, Raveendra NK, Chhabra AK, Verma M (1978) Comparison of BCG inoculation by conventional intradermal and jet methods. Indian Pediatr 15:341–347

Peachman KK, Rao M, Alving CR (2003) Immunization with DNA through the skin. Methods 31:232–242

Perennes F, Marmiroli B, Matteucci M, Tormen M, Vaccari L, Di Fabrizio E (2006) Sharp beveled tip hollow microneedle arrays fabricated by LIGA and 3D soft lithography with polyvinyl alcohol. J Micromech Microeng 16:473–479

Phanuphak P, Khaoplod P, Benjavongkulchai M, Chutivongse S, Wilde H (1990) What happens if intradermal injections of rabies vaccine are partially or entirely injected subcutaneously? Bull WHO 68:83–85

Plotkin S, Orenstein W, Offit P (eds) (2008) Vaccines. Saunders, Philadelphia

Pokorna D, Polakova I, Kindlova M, Duskova M, Ludvikova V, Gabriel P, Kutinova L, Muller M, Smahel M (2009) Vaccination with human papillomavirus type 16-derived peptides using a tattoo device. Vaccine 27:3519–3529

Potthoff A, Schwannecke S, Nabi G, Hoffmann D, Grunwald T, Wildner O, Brockmeyer NH, Uberla K, Tenbusch M (2009) Immunogenicity and efficacy of intradermal tattoo immunization with adenoviral vector vaccines. Vaccine 27:2768–2774

Prausnitz MR (2004) Microneedles for transdermal drug delivery. Adv Drug Deliv Rev 56:581–587

Prausnitz MR, Langer R (2008) Transdermal drug delivery. Nat Biotechnol 26:1261–1268

Prausnitz MR, Bose VG, Langer R, Weaver JC (1993) Electroporation of mammalian skin: a mechanism to enhance transdermal drug delivery. Proc Natl Acad Sci USA 90:10504–10508

Prausnitz MR, Mikszta JA, Cormier M, Andrianov AK (2009) Microneedle-based vaccines. Curr Top Microbiol Immunol 333:369–393

Quaak SGL, van den Berg JH, Toebes M, Schumacher TNM, Haanen J, Beijnen JH, Nuijen B (2008) GMP production of pDERMATT for vaccination against melanoma in a phase I clinical trial. Eur J Pharm Biopharm 70:429–438

Quaak SGL, den Berg JHv, Oosterhuis K, Beijnen JH, Haanen JBAG, Nuijen B (2009) DNA tattoo vaccination: effect on plasmid purity and transfection efficiency of different topoisoforms. J Control Release 139:153–159

Quan FS, Kim YC, Yoo DG, Compans RW, Prausnitz MR, Kang SM (2009) Stabilization of influenza vaccine enhances protection by microneedle delivery in the mouse skin. PLoS One 4:e7152

Quan FS, Kim YC, Vunnava A, Yoo DG, Song JM, Prausnitz MR, Compans RW, Kang SM (2010) Intradermal vaccination with influenza VLPs using microneedles induces superior protection to intramuscular immunization. J Virol 84:7760–7769

Rahman F, Dahmen A, Herzog-Hauff S, Bocher WO, Galle PR, Lohr HF (2000) Cellular and humoral immune responses induced by intradermal or intramuscular vaccination with the major hepatitis B surface antigen. Hepatology 31:521–527

Resik S, Tejeda A, Lago PM, Diaz M, Carmenates A, Sarmiento L, Alemani N, Galindo B, Burton A, Friede M, Landaverde M, Sutter RW (2010) Randomized controlled clinical trial of fractional doses of inactivated poliovirus vaccine administered intradermally by needle-free device in Cuba. J Infect Dis 201:1344–1352

Roberts LK, Barr LJ, Fuller DH, McMahon CW, Leese PT, Jones S (2005) Clinical safety and efficacy of a powdered hepatitis B nucleic acid vaccine delivered to the epidermis by a commercial prototype device. Vaccine 23:4867–4878

Roukens AH, Vossen AC, Bredenbeek PJ, van Dissel JT, Visser LG (2008) Intradermally administered yellow fever vaccine at reduced dose induces a protective immune response: a randomized controlled non-inferiority trial. PLoS One 3:e1993

Roukens AHE, Gelinck LBS, Visser LG (2011) Intradermal vaccination to protect against yellow fever and influenza. Curr Top Microbiol Immunol 351:159–179

Roxhed N, Gasser TC, Griss P, Holzapfel GA, Stemme G (2007) Penetration-enhanced ultrasharp microneedles and prediction on skin interaction for efficient transdermal drug delivery. J MEMS 16:1429–1440

Roy MJ, Wu MS, Barr LJ, Fuller JT, Tussey LG, Speller S, Culp J, Burkholder JK, Swain WF, Dixon RM, Widera G, Vessey R, King A, Ogg G, Gallimore A, Haynes JR, Heydenburg Fuller D (2000) Induction of antigen-specific CD8 + T cells, T helper cells, and protective levels of antibody in humans by particle-mediated administration of a hepatitis B virus DNA vaccine. Vaccine 19:764–778

Samuel BU, Cherian T, Sridharan G, Mukundan P, John TJ (1991) Immune response to intradermally injected inactivated poliovirus vaccine. Lancet 338:343–344

Samuel BU, Cherian T, Rajasingh J, Raghupathy P, John TJ (1992) Immune response of infants to inactivated poliovirus vaccine injected intradermally. Vaccine 10:135

Sangare L, Manhart L, Zehrung D, Wang CC (2009) Intradermal hepatitis B vaccination: a systematic review and meta-analysis. Vaccine 27:1777–1786

Scheuplein RJ, Blank IH (1971) Permeability of the skin. Physiol Rev 51:702–747

Schramm-Baxter J, Mitragotri S (2004) Needle-free jet injections: dependence of jet penetration and dispersion in the skin on jet power. J Control Release 97:527–535

Skountzou I, Quan FS, Jacob J, Compans RW, Kang SM (2006) Transcutaneous immunization with inactivated influenza virus induces protective immune responses. Vaccine 24:6110–6119

Stanfield JP, Bracken PM, Waddell KM, Gall D (1972) Diphtheria–tetanus–pertussis immunization by intradermal jet injection. Brit Med J 2:197–199

Sullivan SP, Murthy N, Prausnitz MR (2008) Minimally invasive protein delivery with rapidly dissolving polymer microneedles. Adv Mat 20:933–938

Sullivan SP, Koutsonanos DG, Del Pilar Martin M, Lee JW, Zarnitsyn V, Choi SO, Murthy N, Compans RW, Skountzou I, Prausnitz MR (2010) Dissolving polymer microneedle patches for influenza vaccination. Nat Med 16:915–920

Sutter R (2009) Status of GPEI research and product development. Manufacturer's Meeting, Geneva 30 Oct 2009.

Takigawa M, Tokura Y, Hashizume H, Yagi H, Seo N (2001) Percutaneous peptide immunization via corneum barrier-disrupted murine skin for experimental tumor immunoprophylaxis. Ann N Y Acad Sci 941:139–146

Tang H, Wang CC, Blankschtein D, Langer R (2002) An investigation of the role of cavitation in low-frequency ultrasound-mediated transdermal drug transport. Pharm Res 19:1160–1169

Tezel A, Mitragotri S (2003) Interactions of inertial cavitation bubbles with stratum corneum lipid bilayers during low-frequency sonophoresis. Biophys J 85:3502–3512

Tezel A, Sens A, Tuchscherer J, Mitragotri S (2001) Frequency dependence of sonophoresis. Pharm Res 18:1694–1700

Tezel A, Sens A, Mitragotri S (2002) Investigations of the role of cavitation in low-frequency sonophoresis using acoustic spectroscopy. J Pharm Sci 91:444–453

Tezel A, Paliwal S, Shen Z, Mitragotri S (2005) Low-frequency ultrasound as a transcutaneous immunization adjuvant. Vaccine 23:3800–3807

Van Damme P, Oosterhuis-Kafeja F, Van der Wielen M, Almagor Y, Sharon O, Levin Y (2009) Safety and efficacy of a novel microneedle device for dose sparing intradermal influenza vaccination in healthy adults. Vaccine 27:454–459

Van den Berg JH, Nuijen B, Beijnen JH, Vincent A, Van Tinteren H, Kluge J, Woerdeman LAE, Hennink WE, Storm G, Schumacher TN, Haanen J (2009) Optimization of intradermal vaccination by DNA tattooing in human skin. Human Gene Ther 20:181–189

Van Kampen KR, Shi Z, Gao P, Zhang J, Foster KW, Chen DT, Marks D, Elmets CA, Tang DC (2005) Safety and immunogenicity of adenovirus-vectored nasal and epicutaneous influenza vaccines in humans. Vaccine 23:1029–1036

Vandermeulen G, Daugimont L, Richiardi H, Vanderhaeghen ML, Lecouturier N, Ucakar B, Preat V (2009) Effect of tape stripping and adjuvants on immune response after intradermal DNA electroporation. Pharm Res 26:1745–1751

Verstrepen BE, Bins AD, Rollier CS, Mooij P, Koopman G, Sheppard NC, Sattentau Q, Wagner R, Wolf H, Schumacher TNM, Heeney JL, Haanen JBAG (2008) Improved HIV-1 specific T-cell responses by short-interval DNA tattooing as compared to intramuscular immunization in non-human primates. Vaccine 26:3346–3351

Wang PM, Cornwell M, Hill J, Prausnitz MR (2006) Precise microinjection into skin using hollow microneedles. J Invest Dermatol 126:1080–1087

Wang PC, Wester BA, Rajaraman S, Paik SJ, Kim SH, Allen MG (2009) Hollow polymer microneedle array fabricated by photolithography process combined with micromolding technique. Annual International Conference of the IEEE Engineering in Medicine and Biology Society, Minneapolis, pp 7026–7029

Warrell MJ (2011) Intradermal rabies vaccination: the evolution and future of pre-and post-exposure prophylaxis. Curr Top Microbiol Immunol 351:139–157

Weniger BG, Papania MJ (2008) Alternative vaccine delivery methods. In: Plotkin SA, Orenstein WA, Offit P (eds) Vaccines. Saunders Elsevier, Philadelphia, pp 1357–1392

Whittle HC, Rowland MG, Mann GF, Lamb WH, Lewis RA (1984) Immunisation of 4–6 month old Gambian infants with Edmonston–Zagreb measles vaccine. Lancet 2:834–837

WHO (2005) WHO expert consultation on rabies. WHO Tech Rep Ser 931:1–88

WHO (2007) Rabies vaccines. WHO position paper. Wkly Epidemiol Rec 82:425–435

WHO (2010) WHO fact sheet: smallpox. WHO, Geneva. http://www.who.int/mediacentre/factsheets/smallpox/en/ 14 Sept 2010

Widera G, Johnson J, Kim L, Libiran L, Nyam K, Daddona PE, Cormier M (2006) Effect of delivery parameters on immunization to ovalbumin following intracutaneous administration by a coated microneedle array patch system. Vaccine 24:1653–1664

Williams J, Fox-Leyva L, Christensen C, Fisher D, Schlicting E, Snowball M, Negus S, Mayers J, Koller R, Stout R (2000) Hepatitis A vaccine administration: comparison between jet-injector and needle injection. Vaccine 18:1939–1943

Zhao YL, Murthy SN, Manjili MH, Guan LJ, Sen A, Hui SW (2006) Induction of cytotoxic T-lymphocytes by electroporation-enhanced needle-free skin immunization. Vaccine 24:1282–1290

Zhu QY, Zarnitsyn VG, Ye L, Wen ZY, Gao YL, Pan L, Skountzou I, Gill HS, Prausnitz MR, Yang CL, Compans RW (2009) Immunization by vaccine-coated microneedle arrays protects against lethal influenza virus challenge. Proc Natl Acad Sci USA 106:7968–7973

Zoulek G, Roggendorf M, Deinhardt F (1984) Immune response to single dose, multisite, intradermal and to intramuscular administration of vaccine against tick-borne encephalitis virus. Lancet 2:584

Zoulek G, Roggendorf M, Deinhardt F, Kunz C (1986) Different immune responses after intradermal and intramuscular administration of vaccine against tick-borne encephalitis virus. J Med Virol 19:55–61

Targeting Skin Dendritic Cells to Improve Intradermal Vaccination

N. Romani, V. Flacher, C. H. Tripp, F. Sparber, S. Ebner and P. Stoitzner

Abstract Vaccinations in medicine are typically administered into the muscle beneath the skin or into the subcutaneous fat. As a consequence, the vaccine is immunologically processed by antigen-presenting cells of the skin or the muscle. Recent evidence suggests that the clinically seldom used intradermal route is effective and possibly even superior to the conventional subcutaneous or intramuscular route. Several types of professional antigen-presenting cells inhabit the healthy skin. Epidermal Langerhans cells (CD207/langerin$^+$), dermal langerin^{neg}, and dermal langerin$^+$ dendritic cells (DC) have been described, the latter subset so far only in mouse skin. In human skin langerin^{neg} dermal DC can be further classified based on their reciprocal expression of CD1a and CD14. The relative contributions of these subsets to the generation of immunity or tolerance are still unclear. Yet, specializations of these different populations have become apparent. Langerhans cells in human skin appear to be specialized for induction of cytotoxic T lymphocytes; human CD14$^+$ dermal DC can promote antibody production by B cells. It is currently attempted to rationally devise and improve vaccines by harnessing such specific properties of skin DC. This could be achieved by specifically targeting functionally diverse skin DC subsets. We discuss here advances in our knowledge on the immunological properties of skin DC and strategies to significantly improve the outcome of vaccinations by applying this knowledge.

N. Romani (✉) · V. Flacher · C. H. Tripp · F. Sparber · S. Ebner · P. Stoitzner
Department of Dermatology and Venereology, Innsbruck Medical University, Anichstrasse 35, 6020 Innsbruck, Austria
e-mail: nikolaus.romani@i-med.ac.at

N. Romani · C. H. Tripp · S. Ebner
Oncotyrol—Center for Personalized Cancer Medicine, Innsbruck, Austria

Current Topics in Microbiology and Immunology (2012) 351: 113–138
DOI: 10.1007/82_2010_118

Published Online: 21 January 2011

Contents

1 Modern Vaccine Science—Devising Rational Vaccines

Vaccinations in medicine are a success story. They are well established and well investigated. The traditional vaccines induce robust immunity against bacterial and viral microbes, thereby preventing the outbreak of infectious diseases. The commonly applied vaccines, which are used worldwide, were developed by microbiologists. Louis Pasteur discovered that distinct microbes cause diseases and that attenuated microbes can induce long-lived protection against a subsequent infection by the pathogenic, i.e., non-attenuated form of that organism. This was long before there was any clear understanding of cellular, let alone molecular mechanisms of vaccine immunity, such as the decisive role that dendritic cells (DC) have in this process (Steinman 2008b). The twentieth century brought major advances in our knowledge and understanding of the immune system. This initiated a new period of vaccine research that is based on our understanding and exploitation of key immune principles rather than on the empirical approach.

A vaccine can be defined as *a formulation that induces specific, non-toxic, and long-lasting immune responses to prevent or treat disease* (Steinman 2008b). Typically, this was, and still is, an infectious disease. Present vaccine research attempts to widen the spectrum of antigens, against which one could vaccinate, and include antigens specific for cancer, autoimmunity, or allergy (Pulendran and Ahmed 2006). Thus, in the future vaccines will not only serve to enhance immunity in the classical sense, but hopefully also to regulate or dampen it or even induce immunological tolerance in patients, as it would be desired in autoimmune diseases. DC are the prime inducers and regulators of immunity and tolerance. They are critical in designing of modern vaccines and are, therefore, being increasingly recognized in this context (Banchereau et al. 2009; Steinman 2008a; Steinman and Banchereau 2007). It is important to study these cells in vivo in order to move beyond traditional approaches and devise vaccines that directly take advantage of the specialized properties of DC to control immunity (Steinman 2008b). Thus, current vaccinology is characterized by the continuing use of the established and undisputed classical vaccines and by a wide open field of research that aims at rationally utilizing immunological knowledge to make vaccines helpful in a much wider spectrum of diseases than today.

2 Skin Dendritic Cells are Recipients of Intradermal Vaccines

Vaccines are commonly administered into the skin by injection. Most vaccines in humans, however, are deposited into the subcutaneous fat or into the muscle beneath the skin. Relatively few vaccines chose the route into the dermis (Nicolas and Guy, 2008). This comes a bit as a surprise to the dermato-immunologist, who has been studying for many years the prominent, though not completely understood, network of DC in the dermis and epidermis. These two layers of the skin are densely inhabited by different subsets of DC. In contrast, SC fat and muscle tissue (Casares et al. 1997; Dupuis et al. 1998; Hart and Fabre 1981) contain relatively few, not well-investigated DC. This conceptual discrepancy reflects the above-described fields of vaccinology, namely, the traditional, empirical approach and the modern, rational approach. A recent example for an intradermal (ID) vaccine is a newly developed influenza vaccine that is administered into the dermis and that was shown to elicit good immune responses (Arnou et al. 2009). Less well-characterized and hardly applied clinically is the topical route, often called transcutaneous (Frech et al. 2008; Warger et al. 2007) or epicutaneous. Each of these routes of application (intramuscular, subcutaneous, ID, and epicutaneous) requires the presence of DC in the tissue that take up the vaccine, process it, transport it, and present it to T lymphocytes in the draining lymphoid organs. Different subsets of skin DC have been described over the years, starting from epidermal Langerhans cells already in the nineteenth century (Langerhans, 1868) to dermal langerin$^+$ DC only few years ago (Bursch et al. 2007; Ginhoux et al. 2007; Poulin et al. 2007). For more in-depth reviews about skin DC, in particular Langerhans cells, the reader is referred to companion articles by Ginhoux et al. (2010) and Teunissen et al. (2011) in this issue of *Current Topics in Microbiology and Immunology*, to a few recent reviews (Dupasquier et al. 2008; Merad et al. 2008; Romani et al. 2008, 2010a; Zaba et al. 2009), and to an entire issue of *Immunology and Cell Biology* (Special Feature: Understanding the biology and function of Langerhans cells; volume 88 issue 4, 2010).

2.1 Langerhans Cells

The classical skin DC is the Langerhans cell (LC) of the epidermis (Romani et al. 2010a). This cell type has long been known and it is well characterized. LC form a

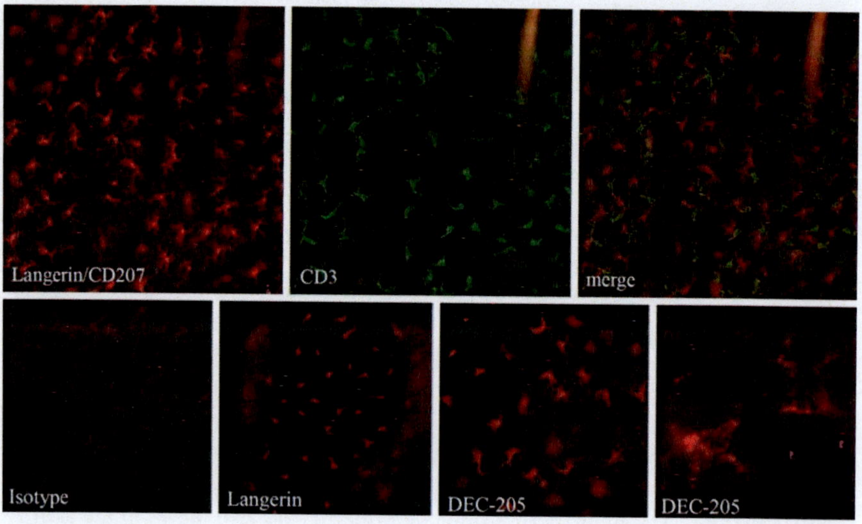

Fig. 1 In the *upper row,* LC are visualized within epidermal sheets from murine skin by immunolabeling with anti-langerin antibody (*red fluorescence*). Dendritic epidermal T cells are identified by anti-CD3 antibodies (*green fluorescence*). The *bottom row* demonstrates how well murine LC can be targeted with antibodies injected into the dermis of the ear (anti-langerin, anti-DEC-205, isotype control). Epidermal sheets were prepared 4 days after the injection and stained with a fluorochrome-coupled anti-rat Ig antibody. Note that an unrelated antibody (isotype) does not bind to the LC whereas anti-langerin and anti-DEC-205 antibodies readily find their way into the epidermis and are taken up by LC. The picture to the far right is a higher magnification of DEC-205-targeted LC in situ. Intracellular vesicles containing the targeting antibody can be appreciated

network that spans our entire body (Fig. 1). They occur also in mucosae (Iwasaki 2007), including the oral/buccal (Cutler and Jotwani 2006) and nasal (Allam et al. 2006) mucosae, which occasionally serve as a site for vaccination. Examples are the well-known oral vaccination against polio or the less established intranasal vaccination against influenza (aerosol or powder administration) (Deans et al. 2010; Hickey and Garmise 2009). It is obvious that in these non-cornified epithelia LC most likely get in contact with the vaccine. Indeed, skin DC in the mouse, possibly including LC express CD155, the receptor for polio virus and CD155 knock-out mice, mount reduced IgG and IgA responses (Maier et al. 2007). This suggests that LC may play an important role in oral vaccination.

2.2 Dermal Langerin^{negative} Dendritic Cells

Healthy human and murine skin harbors dermal DC that do not express langerin/CD207 (Dupasquier et al. 2008). They were first unequivocally identified by studying human and murine skin explant cultures, a method to obtain *mature* skin

DC, developed by the group of Jonathan Austyn 20 years ago (Larsen et al. 1990). Conspicuous cells emigrated from the explants over a culture period of 2–4 days. Their typical morphology (thin cytoplasmic processes, "veils", see Fig. 2), their strong T cell stimulatory capacity in allogeneic mixed leukocyte reactions, and the absence of macrophage markers such as CD14, CD68, or F4/80 (in the mouse) proved their DC nature (Ebner et al. 1998; Lenz et al. 1993; Nestle et al. 1993). This clear picture contrasts with the much more complex situation in situ. There was, and still is, quite some uncertainty as to the relative proportions of DC and macrophages in the dermis. Important studies by the groups of Michelle Lowes in human skin (Zaba et al. 2007; Zaba et al. 2009) and Pieter Leenen in murine skin (Dupasquier et al. 2004, 2008) clarified the issue to a large extent. This work showed and emphasized that the healthy dermis generally contains more macrophages than DC. In human skin, macrophages were identified by virtue of their expression of CD163, a scavenger receptor (Zaba et al. 2007). $CD163^+$ dermal cells did not co-express the DC-specific molecules CD1c or CD11c. High levels of

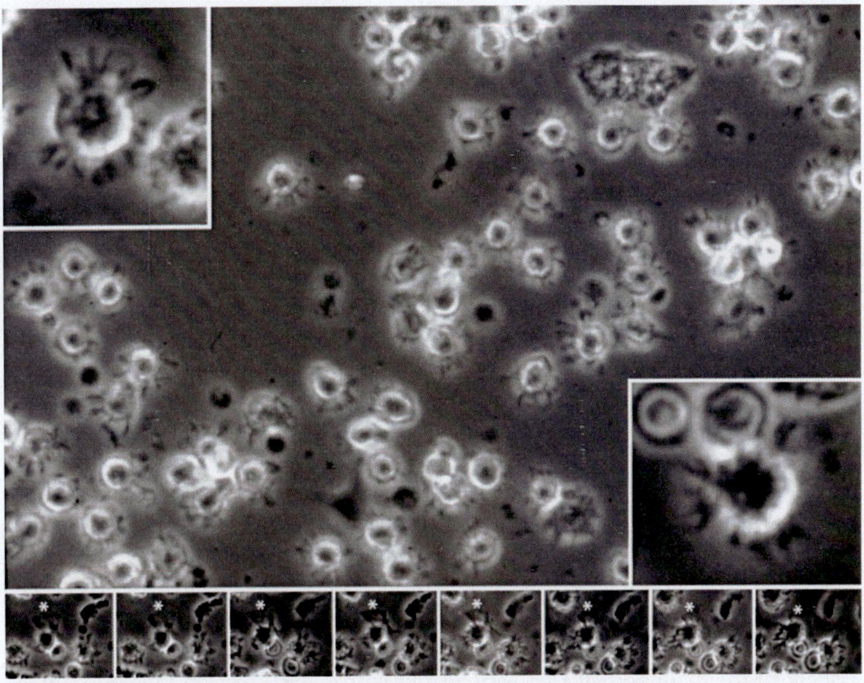

Fig. 2 Human dermal DC obtained by emigration from dermal explants. This means that epidermis and dermis were separated from each other *before* the onset of culture. Phase contrast photographs of cells that migrated out of the explants into the culture medium over a period of 3 days. Note the typical morphology of mature DC with thin cytoplasmic processes ("veils"), best visible in the two inserts. The processes are motile as can be seen in the bottom row of photographs that were taken about 15 s apart from each other. Please note the shape change of one exemplary "veil" under the *white asterisk*

autofluorescence are also useful to discriminate dermal macrophages from dermal DC (Haniffa et al. 2009). Macrophages in mouse dermis were characterized by expression of CD301, a galactose-/N-acetylgalactosamine-specific C-type lectin receptor (Dupasquier et al. 2004). Haniffa et al. have recently unraveled an important role for these dermal macrophages in sustaining graft-versus-host disease in human transplant patients (Haniffa et al. 2009). Phenotypical markers such as DC-SIGN/CD209, which were previously thought to be specific for (dermal) DC, are also expressed on macrophages (Granelli-Piperno et al. 2005; Zaba et al. 2007) and, therefore, confounded analyses for some time.

In spite of this progress the relationship between macrophages and DC in the dermis is still not entirely clear. As mentioned, there are distinct phenotypical differences between DC and macrophages in situ. In skin explant cultures, however, the population of migrated dermal DC appears relatively homogenous. The majority of these mature human DC express high levels of MHC class II, CD86, CD80, CD40, CD83, CD205, and CD208/DC-LAMP but no CD14 (Ebner et al. 2004). There is only a small subset of $CD14^{+}$ cells that is negative for CD205 and DC-LAMP. These are probably macrophages. With regard to CD14 and CD1a expression, these observations in skin explant cultures are similar to what was found in populations that had been directly isolated from human dermal tissue by enzymatic treatment. Dermal DC could be further subdivided into a quantitatively minor population expressing CD14 but not CD1a and a major population characterized by strong CD1a but not CD14 expression (Angel et al. 2007, 2009). In essence, this was already anticipated by Nestle et al. (1993). Whereas macrophages outnumber DC in the dermis of the mouse (Dupasquier et al. 2004) or are at least present in almost equal numbers in human dermis (Zaba et al. 2007) in situ, cells with a clear DC phenotype and morphology are more numerous in the migrant ("crawl-out") populations. Thus, these proportions become inverted. This raises the question whether macrophages may be more firmly anchored in the dermal connective tissue and stay behind, as indicated in a recent study by Haniffa et al. (2009). Alternatively, intrinsic differences in molecules involved in migration [chemokine receptors, matrix metalloproteinases (Ratzinger et al. 2002), etc.] could account for the discrepancy between in vivo and ex vivo proportions of macrophages and DC. Finally, the strong inflammatory milieu in these explant cultures may make some or many macrophages transform into DC. Such a transformation might happen as macrophages migrate across endothelial borders into lymph vessels, as it was shown for skin DC (Randolph et al. 2008; Romani et al. 2001). Transmigration across endothelial barriers of blood vessels can indeed mediate transformation of monocytes into DC in vitro (Randolph et al. 1998) and in vivo (Randolph et al. 1999). Very recent evidence further supports the transition from monocytes to DC in vivo: DC-SIGN/CD209-expressing DCs arise in mouse lymph nodes in response to LPS. They were shown to derive from monocytes (Cheong et al. 2010). What stands against the validity of this notion in the context of skin, at least at first glance, is the observation by Förster's team, that in skin explant cultures many DC probably migrate into the culture medium without ever entering lymph vessels. This was inferred from skin explant cultures in CCR7 knock-out mice where no DC-filled lymph

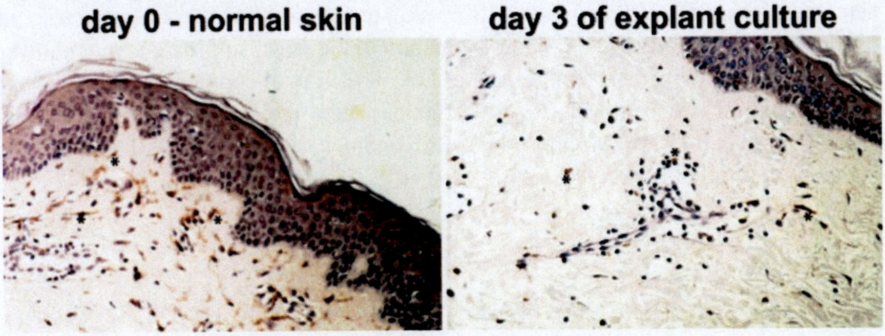

Fig. 3 Human skin before (*left*) and after a 3-day skin explant culture (*right*). Dermal macrophages were visualized with an immunoperoxidase technique using antibodies against Factor XIIIa, a marker for these cells (Zaba et al. 2007). Positive cells can be identified by the brown reaction product (few examples marked with an *asterisk*). Note that after 3 days of culture the numbers of dermal macrophages are markedly reduced

vessels ["cords" (Larsen et al. 1990; Lukas et al. 1996; Weinlich et al. 1998)] could be found but yet, many more DC migrated into the culture medium (Ohl et al. 2004). However, these authors also noted that in the CCR7 knock-out mice migration of LC into the draining lymph nodes was severely inhibited indicating that in the intact organism the majority of cells migrate indeed via lymph vessels, and therefore, such a transformation could theoretically take place. In support of this hypothesis are unpublished observations from our lab. We found that cells expressing typical macrophage markers such as FXIIIa (Zaba et al. 2007) or CD68 became less in numbers during an explant culture indicating that they physically leave the dermis (Fig. 3). In conclusion, the interrelationship of macrophages and DC in the dermis is not yet resolved and clearly needs more study.

2.3 Dermal Langerin$^+$ Dendritic Cells

Few scattered langerin$^+$ cells have been observed in healthy human skin ever since antibodies against langerin were available, i.e., the antibody against the "lag" antigen (Kashihara et al. 1986), and antibodies against langerin/CD207 (Valladeau et al. 1999). Little attention was payed to these cells, mainly because they were so very few in numbers as compared to LC, but also because it seemed clear that they were epidermal LC in transit to the lymph nodes. Only recently this issue was revisited using modern methodologies such as bone marrow chimeric mice (Merad et al. 2008), LC ablation models (Kaplan et al. 2008), and langerin-EGFP transgenic mice (Kissenpfennig et al. 2005). It turned out that these langerin$^+$ cells in the dermis were, at least in part, a dermis-resident population, unrelated to LC and named "dermal langerin$^+$ DC" (Bursch et al. 2007; Ginhoux et al. 2007; Poulin et al. 2007). As opposed to the scarcity of dermal langerin$^+$ DC in situ, they can be readily detected in the migrated populations from skin explant cultures or, even more so, in the draining lymphoid organs. Their frequency in the dermis of mice is much lower than the frequency of langerin^{neg} dermal DC. The human counterpart for this very rare population is currently being investigated; there are hints that human dermis also harbors such a subset (reported in ref (Romani et al. 2010a) and discussed in a companion article by Teunissen et al. (2011).

2.4 *Which Subset of Skin Dendritic Cells is the Major Recipient of an Intradermal Vaccine?*

At first glance it would seem logical that dermal DC would pick up most of the ID injected antigen. It should be mentioned up front that this issue has not been studied systematically. Especially little is known in this regard about human skin. Nevertheless, some interesting pieces of knowledge have emerged from old and recent studies. Using an antibody (against MHC class II) as a protein antigen, Aberer et al. (1986) noted, somewhat surprisingly, that after intraperitoneal injection of the protein even epidermal LC had captured the protein. They detected this by simply labeling epidermal sheets from such treated mice with a fluorescently labeled secondary antibody. This underscored that a vaccine can easily reach LC "from within". Recently, Flacher et al. (2010) addressed this question in an experimental setting that was more realistic with regard to clinical vaccinations. A protein antigen (again an antibody directed to an endocytic receptor on the surface of LC), which was injected into the dermis of mice (into the ear pinna), was readily taken up by epidermal LC, again emphasizing that LC are most likely involved in ID vaccination, even though the vaccine is not placed directly into the habitat of these cells. Similarly, this antigen also reached human LC when placed into a skin explant culture (Flacher et al. 2010). The mechanism by which protein antigen crosses the basement membrane between the dermis and the epidermis was not studied. Presumably it is diffusion. However, an active mechanism whereby LC "reach out" into the dermis in order to fetch the antigen cannot be ruled out. This was shown for gut DC that extend their "arms" into the lumen of the gut to grab bacteria (Rescigno et al. 2001). It was also observed with LC that reach "up" into the horny layer (stratum corneum) of the epidermis where they might sample and take up microbes (Kubo et al. 2009). As expected, ID-injected protein antigen is readily taken up by both langerin^{neg} and langerin^{+} dermal DC (Flacher et al. 2010). Thus, it seems that in ID vaccination all subsets of skin DC gain access to the antigen and, therefore, contribute to the response.

There is one important caveat, though, to this conclusion. The experiments described above were performed with antibodies recognizing cell surface molecules on LC, i.e., MHC class II and the endocytic C-type lectin receptors DEC-205/CD205 and langerin/CD207. Control antibodies that did not have a binding partner on the surface of the LC, e.g., anti-langerin antibody 929F3, which recognizes only the intracellular domain of langerin, did not reach LC in detectable quantities (Flacher et al. 2010). On the one hand, this highlights the potential of targeting antigens selectively to receptors on skin DC [as discussed below and reviewed in ref. (Romani et al. 2010c)]. On the other hand, it leaves the question open, how LC would contribute when a conventional protein antigen, which is not a LC-binding antibody, is injected into the skin. Again, it would be expected that dermal DC take up this antigen. However, in a skin explant model where the fluorescently conjugated model protein ovalbumin (OVA) was offered in the culture medium, we could expectedly show uptake into langerin^{+} as well as langerin^{neg} dermal DC. But also LC in situ took up readily detectable quantities of OVA (Sparber et al. 2010). Compared to antigen conjugated to surface receptors on LC, however, at least 100-times more native protein needed to be given (Flacher et al. 2010). Also when injected ID did epidermal LC capture the protein antigen and carry it to the lymph node (Sparber et al. 2010).

Taken together, the evidence points to an involvement of all subsets of skin DC, including LC, in ID vaccination. The relative contributions of the different subsets, in particular of LC, may critically depend on the quantity of ID-injected antigen but also on the expression of receptors involved in internalization (see below).

3 Functional Repertoire of Skin Dendritic Cells

About a decade ago there was no doubt in the field that LC and dermal DC were always immunogenic in vivo. This conclusion was based on the manifold evidence that they are strongly immunostimulatory in in vitro experimental settings (Romani et al. 1989; Schuler and Steinman 1985; Stingl et al. 1980). LC were regarded as prototype DC that served as the "role model" for all other DC. This concept was frequently called the "Langerhans cell paradigm" (Girolomoni et al. 2002; Wilson and Villadangos 2004). This paradigm needed to be revisited in response to two important findings. (1) It was recognized that DC not only induce immunity but also serve to establish and maintain tolerance (Steinman et al. 2003; Steinman and Nussenzweig 2002). This occurs when they present antigen in the steady state, i.e., in the absence of full maturation. (2) Furthermore, herpes virus infection models and transgenic antigen expression models in mice showed that LC do not under all circumstances present antigens that they have acquired in the skin in the draining lymph nodes in vivo; other DC including dermal langerin^{+} DC can do the (cross-) presentation (Allan et al. 2003; Bedoui et al. 2009; Heath and Carbone 2009; Henri et al. 2010). Research into the in vivo functions of LC is presently in full bloom (Romani et al. 2010b), taking advantage of modern methodology, foremost of mouse models where langerin^{+} cells can be selectively depleted from the living mouse [reviewed in (Kaplan et al. 2008)].

Early investigations of LC-like (CD1a and langerin-expressing) and non-LC-like (CD14-expressing, interstitial type, dermal type) DC grown from human CD34^{+} hematopoietic stem cells highlighted possible functional differences between the different types of skin DC for the first time. LC-like DC take up less endocytic tracers such as fluorescein isothiocyanate dextran or peroxidase. Another difference is the failure of LC-like DC to induce naive B cells to differentiate into IgM-secreting cells, in response to CD40 triggering and interleukin-2 (IL-2), as opposed to interstitial type DC (Caux et al. 1997). This was essentially verified with LC and CD14^{+} dermal DC directly isolated from human skin. The former subset was superior in cross-priming CD8^{+} T cells, and the latter subset was specialized to prime CD4^{+} helper T cells that in turn induced B cells to become antibody producing cells (Klechevsky et al. 2008). As pointed out above, the CD14^{+} subset of dermal DC comprises only about a tenth of all langerin^{neg} dermal DC (Banchereau et al. 2009). The majority of langerin^{neg} dermal DC, i.e., CD14^{neg}/CD1a^{+} cells, appear to be functionally in between LC and the CD14^{+} subset (Klechevsky et al. 2008). It remains unclear at this point how this could relate to ID vaccination, notably because the means of antigen uptake by DC in situ or by DC cultured ex vivo are likely to differ fundamentally. Nevertheless, these in vitro data correspond to in vivo observations in mice, where skin-derived dermal DC localized close to the B cell follicles in the outer paracortex of the lymph node. LC, in contrast, arrived and settled in the inner paracortex, intermingled with lymph node-resident langerin^{+} cells (Kissenpfennig et al. 2005). It is not known, however, whether these dermal DC correspond to the human dermal DC subset that promotes the humoral response, i.e., the CD14^{+} subpopulation. Yet, these findings highlight that a "division of labor" may indeed be operative in vivo.

At present, virtually all clinical trials that attempt to harness the immunogenic potential of DC are vaccination studies against cancer. They aim primarily at generating powerful cytotoxic T lymphocytes. Some recent observations are of importance in this regard. Several groups could show that LC, as opposed to dermal DC, are especially capable of inducing cytotoxic T lymphocytes. This was first shown with human LC-like DC derived from CD34^{+} stem cells (Ratzinger et al. 2004). Importantly, these data were recently confirmed using human LC isolated from the epidermis; LC were indeed more potent to induce CD8^{+} T cells that contained increased levels of lytic molecules (perforin, granzymes) and that efficiently killed tumor cell lines. LC-derived IL-15 appeared to be a critical factor (Klechevsky et al. 2008; Ueno et al. 2010). Of note, we found mature human LC, obtained by migration from cultured epidermal sheets, to induce substantial levels of IFN-γ secretion in naive allogeneic CD4^{+} helper T cells (Ebner et al. 2007), surprisingly without detectable secretion of bioactive IL-12 p70 (Ebner et al. 2001). Also murine epidermal LC clearly have the capacity to elicit IFN-γ producing T cells (Koch et al. unpublished data; Table 1) in spite of making almost no bioactive IL-12 (Heufler et al. 1996). Studies in a mouse tumor model confirmed and emphasized that LC (and possibly also dermal langerin^{+} DC) are essential for anti-tumor immunity in vivo. Protection from an experimental tumor (B16 melanoma) was lost when LC and dermal langerin^{+} DC had been ablated (Stoitzner et al. 2008) by means of the diphtheria toxin receptor knock-in technology (Kaplan et al. 2008).

Table 1 Induction of a Th1 cytokine secretion pattern in T lymphocytes by murine Langerhans cells

	10,000	3,000	1,000	300	LC/well
	15,900	10,900	7,130	4,450	IFNγ (pg/ml)
Anti-IL-12	1,060	940	800	390	IFNγ (pg/ml)
	55	61	40	45	IL-4 (pg/ml)
Anti-IL-12	81	62	55	55	IL-4 (pg/ml)

Resting T lymphocytes of C57BL/6 mice were stimulated by graded doses of mature epidermal Langerhans cells (LC) from BALB/c mice in an allogeneic mixed leukocyte reaction. Resulting T cell blasts were restimulated for three additional rounds with fresh batches of mature LC. Supernatants of the forth allogeneic mixed leukocyte reaction were tested for the presence of secreted T cell cytokines by ELISA. Note that LC induced strong secretion of IFN-γ but virtually no IL-4. IFN-γ production was inhibited when anti-IL-12 antibodies were continuously present in the cultures (Koch et al. unpublished data)

In conclusion, it is important and promising to rationally address DC subsets of the skin, especially LC, for purposes of vaccination (Ueno et al. 2010). Depending on the subset that contributes most, the response will be dominated by cytotoxic T cells, and thus be useful for vaccinating against cancer, or by a humoral response and thus be beneficial for vaccination against infectious agents. LC appear to be responsible for the development of cytotoxicity, and CD14^{+} dermal DC for the generation of an antibody response. Clearly, in reality the picture is not as simple as that. Yet, these data form a good basis to further explore the relative roles of skin DC in ID vaccination. One elegant approach to address this issue in vivo is to target antigens to one subset or another (see Sect. 4.1.5).

4 Harnessing the Distinct Properties of Skin Dendritic Cells for Intradermal Vaccination

4.1 Augment Lymphocyte Responses by Targeting Vaccine to Specific Antigen Uptake Receptors on Skin Dendritic Cells

4.1.1 What is "Antigen Targeting"?

DC are equipped with a wide range of receptors that facilitate the uptake of pathogens, including the so-called "C-type lectin receptors". They recognize pathogen-associated molecular patterns (Figdor et al. 2002). Important examples are DEC-205/CD205, langerin/CD207 (Fig. 1), DC-SIGN/CD209, Dectin, and DCIR2. Groundbreaking studies from the groups of Steinman and Nussenzweig at Rockefeller University labs has revealed that immune responses can be dramatically enhanced when an antigen is delivered ("targeted") directly and selectively to DC rather than being "only" injected into the dermis or under the skin (subcutaneously or intramuscular, as in conventional vaccinations or in footpad injections in mice). In other words, the vaccine obtains an "address tag" in the form of a specific antibody against a C-type lectin receptor. Thereby, the antigen or vaccine is guided directly and exclusively to the DC that expresses the respective C-type lectin receptor on its surface. This is achieved by coupling protein or peptide antigens to monoclonal antibodies against C-type lectin receptors. Researchers employ chemical conjugation methods or, preferrably, the genetic engineering approach. Antibodies to different C-type lectin receptors for conjugation are used as whole antibodies (Idoyaga et al. 2008) or as single chain fragments (Birkholz et al. 2010; Nchinda et al. 2008). This strategy is currently being extended beyond the widely used model antigen OVA to other antigens like hen egg lysozyme/HEL (Hawiger et al. 2001), or keyhole limpet hemocyanin/KLH (Tacken et al. 2005). Data from the OVA model must always be judged with caution, and premature generalizations must be avoided. OVA peptide-specific TCR transgenic T cells, in particular the $CD8^+$ T cells ("OT-I cells") are extremely sensitive to TCR stimulation in an unphysiological manner: they already respond to tiny amounts of antigen in the picomolar range (Choi et al. 2009). Therefore, the supplementation of the experimental OVA model with other models is an indispensable goal, even though the OVA model has yielded and is still yielding important insights. Importantly, a number of antigens relevant for clinical studies have now been successfully used in this approach, including HIV gag (Nchinda et al. 2008; Trumpfheller et al. 2008), a mouse melanoma tumor antigen (Mahnke et al. 2005) or the human tumor antigens mesothelin (Wang et al. 2009) and MAGE-A3 (Birkholz et al. 2010).

The first hints for the potential to enhance immune responses by addressing C-type lectin receptors came from the initial studies of the cell biology of antigen uptake into DC via such receptors (Mahnke et al. 2000). Mahnke et al. investigated the fate of immunoglobulin (Ig) binding to chimeric Fc receptors where the cytosolic domain of the Fc receptor was replaced by the cytosolic portion of two different C-type lectin receptors. When Ig was given to DC expressing the cytosolic part of the DEC-205 receptor, its uptake was strongly enhanced. Moreover, in contrast to targeting via the macrophage mannose receptor, antigens were specifically routed to late endosomes or lysosomes that contained abundantly MHC class II molecules. This resulted in a markedly (up to 100-fold) augmented T cell response in vitro (Mahnke et al. 2000). These seminal observations led to the series of in vivo *studies* described below.

4.1.2 Targeting Dendritic Cells in the Steady State

Immunization of mice with anti-DEC-205 antigen conjugates (OVA or hen egg lysozyme) in the absence of DC maturation stimuli (such as CD40 ligation or poly(I:C)), i.e., in the steady state, led to T cell unresponsiveness in both the $CD4^+$ (Hawiger et al. 2001) and the $CD8^+$ (Bonifaz et al. 2002) T cell compartment. Injection of the conjugates into the footpads under these experimental conditions induced an initial wave of T cell division. Importantly, proliferation was orders of magnitude greater than the proliferation in response to the free, unconjugated antigen. However, this proliferation was not sustained but, rather, T cell numbers dropped, and the remaining T cells did not respond any longer to a standard immunization protocol using complete Freund's adjuvant. This indicated that peripheral tolerance had developed in response to the steady-state administration of the antigen–antibody conjugate (Steinman et al. 2003). These findings were validated in a mouse model for type I autoimmune diabetes where both onset and progression of the disease could be inhibited by treatment with anti-DEC-205-conjugated antigen (Bruder et al. 2005; Mukhopadhaya et al. 2008). The underlying mechanism for tolerance induction appears to be not only deletion and anergy, as shown in the original study (Bonifaz et al. 2002; Hawiger et al. 2001), but also induction of regulatory T cells (Yamazaki et al. 2008).

4.1.3 Targeting Dendritic Cells Under Inflammatory/Immunogenic Conditions

In the above-described studies the outcome in terms of T cell responses changed dramatically when DC maturation stimuli were added at the time of immunization together with the anti-DEC-205–antigen conjugate. Again, T cell proliferation in vivo increased several orders of magnitude as compared with immunization with the same amount of unconjugated antigen, be it a peptide (Hawiger et al. 2001) or the whole antigenic protein (Bonifaz et al. 2002). Importantly, the augmented massive T cell proliferation translated into markedly improved anti-tumor immunity in an experimental model in vivo. The very infrequent naive antigen-specific T cells, which exist in a non-immune mouse, could only be primed if the subcutaneously (footpad) injected antigen was coupled to an anti-DEC-205 antibody and a strong DC maturation stimulus (CD40 ligation) was co-administered. Uncoupled antigen plus/minus CD40 ligation, as well as immunization with antigen-pulsed cultured DC, did not lead to efficient priming of naïve T cells in this setting (Bonifaz et al. 2004). Alternatively, DC maturation and subsequent responses could be achieved by TLR agonists, such as poly(I:C) (Trumpfheller et al. 2008). This further highlights the potential of antigen targeting also for vaccinations in humans where vaccine-specific T cells would be equally scarce and difficult to be activated in sufficient numbers, enough to obtain clinical effects. Not unexpectedly, the increased stimulation of helper T cells by the anti-DEC-205-antigen conjugates led to amplified antibody responses in mice (Boscardin et al. 2006). These data emphasize that it is also feasible to harness antigen targeting for improving humoral immune responses in vaccinations.

4.1.4 Targeting Different Receptors on the Surface of Dendritic Cells

Conceptually, two scenarios have to be considered. (1) A given subset of DC expresses simultaneously different targetable endocytic receptors. Immune responses may be influenced depending on which of these receptors is targeted. Examples are described below. (2) Subsets of DC often express different, non-overlapping targetable receptors. Immune responses may be influenced depending on which DC subset receives the antigen. This will be illustrated in Sect. 4.1.5.

The type of targeted endocytic receptor can influence the quantity and quality of resulting immune responses. This became evident in the original studies by Mahnke et al. (2000) who used mouse bone marrow-derived DC that expressed both DEC-205 and macrophage mannose receptor on their surfaces. Yet, antigen targeted to either of these two receptors was taken up differently, routed differently, and enhanced T cell responses were only observed with DEC-205-targeted antigen. A more recent, similar example was provided by Bozzacco et al. (Bozzacco et al. 2007) who compared targeting an HIV antigen (p24 gag) to human DC with anti-DEC-205 vis-à-vis anti-DC-SIGN antibodies. Both receptors are expressed on the same DC at similar levels (Ebner et al. 2004). Yet, the anti-DEC-205-conjugated antigen was more effectively cross-presented than anti-DC-SIGN-conjugated antigen, indicating different intracellular processing.

With special regard to the skin, we found pronounced differences in the handling of the model antigen OVA depending on whether it was offered to epidermal LC by ID injection as an anti-DEC-205/OVA conjugate or an anti-langerin/OVA conjugate. Both receptors are expressed on the surface of murine LC (Cheong et al. 2007; Inaba et al. 1995) and both receptors can be successfully targeted by the respective antibodies (Flacher et al. 2010)(Fig. 1). Idoyaga et al. observed previously that $CD4^{+}$ and $CD8^{+}$ T cells proliferated in vivo in the draining lymph nodes following targeting of DEC-205 or langerin receptors by SC injection of the antigen conjugates into the footpads of mice (Idoyaga et al. 2008). On the other hand, when we "loaded" LC in vivo with antigen via DEC-205 or langerin by ID injection into the ear, $CD4^{+}$ and $CD8^{+}$ T cell proliferation in vitro was only induced by LC that had taken up the antigen via the DEC-205 receptor. Targeting the antigen to the langerin receptor did not result in $CD4^{+}$ and $CD8^{+}$ T cell division. This unexpected discrepancy probably reflects the importance of other $langerin^{+}$ DC subsets present in the dermis or in lymph nodes draining the immunization site (see below). These other subsets were *not* present in these experimental settings (Flacher et al. 2010).

4.1.5 Delivering the Vaccine to Selected Dendritic Cell Subsets by Targeting Differentially Expressed Surface Receptors

As discussed above, antigen targeting allows to manipulate the antigen processing and presentation capacity of a given DC such that resulting T cell responses can differ in quantitative and qualitative terms. In the context of most vaccination schemes, including ID vaccination, the injected antigen can be sequestered by different subsets of DC. In the case of skin these are LC and $langerin^{neg}$ and $langerin^{+}$ dermal DC. Here, antigen targeting allows to address the vaccine to defined subsets of DCs. For instance, ID targeting via langerin would bring the antigen to LC and langerin$^+$ dermal DC but leave out langerin^{neg} DC (Flacher et al. 2010). Targeting to a putative C-type lectin receptor expressed exclusively by langerin^{neg} dermal DC could be an alternative. Unfortunately, such a molecule has not been found yet. Future research will teach us about pros and cons for one or the other approach.

The importance of delivering vaccine antigens to defined DC subsets was highlighted in the first thorough side-by-side comparison of different targeting strategies by Dudziak et al. (2007). They looked at immune responses induced by immunization with antigens conjugated to antibodies against DEC-205 versus DCIR2 (dendritic cell inhibitory receptor-2; "33D1 antigen") that are expressed by CD8$^+$ and CD8^{neg} DC in the spleen of mice, respectively. Immunization via DEC-205 favored CD8$^+$ T cell responses whereas DCIR2 targeting preferentially induced CD4$^+$ T cell responses. Gene expression analyses indeed showed that CD8$^+$/DEC-205$^+$ DC expressed more genes associated with processing for the MHC class I pathway (TAP, calreticulin, etc.) and CD8^{neg}/DCIR2$^+$ DC expressed more genes associated with processing for the MHC class II pathway (cathepsins, etc.) (Dudziak et al. 2007). At another level, it was shown that the selective delivery of antigen to the CD8$^+$/DEC-205$^+$ and CD8^{neg}/DCIR2$^+$ DC subsets of spleen DC by means of the respective antigen–antibody conjugates in the absence of DC maturation signal, led to the de novo induction of FoxP3$^+$ regulatory T cells and to the expansion of preexisting FoxP3$^+$ regulatory T cells, respectively (Yamazaki et al. 2008; Yamazaki and Steinman 2009).

Finally, the development of monoclonal antibodies recognizing the extracellular domain of the langerin (CD207 (Valladeau et al. 2000)) molecule (Cheong et al. 2007) opened the way to study antigen targeting to this molecule expressed on important skin DC, particularly on LC. Given the pronounced properties of LC in the induction of cytotoxic responses (see above), targeting this receptor is of high interest. Initial analyses revealed many similarities in targeting properties to DEC-205 and only subtle differences between DEC-205 and langerin targeting (Idoyaga et al. 2008). The SC route (footpad) of immunization was used in these experiments, rather than the ID one. The splenic CD8α^+ DC subset, which is the key subset responsible for cross-presentation in vivo (Heath et al. 2004), specifically co-expresses the langerin receptor (Douillard et al. 2005; Idoyaga et al. 2009; McLellan et al. 2002). It will be interesting to study antigen targeting to this important population of DC. Recent data suggest that, indeed, cross-presenting activity is restricted to that CD8α^+/langerin$^+$ DC population in mouse spleen (Farrand et al. 2009).

4.1.6 Targeting Antigens Specifically on Skin Dendritic Cells

Which endocytic receptors on skin DC could be of importance for antigen targeting? For this it is important to determine in detail the expression patterns of the various endocytic receptors on skin DC. These patterns are still incompletely known.

Langerhans cells. They are phenotypically well characterized both in mouse and human skin, and their identifying receptor langerin and the prototype targeting receptor DEC-205 have been dealt with above. Both are expressed on the cell surface of LC (Cheong et al. 2007; Ebner et al. 2004; Inaba et al. 1995; Zaba et al. 2007) (Fig. 1). In addition, they express Dectin-1 (Ariizumi et al. 2000b) and Dectin-2 (Ariizumi et al. 2000a). Antigen targeting to both molecules was shown to elicit stronger responses than immunization with equal amounts of free antigen (Carter et al. 2006a, 2006b). The DCIR2 molecule is absent from murine LC (Witmer-Pack et al. 1987). For human LC this has not yet been determined.

Dermal DC. Most phenotypical data in the dermis do not (yet) take into account the newly described subsets of dermal DC. The "classical", langerin^{neg} dermal DC express DEC-205 both in human (Ebner et al. 2004; Zaba et al. 2007) and in mouse skin (Henri et al. 2001; Lenz et al. 1993; Nagao et al. 2009). Interestingly, however, unequivocal cell surface expression on immature murine dermal DC has not been demonstrated, not least due to the trypsin sensitivity of this molecule (Inaba et al. 1995). Yet, two features became clear from these studies. DEC-205 is up-regulated on dermal DC, but even then, surface expression is lower than on LC. Finally, the ability to target dermal langerin^{neg} DC with anti-DEC-205 antibodies strongly argues for a functional level of surface expression (Flacher et al. 2010). The other subset of dermal DC, namely, langerin^{+} dermal DC expresses DEC-205 at levels similar to LC and can readily be targeted with anti-DEC-205 [Flacher et al. unpublished observations and (Flacher et al. 2010)]. DC-SIGN, which was initially regarded as a marker for dermal DC (Ebner et al. 2004), occurs more abundantly on macrophages in the dermis as identified by CD14 (Klechevsky et al. 2008; Turville et al. 2002) or CD163 (Zaba et al. 2007) expression. Thinking of vaccinations that aim at generating robust antibody responses, one could envisage to target antigen to dermal DC, namely, the CD14^{+} subset, in order to exploit the capacity of that subset to promote immunoglobulin production (Banchereau et al. 2009). CD36, the thrombospondin receptor and a scavenger receptor might be a candidate since this molecule is specifically expressed on dermal DC (Lenz et al. 1993), and there is evidence that targeting CD36 may also improve immune responses (Tagliani et al. 2008).

The expression on skin DC of additional interesting candidates for targeting such as Clec9 (Caminschi et al. 2008), Clec12 (Lahoud et al. 2009), Lox (Delneste et al. 2002), and others (reviewed recently by Caminschi et al. 2009) has not yet been investigated. Molecules beyond the field of C-type lectin receptors may also be interesting candidates. For instance, improved immune responses have been reported for antigens that were more broadly targeted to MHC molecules (by means of a novel construct based on an MHC-binding superantigen, not with antibodies) (Dickgreber et al. 2009).

In closing, it should be emphasized once more that virtually all studies hitherto used the subcutaneous route of immunization rather than the ID one. Given the likely differences in DC subset composition between the subcutis and the dermis, it will be necessary to study in detail targeting the various endocytic receptors in ID vaccination.

4.2 Augment and Broaden Responses by Including Innate Lymphocyte Responses

Antigen targeting via endocytic receptors on DC aims at improving $CD4^{+}$ and $CD8^{+}$ T cell responses. Cytotoxic T lymphocytes are undoubtedly the immune system's strongest weapon against cancer. However, there are other important innate lymphocytes that are also critically involved in immune defense reactions and that should also take part in vaccine-induced immune responses. NKT cells are important in two ways. First, they can serve as potent cytotoxic effector cells (Cerundolo et al. 2009; Godfrey et al. 2010; Neparidze and Dhodapkar 2009). Second, the mutual cross-talk between NKT cells and DC leads to activation and full maturation of both cells types. The glycolipid alpha-galactosylceramide (alpha-GalCer) is the molecular link between the two cell types. It is presented by DC on their CD1d molecules and thereby mediates the activation and numerical expansion of NKT cells (Fujii et al. 2002). These activated NKT cells, in turn, bring about full maturation of DC (Fujii et al. 2003). These cellular interactions are the likely basis for the observed clinical benefit when using alpha-GalCer as an adjuvant in the treatment of cancer (Chang et al. 2005; Neparidze and Dhodapkar 2009). This approach appears so promising that in a recent review article Fujji and Steinman "*urge development of the DC-NKT axis to provide innate and adaptive immunity to human cancers* (Fujii et al. 2007)".

How can ID vaccination harness the potential of NKT cells? We have recently studied this question in some detail in the mouse (Tripp et al. 2009). The initial observation was that cutaneous DC express and upregulate CD1d on their surface in situ and ex vivo. At least half of the LC and dermal DC (including dermal langerin^{+} DC) express CD1d on their surface upon emigration from skin explants. In the skin-draining lymph nodes nearly all DC derived from the skin were positive for CD1d besides all lymph node-resident DC subsets. Corresponding to this finding, skin and lymph node-derived DC were able to present the synthetic glycolipid alpha-GalCer to an NKT cell hybridoma in vitro. Moreover, ID-injected alpha-GalCer was incorporated and presented by migratory DC. The adjuvant effect of ID-injected alpha-GalCer was not via a migration stimulus or the induction of maturation markers on lymph node DC, but rather led to an enhancement of CD40 expression on distant, more immature spleen DC. Furthermore, alpha-GalCer activated B and T cells in lymph node and spleen to upregulate CD69. The effects observed in the spleen indicate that ID-injected alpha-GalCer exerts its effect systemically, at least in the small body of a mouse. However, the stimulation of antigen-specific $CD8^{+}$ T cells happened in a locally restricted way. ID immunization activated cytotoxic T cells only in the lymph nodes, in contrast to the intravenous route which mainly provoked T cell responses in the spleen. Most importantly, ID treatment of mice demonstrated that the combination of a protein antigen plus alpha-GalCer can improve the survival of mice bearing B16 melanoma tumors. Thus, alpha-GalCer proved to be a promising adjuvant not just for intravenous immunization but also for the ID route. A surprising finding of this study was that migratory skin DC are not mandatory to mediate the effect of ID immunization with protein antigen plus alpha-GalCer. When we prevented the participation of migratory skin DC by depletion of langerin^{+} DC subsets (using the diphtheria toxin ablation technique (Kaplan et al. 2008)) or by removal of the immunization site within 4 h, activation of cytotoxic T cells was still induced. This indicates that most of the ID-injected antigen and adjuvant diffused through lymph and blood to lymphatic organs where resident DC could stimulate cytotoxic T cell responses. In an attempt to increase T cell responses even more, we compared side-by-side unconjugated and anti-DEC-205-conjugated antigen in combination with alpha-GalCer. We observed that 1,000-times less of the conjugated antigen was sufficient to achieve equivalent anti-tumor responses in the B16 model (Tripp, unpublished observations). This is of importance in regard to the immense costs of producing antigens in good-manufacturing practice (GMP) quality (Ueno et al. 2010). With regard to ID vaccination in man, it is important that dermal DC in human skin express CD1d and could, therefore, be targeted with alpha-GalCer expressed on dermal dendritic DC (Gerlini et al. 2001). In conclusion, the synthetic glycolipid alpha-GalCer proved to be a potent adjuvant for ID immunization with protein antigen and might be a promising adjuvant for targeted immunotherapies.

5 Concluding Remarks

ID injection of an antigen is an old technique as illustrated by the classical tuberculin test. Novel influenza vaccines that are ID injected have only recently been introduced on the market (Deans et al. 2010). They were developed in the classical way, mainly based on empirical knowledge. Researchers are now trying to improve ID vaccination rationally by harnessing the specific properties of skin DC as they become known bit by bit. Targeting of antigens to defined, functionally distinct subsets of skin DC and addressing innate lymphocytes as additional, powerful effector cells are two promising strategies to further establish this route of immunization and, in the more distant future, also tolerization. This should ultimately lead to more effective protective as well as therapeutic vaccines.

Acknowledgments This study has continuously been supported by the Austrian Science Fund (currently, FWF project P21487 to P. Stoitzner). NR, CHT, and SE are further supported by the COMET Center ONCOTYROL and funded by the Federal Ministry for Transport Innovation & Technology (BMVIT) and the Federal Ministry of Economics & Labour/the Federal Ministry of Economy, Family & Youth (BMWA/BMWFJ), the Tiroler Zukunftsstiftung (TZS). We appreciate the participation of the TILAK hospital holding company, who serves as a partner the Oncotyrol research program. FS is supported by a grant (#11) of the IFTZ (Integriertes Forschungs- und Therapiezentrum) at Innsbruck Medical University.

References

Aberer W, Kruisbeek AM, Shimada S, Katz SI (1986) In vivo treatment with anti-I-A antibodies: differential effects on Ia antigens and antigen-presenting cell function of spleen cells and epidermal Langerhans cells. J Immunol 136:830–836

Allam JP, Niederhagen B, Bucheler M, Appel T, Betten H, Bieber T, Berge S, Novak N (2006) Comparative analysis of nasal and oral mucosa dendritic cells. Allergy 61:166–172

Allan RS, Smith CM, Belz GT, Van Lint AL, Wakim LM, Heath WR, Carbone FR (2003) Epidermal viral immunity induced by $CD8\alpha^+$ dendritic cells but not by Langerhans cells. Science 301:1925–1928

Angel CE, Lala A, Chen CJ, Edgar SG, Ostrovsky LL, Dunbar PR (2007) $CD14^+$ antigen-presenting cells in human dermis are less mature than their $CD1a^+$ counterparts. Int Immunol 19:1271–1279

Angel CE, Chen CJ, Horlacher OC, Winkler S, John T, Browning J, MacGregor D, Cebon J, Dunbar PR (2009) Distinctive localization of antigen-presenting cells in human lymph nodes. Blood 113:1257–1267

Ariizumi K, Shen GL, Shikano S, Ritter R, III, Zukas P, Edelbaum D, Morita A, Takashima A (2000a) Cloning of a second dendritic cell-associated C-type lectin (Dectin-2) and its alternatively spliced isoforms. J Biol Chem 275:11957–11963

Ariizumi K, Shen GL, Shikano S, Xu S, Ritter R, III, Kumamoto T, Edelbaum D, Morita A, Bergstresser PR, Takashima A (2000b) Identification of a novel, dendritic cell-associated molecule, dectin-1, by subtractive cDNA cloning. J Biol Chem 275:20157–20167

Arnou R, Icardi G, De Decker M, Ambrozaitis A, Kazek MP, Weber F, Van Damme P (2009) Intradermal influenza vaccine for older adults: a randomized controlled multicenter phase III study. Vaccine 27:7304–7312

Banchereau J, Klechevsky E, Schmitt N, Morita R, Palucka K, Ueno H (2009) Harnessing human dendritic cell subsets to design novel vaccines. Ann N Y Acad Sci 1174:24–32

Bedoui S, Whitney PG, Waithman J, Eidsmo L, Wakim L, Caminschi I, Allan RS, Wojtasiak M, Shortman K, Carbone FR, Brooks AG, Heath WR (2009) Cross-presentation of viral and self antigens by skin-derived $CD103^+$ dendritic cells. Nat Immunol 10:488–495

Birkholz K, Schwenkert M, Kellner C, Gross S, Fey G, Schuler-Thurner B, Schuler G, Schaft N, Dörrie J (2010) Targeting of DEC-205 on human dendritic cells results in efficient MHC class II-restricted antigen presentation. Blood 116:2277–2285

Bonifaz L, Bonnyay D, Mahnke K, Rivera M, Nussenzweig MC, Steinman RM (2002) Efficient targeting of protein antigen to the dendritic cell receptor DEC-205 in the steady state leads to antigen presentation on major histocompatibility complex class I products and peripheral $CD8^+$ T cell tolerance. J Exp Med 196:1627–1638

Bonifaz LC, Bonnyay DP, Charalambous A, Darguste DI, Fujii SI, Soares H, Brimnes MK, Moltedo B, Moran TM, Steinman RM (2004) In vivo targeting of antigens to maturing dendritic cells via the DEC-205 receptor improves T cell vaccination. J Exp Med 199:815–824

Boscardin SB, Hafalla JCR, Masilamani RF, Kamphorst AO, Zebroski HA, Rai U, Morrot A, Zavala F, Steinman RM, Nussenzweig RS, Nussenzweig MC (2006) Antigen targeting to dendritic cells elicits long-lived T cell help for antibody responses. J Exp Med 203:599–606

Bozzacco L, Trumpfheller C, Siegal FP, Mehandru S, Markowitz M, Carrington M, Nussenzweig MC, Piperno AG, Steinman RM (2007) DEC-205 receptor on dendritic cells mediates presentation of HIV gag protein to $CD8^+$ T cells in a spectrum of human MHC I haplotypes. Proc Natl Acad Sci USA 104:1289–1294

Bruder D, Westendorf AM, Hansen W, Prettin S, Gruber AD, Qian YJ, Von Boehmer H, Mahnke K, Buer J (2005) On the edge of autoimmunity—T-cell stimulation by steady-state dendritic cells prevents autoimmune diabetes. Diabetes 54:3395–3401

Bursch LS, Wang L, Igyarto B, Kissenpfennig A, Malissen B, Kaplan DH, Hogquist KA (2007) Identification of a novel population of langerin + dendritic cells. J Exp Med 204:3147–3156

Caminschi I, Proietto AI, Ahmet F, Kitsoulis S, Teh JS, Lo JCY, Rizzitelli A, Wu L, Vremec D, Van Dommelen SLH, Campbell IK, Maraskovsky E, Braley H, Davey GM, Mottram P, van de Velde N, Jensen K, Lew AM, Wright MD, Heath WR, Shortman K, Lahoud M (2008) The dendritic cell subtype-restricted C-type lectin Clec9A is a target for vaccine enhancement. Blood 112:3264–3273

Caminschi I, Lahoud MH, Shortman K (2009) Enhancing immune responses by targeting antigen to DC. Eur J Immunol 39:931–938

Carter RW, Thompson C, Reid DM, Wong SY, Tough DF (2006a) Preferential induction of $CD4^+$ T cell responses through in vivo targeting of antigen to dendritic cell-associated C-type lectin-1. J Immunol 177:2276–2284

Carter RW, Thompson C, Reid DM, Wong SYC, Tough DF (2006b) Induction of $CD8^+$ T cell responses through targeting of antigen to Dectin-2. Cell Immunol 239:87–91

Casares S, Inaba K, Brumeanu TD, Steinman RM, Bona CA (1997) Antigen presentation by dendritic cells after immunization with DNA encoding a major histocompatibility complex class II-restricted viral epitope. J Exp Med 186:1481–1486

Caux C, Massacrier C, Vanbervliet B, Dubois B, Durand I, Cella M, Lanzavecchia A, Banchereau J (1997) $CD34^+$ hematopoietic progenitors from human cord blood differentiate along two independent dendritic cell pathways in response to granulocyte-macrophage colony-stimulating factor plus tumor necrosis factor α. 2. Functional analysis. Blood 90:1458–1470

Cerundolo V, Silk JD, Masri SH, Salio M (2009) Harnessing invariant NKT cells in vaccination strategies. Nat Rev Immunol 9:28–38

Chang DH, Osman K, Connolly J, Kukreja A, Krasovsky J, Pack M, Hutchinson A, Geller M, Liu N, Annable R, Shay J, Kirchhoff K, Nishi N, Ando Y, Hayashi K, Hassoun H, Steinman RM, Dhodapkar MV (2005) Sustained expansion of NKT cells and antigen-specific T cells after injection of α-galactosyl-ceramide loaded mature dendritic cells in cancer patients. J Exp Med 201:1503–1517

Cheong C, Idoyaga J, Do Y, Pack M, Park SH, Lee H, Kang YS, Choi JH, Kim JY, Bonito A, Inaba K, Yamazaki S, Steinman RM, Park CG (2007) Production of monoclonal antibodies that recognize the extracellular domain of mouse Langerin/CD207. J Immunol Methods 324:48–62

Cheong C, Matos I, Choi J-H, Dandamudi DB,Shrestha E, Longhi MP, Jeffrey KL, Anthony RM, Kluger C, Nchinda G, Koh H, Rodriguez A, Idoyaga J, Pack M, Velinzon K, Park CG, Steinman RM (2010) Microbial stimulation fully differentiates monocytes to DC-SIGN/$CD209^+$ dendritic cells for immune T cell areas. Cell 143:416–429

Choi JH, Do Y, Cheong C, Koh H, Boscardin SB, Oh YS, Bozzacco L, Trumpfheller C, Park CG, Steinman RM (2009) Identification of antigen-presenting dendritic cells in mouse aorta and cardiac valves. J Exp Med 206:497–505

Cutler CW, Jotwani R (2006) Dendritic cells at the oral mucosal interface. J Dent Res 85:678–689

Deans GD, Stiver HG, McElhaney JE (2010) Influenza vaccines provide diminished protection but are cost-saving in older adults. J Intern Med 267:220–227

Delneste Y, Magistrelli G, Gauchat JF, Haeuw JF, Aubry JP, Nakamura K, Kawakami-Honda N, Goetsch L, Sawamura T, Bonnefoy JY, Jeannin P (2002) Involvement of LOX-1 in dendritic cell-mediated antigen cross-presentation. Immunity 17:353–362

Dickgreber N, Stoitzner P, Bai Y, Price KM, Farrand KJ, Manning K, Angel CE, Dunbar PR, Ronchese F, Fraser JD, Backstrom BT, Hermans IF (2009) Targeting antigen to MHC class II molecules promotes efficient cross-presentation and enhances immunotherapy. J Immunol 182:1260–1269

Douillard P, Stoitzner P, Tripp CH, Clair-Moninot V, Ait-Yahia S, McLellan A, Eggert A, Romani N, Saeland S (2005) Mouse lymphoid tissue contains distinct subsets of Langerin/$CD207^+$ dendritic cells, only one of which represents epidermal-derived Langerhans cells. J Invest Dermatol 125:983–994

Dudziak D, Kamphorst AO, Heidkamp GF, Buchholz VR, Trumpfheller C, Yamazaki S, Cheong C, Liu K, Lee HW, Park CG, Steinman RM, Nussenzweig MC (2007) Differential antigen processing by dendritic cell subsets in vivo. Science 315:107–111

Dupasquier M, Stoitzner P, Van Oudenaren A, Romani N, Leenen PJM (2004) Macrophages and dendritic cells constitute a major subpopulation of cells in the mouse dermis. J Invest Dermatol 123:876–879

Dupasquier M, Prens EP, Leenen PJM (2008) Dermal mononuclear phagocytes. In: Saeland S (ed) Recent advances in skin immunology. Research Signpost, Trivandrum, India pp 75–104

Dupuis M, Murphy TJ, Higgins D, Ugozzoli M, Van Nest G, Ott G, McDonald DM (1998) Dendritic cells internalize vaccine adjuvant after intramuscular injection. Cell Immunol 186:18–27

Ebner S, Lenz A, Reider D, Fritsch P, Schuler G, Romani N (1998) Expression of maturation-/migration-related molecules on human dendritic cells from blood and skin. Immunobiology 198:568–587

Ebner S, Ratzinger G, Krösbacher B, Schmuth M, Weiss A, Reider D, Kroczek RA, Herold M, Heufler C, Fritsch P, Romani N (2001) Production of IL-12 by human monocyte-derived dendritic cells is optimal when the stimulus is given at the onset of maturation, and is further enhanced by IL-4. J Immunol 166:633–641

Ebner S, Ehammer Z, Holzmann S, Schwingshackl P, Forstner M, Stoitzner P, Huemer GM, Fritsch P, Romani N (2004) Expression of C-type lectin receptors by subsets of dendritic cells in human skin. Int Immunol 16:877–887

Ebner S, Nguyen VA, Forstner M, Wang YH, Wolfram D, Liu Y-J, Romani N (2007) Thymic stromal lymphopoietin converts human epidermal Langerhans cells into antigen presenting cells that induce pro-allergic T cells. J Allergy Clin Immunol 119:982–990

Farrand KJ, Dickgreber N, Stoitzner P, Ronchese F, Petersen TR, Hermans IF (2009) Langerin + CD8α + dendritic cells are critical for cross-priming and IL-12 production in response to systemic antigens. J Immunol 183:7732–7742

Figdor CG, Van Kooyk Y, Adema GJ (2002) C-type lectin receptors on dendritic cells and Langerhans cells. Nat Rev Immunol 2:77–84

Flacher V, Tripp CH, Stoitzner P, Haid B, Ebner S, Del Frari B, Koch F, Park CG, Steinman RM, Idoyaga J, Romani N (2010) Epidermal Langerhans cells rapidly capture and present antigens from C-type lectin-targeting antibodies deposited in the dermis. J Invest Dermatol 130:755–762

Frech SA, Dupont HL, Bourgeois AL, McKenzie R, Belkind-Gerson J, Figueroa JF, Okhuysen PC, Guerrero NH, Martinez-Sandoval FG, Melendez-Romero JH, Jiang ZD, Asturias EJ, Halpern J, Torres OR, Hoffman AS, Villar CP, Kassem RN, Flyer DC, Andersen BH, Kazempour K, Breisch SA, Glenn GM (2008) Use of a patch containing heat-labile toxin from *Escherichia coli* against travellers' diarrhoea: a phase II, randomised, double-blind, placebo-controlled field trial. Lancet 371:2019–2025

Fujii S, Shimizu K, Kronenberg M, Steinman RM (2002) Prolonged IFN-gamma-producing NKT response induced with alpha- galactosylceramide-loaded DCs. Nat Immunol 3:867–874

Fujii S, Shimizu K, Smith C, Bonifaz L, Steinman RM (2003) Activation of natural killer T cells by α-galactosylceramide rapidly induces the full maturation of dendritic cells in vivo and thereby acts as an adjuvant for combined CD4 and CD8 T cell immunity to a coadministered protein. J Exp Med 198:267–279

Fujii S, Shimizu K, Hemmi H, Steinman RM (2007) Innate Valpha14(+) natural killer T cells mature dendritic cells, leading to strong adaptive immunity. Immunol Rev 220:183–198

Gerlini G, Hefti HP, Kleinhans M, Nickoloff BJ, Burg G, Nestle FO (2001) CD1d is expressed on dermal dendritic cells and monocyte-derived dendritic cells. J Invest Dermatol 117:576–582

Ginhoux F, Collin M, Bogunovic M, Abel M, Leboef M, Helft J, Ochando JC, Kissenpfennig A, Malissen B, Grisotto M, Snoeck H, Randolph GJ, Merad M (2007) Blood-derived dermal langerin + dendritic cells survey the skin in the steady state. J Exp Med 204:3133–3146

Ginhoux F, Ng LG, Merad M (2010) Understanding the murine cutaneous dendritic cell network to improve intradermal vaccination strategies. Curr Top Microbiol Immunol 351:1–24

Girolomoni G, Caux C, Lebecque S, Dezutter-Dambuyant C, Ricciardi-Castagnoli P (2002) Langerhans cells: still a fundamental paradigm for studying the immunobiology of dendritic cells. Trends Immunol 23:6–8

Godfrey DI, Stankovic S, Baxter AG (2010) Raising the NKT cell family. Nat Immunol 11:197–206

Granelli-Piperno A, Pritsker A, Pack M, Shimeliovich I, Arrighi JF, Park CG, Trumpfheller C, Piguet V, Moran TM, Steinman RM (2005) Dendritic cell-specific intercellular adhesion molecule 3-grabbing nonintegrin/CD209 is abundant on macrophages in the normal human lymph node and is not required for dendritic cell stimulation of the mixed leukocyte reaction. J Immunol 175:4265–4273

Haniffa M, Ginhoux F, Wang XN, Bigley V, Abel M, Dimmick I, Bullock S, Grisotto M, Booth T, Taub P, Hilkens C, Merad M, Collin M (2009) Differential rates of replacement of human dermal dendritic cells and macrophages during hematopoietic stem cell transplantation. J Exp Med 206:371–385

Hart DNJ, Fabre JW (1981) Demonstration and characterization of Ia-positive dendritic cells in the interstitial connective tissues of rat heart and other tissues, but not brain. J Exp Med 154:347–361

Hawiger D, Inaba K, Dorsett Y, Guo M, Mahnke K, Rivera M, Ravetch JV, Steinman RM, Nussenzweig MC (2001) Dendritic cells induce peripheral T cell unresponsiveness under steady state conditions in vivo. J Exp Med 194:769–779

Heath WR, Carbone FR (2009) Dendritic cell subsets in primary and secondary T cell responses at body surfaces. Nat Immunol 10:1237–1244

Heath WR, Belz GT, Behrens GM, Smith CM, Forehan SP, Parish IA, Davey GM, Wilson NS, Carbone FR, Villadangos J (2004) Cross-presentation, dendritic cell subsets, and the generation of immunity to cellular antigens. Immunol Rev 199:9–26

Henri S, Vremec D, Kamath A, Waithman J, Williams S, Benoist C, Burnham K, Saeland S, Handman E, Shortman K (2001) The dendritic cell populations of mouse lymph nodes. J Immunol 167:741–748

Henri S, Poulin LF, Tamoutounour S, Ardufn L, Guilliams M, de Bovis B, Devilard E, Viret C, Azukizawa H, Kissenpfennig A, Malissen B (2010) $CD207^+$ $CD103^+$ dermal dendritic cells cross-present keratinocyte-derived antigens irrespective of the presence of Langerhans cells. J Exp Med 207:189–206

Heufler C, Koch F, Stanzl U, Topar G, Wysocka M, Trinchieri G, Enk A, Steinman RM, Romani N, Schuler G (1996) Interleukin-12 is produced by dendritic cells and mediates T helper 1 development as well as interferon-gamma production by T helper 1 cells. Eur J Immunol 26:659–668

Hickey AJ, Garmise RJ (2009) Dry powder nasal vaccines as an alternative to needle-based delivery. Crit Rev Ther Drug Carrier Syst 26:1–27

Idoyaga J, Cheong C, Suda K, Suda N, Kim JY, Lee H, Park CG, Steinman RM (2008) The Langerin/CD207 receptor on dendritic cells mediates efficient antigen presentation on MHC I and MHC II products in vivo. J Immunol 180:3647–3650

Idoyaga J, Suda N, Suda K, Park CG, Steinman RM (2009) Antibody to Langerin/CD207 localizes large numbers of $CD8\alpha^+$ dendritic cells to the marginal zone of mouse spleen. Proc Natl Acad Sci USA 106:1524–1529

Inaba K, Swiggard WJ, Inaba M, Meltzer J, Mirza A, Sasagawa T, Nussenzweig MC, Steinman RM (1995) Tissue distribution of the DEC-205 protein that is detected by the monoclonal antibody NLDC-145. I. Expression on dendritic cells and other subsets of mouse leukocytes. Cell Immunol 163:148–156

Iwasaki A (2007) Mucosal dendritic cells. Annu Rev Immunol 25:381–418

Kaplan DH, Kissenpfennig A, Clausen BE (2008) Insights into Langerhans cell function from Langerhans cell ablation models. Eur J Immunol 38:2369–2376

Kashihara M, Ueda M, Horiguchi Y, Furukawa F, Hanaoka M, Imamura S (1986) A monoclonal antibody specifically reactive to human Langerhans cells. J Invest Dermatol 87:602–612

Kissenpfennig A, Henri S, Dubois B, Laplace-Builhé C, Perrin P, Romani N, Tripp CH, Douillard P, Leserman L, Kaiserlian D, Saeland S, Davoust J, Malissen B (2005) Dynamics and function of Langerhans cells in vivo: dermal dendritic cells colonize lymph node areas distinct from slower migrating Langerhans cells. Immunity 22:643–654

Klechevsky E, Morita R, Liu M, Cao Y, Coquery S, Thompson-Snipes L, Briere F, Chaussabel D, Zurawski G, Palucka AK, Reiter Y, Banchereau J, Ueno H (2008) Functional specializations of human epidermal Langerhans cells and CD14$^+$ dermal dendritic cells. Immunity 29:497–510

Kubo A, Nagao K, Yokouchi M, Sasaki H, Amagai M (2009) External antigen uptake by Langerhans cells with reorganization of epidermal tight junction barriers. J Exp Med 206:2937–2946

Lahoud MH, Proietto AI, Ahmet F, Kitsoulis S, Eidsmo L, Wu L, Sathe P, Pietersz S, Chang HW, Walker ID, Maraskovsky E, Braley H, Lew AM, Wright MD, Heath WR, Shortman K, Caminschi I (2009) The C-type lectin Clec12A present on mouse and human dendritic cells can serve as a target for antigen delivery and enhancement of antibody responses. J Immunol 182:7587–7594

Langerhans P (1868) Über die Nerven der menschlichen Haut. Virchows Arch [A] 44:325–337

Larsen CP, Steinman RM, Witmer-Pack M, Hankins DF, Morris PJ, Austyn JM (1990) Migration and maturation of Langerhans cells in skin transplants and explants. J Exp Med 172:1483–1493

Lenz A, Heine M, Schuler G, Romani N (1993) Human and murine dermis contain dendritic cells. Isolation by means of a novel method and phenotypical and functional characterization. J Clin Invest 92:2587–2596

Lukas M, Stössel H, Hefel L, Imamura S, Fritsch P, Sepp NT, Schuler G, Romani N (1996) Human cutaneous dendritic cells migrate through dermal lymphatic vessels in a skin organ culture model. J Invest Dermatol 106:1293–1299

Mahnke K, Guo M, Lee S, Sepulveda H, Swain SL, Nussenzweig M, Steinman RM (2000) The dendritic cell receptor for endocytosis, DEC-205, can recycle and enhance antigen presentation via major histocompatibility complex class II-positive lysosomal compartments. J Cell Biol 151:673–683

Mahnke K, Qian YJ, Fondel S, Brueck J, Becker C, Enk AH (2005) Targeting of antigens to activated dendritic cells in vivo cures metastatic melanoma in mice. Cancer Res 65:7007–7012

Maier MK, Seth S, Czeloth N, Qiu Q, Ravens I, Kremmer E, Ebel M, Müller W, Pabst O, Förster R, Bernhardt G (2007) The adhesion receptor CD155 determines the magnitude of humoral immune responses against orally ingested antigens. Eur J Immunol 37:2214–2225

McLellan AD, Kapp M, Eggert A, Linden C, Bommhardt U, Bröcker EB, Kämmerer U, Kämpgen E (2002) Anatomic location and T-cell stimulatory functions of mouse dendritic cell subsets defined by CD4 and CD8 expression. Blood 99:2084–2093

Merad M, Ginhoux F, Collin M (2008) Origin, homeostasis and function of Langerhans cells and other langerin-expressing dendritic cells. Nat Rev Immunol 8:935–947

Mukhopadhaya A, Hanafusa T, Jarchum I, Chen YG, Iwai Y, Serreze DV, Steinman RM, Tarbell KV, DiLorenzo TP (2008) Selective delivery of beta cell antigen to dendritic cells in vivo leads to deletion and tolerance of autoreactive CD8$^+$ T cells in NOD mice. Proc Natl Acad Sci USA 105:6374–6379

Nagao K, Ginhoux F, Leitner WW, Motegi S, Bennett CL, Clausen BE, Merad M, Udey MC (2009) Murine epidermal Langerhans cells and langerin-expressing dermal dendritic cells are unrelated and exhibit distinct functions. Proc Natl Acad Sci USA 106:3312–3317

Nchinda G, Kuroiwa J, Oks M, Trumpfheller C, Park CG, Huang Y, Hannaman D, Schlesinger SJ, Mizenina O, Nussenzweig MC, Uberla K, Steinman RM (2008) The efficacy of DNA vaccination is enhanced in mice by targeting the encoded protein to dendritic cells. J Clin Invest 118:1427–1436

Neparidze N, Dhodapkar MV (2009) Harnessing CD1d-restricted T cells toward antitumor immunity in humans. Ann N Y Acad Sci 1174:61–67

Nestle FO, Zheng X-G, Thompson CB, Turka LA, Nickoloff BJ (1993) Characterization of dermal dendritic cells obtained from normal human skin reveals phenotypic and functionally distinctive subsets. J Immunol 151:6535–6545

Nicolas JF, Guy B (2008) Intradermal, epidermal and transcutaneous vaccination: from immunology to clinical practice. Expert Rev Vaccines 7:1201–1214

Ohl L, Mohaupt M, Czeloth N, Hintzen G, Kiafard Z, Zwirner J, Blankenstein T, Henning G, Förster R (2004) CCR7 governs skin dendritic cell migration under inflammatory and steady-state conditions. Immunity 21:279–288

Poulin LF, Henri S, de Bovis B, Devilard E, Kissenpfennig A, Malissen B (2007) The dermis contains langerin^{+} dendritic cells that develop and function independently of epidermal Langerhans cells. J Exp Med 204:3119–3131

Pulendran B, Ahmed R (2006) Translating innate immunity into immunological memory: implications for vaccine development. Cell 124:849–863

Randolph GJ, Beaulieu S, Lebecque S, Steinman RM, Muller WA (1998) Differentiation of monocytes into dendritic cells in a model of transendothelial trafficking. Science 282:480–483

Randolph GJ, Inaba K, Robbiani DF, Steinman RM, Muller WA (1999) Differentiation of phagocytic monocytes into lymph node dendritic cells in vivo. Immunity 11:753–761

Randolph GJ, Ochando J, Partida-Sánchez S (2008) Migration of dendritic cell subsets and their precursors. Annu Rev Immunol 26:293–316

Ratzinger G, Stoitzner P, Ebner S, Lutz MB, Layton GT, Rainer C, Senior RM, Shipley JM, Fritsch P, Schuler G, Romani N (2002) Matrix metalloproteinases 9 and 2 are necessary for the migration of Langerhans cells and dermal dendritic cells from human and murine skin. J Immunol 168:4361–4371

Ratzinger G, Baggers J, de Cos MA, Yuan J, Dao T, Reagan JL, Münz C, Heller G, Young JW (2004) Mature human Langerhans cells derived from CD34^{+} hemopoietic progenitors stimulate greater cytolytic T lymphocyte activity in the absence of bioactive IL-12p70, by either single peptide presentation or cross-priming, than do dermal-interstitial or monocyte-derived dendritic cells. J Immunol 173:2780–2791

Rescigno M, Urbano M, Valzasina B, Francolini M, Rotta G, Bonasio R, Granucci F, Kraehenbuhl JP, Ricciardi-Castagnoli P (2001) Dendritic cells express tight junction proteins and penetrate gut epithelial monolayers to sample bacteria. Nat Immunol 2:361–367

Romani N, Lenz A, Glassel H, Stössel H, Stanzl U, Majdic O, Fritsch P, Schuler G (1989) Cultured human Langerhans cells resemble lymphoid dendritic cells in phenotype and function. J Invest Dermatol 93:600–609

Romani N, Ratzinger G, Pfaller K, Salvenmoser W, Stössel H, Koch F, Stoitzner P (2001) Migration of dendritic cells into lymphatics—the Langerhans cell example: routes, regulation, and relevance. Int Rev Cytol 207:237–270

Romani N, Ebner S, Flacher V, Tripp CH, Heufler C, Clausen BE, Stoitzner P (2008) Langerhans cells—dendritic cells of the epidermis and other epithelia. In: Saeland S (ed) Recent advances in skin immunology. Research Signpost, Trivandrum, India pp 27–73

Romani N, Clausen BE, Stoitzner P (2010a) Langerhans cells and more: langerin-expressing dendritic cell subsets in the skin. Immunol Rev 234:120–141

Romani N, Merad M, Stingl G, Stoitzner P (2010b) Langerhans cells at the interface of medicine, science, and industry. J Invest Dermatol 130:331–335

Romani N, Thurnher M, Idoyaga J, Steinman RM, Flacher V (2010c) Targeting of antigens to skin dendritic cells: possibilities to enhance vaccine efficacy. Immunol Cell Biol 88:424–430

Schuler G, Steinman RM (1985) Murine epidermal Langerhans cells mature into potent immunostimulatory dendritic cells in vitro. J Exp Med 161:526–546

Sparber F, Tripp CH, Hermann M, Romani N, Stoitzner P (2010) Langerhans cells and dermal dendritic cells capture protein antigens in the skin: possible targets for vaccination through skin. Immunobiology 215:770–779

Steinman RM (2008a) Dendritic cells and vaccines. Proc Bayl Univ Med Cent 21:3–8

Steinman RM (2008b) Dendritic cells in vivo: a key target for a new vaccine science. Immunity 29:319–324

Steinman RM, Banchereau J (2007) Taking dendritic cells into medicine. Nature 449:419–426
Steinman RM, Nussenzweig MC (2002) Avoiding horror autotoxicus: the importance of dendritic cells in peripheral T cell tolerance. Proc Natl Acad Sci USA 99:351–358
Steinman RM, Hawiger D, Nussenzweig MC (2003) Tolerogenic dendritic cells. Annu Rev Immunol 21:685–711
Stingl G, Tamaki K, Katz SI (1980) Origin and function of epidermal Langerhans cells. Immunol Rev 53:149–174
Stoitzner P, Green LK, Jung JY, Price KM, Tripp CH, Malissen B, Kissenpfennig A, Hermans IF, Ronchese F (2008) Tumor immunotherapy by epicutaneous immunization requires Langerhans cells. J Immunol 180:1991–1998
Tacken PJ, De Vries IJM, Gijzen K, Joosten B, Wu DY, Rother RP, Faas SJ, Punt CJA, Torensma R, Adema GJ, Figdor CG (2005) Effective induction of naive and recall T-cell responses by targeting antigen to human dendritic cells via a humanized anti-DC-SIGN antibody. Blood 106:1278–1285
Tagliani E, Guermonprez P, Sepulveda J, Lopez-Bravo M, Ardavin C, Amigorena S, Benvenuti F, Burrone OR (2008) Selection of an antibody library identifies a pathway to induce immunity by targeting CD36 on steady-state CD8α + dendritic cells. J Immunol 180:3201–3209
Teunissen MBM, Haniffa M, Collin MP (2011) Insight into the immunobiology of human skin and functional specialization of skin dendritic cell subsets to innovate intradermal vaccination design. Curr Top Microbiol Immunol 351:25–76
Tripp CH, Sparber F, Hermans IF, Romani N, Stoitzner P (2009) Glycolipids injected into the skin are presented to NKT cells in the draining lymph node independently of migratory skin dendritic cells. J Immunol 182:7644–7654
Trumpfheller C, Caskey M, Nchinda G, Longhi MP, Mizenina O, Huang Y, Schlesinger SJ, Colonna M, Steinman RM (2008) The microbial mimic poly IC induces durable and protective $CD4^+$ T cell immunity together with a dendritic cell targeted vaccine. Proc Natl Acad Sci USA 105:2574–2579
Turville SG, Cameron PU, Handley A, Lin G, Pohlmann S, Doms RW, Cunningham AL (2002) Diversity of receptors binding HIV on dendritic cell subsets. Nat Immunol 3:975–983
Ueno H, Schmitt N, Klechevsky E, Pedroza-Gonzalez A, Matsui T, Zurawski G, Oh S, Fay J, Pascual V, Banchereau J, Palucka K (2010) Harnessing human dendritic cell subsets for medicine. Immunol Rev 234:199–212
Valladeau J, Duvert-Frances V, Pin JJ, Dezutter-Dambuyant C, Vincent C, Massacrier C, Vincent J, Yoneda K, Banchereau J, Caux C, Davoust J, Saeland S (1999) The monoclonal antibody DCGM4 recognizes Langerin, a protein specific of Langerhans cells, and is rapidly internalized from the cell surface. Eur J Immunol 29:2695–2704
Valladeau J, Ravel O, Dezutter-Dambuyant C, Moore K, Kleijmeer M, Liu Y, Duvert-Frances V, Vincent C, Schmitt D, Davoust J, Caux C, Lebecque S, Saeland S (2000) Langerin, a novel C-type lectin specific to Langerhans cells, is an endocytic receptor that induces the formation of Birbeck granules. Immunity 12:71–81
Wang B, Kuroiwa JM, He LZ, Charalambous A, Keler T, Steinman RM (2009) The human cancer antigen mesothelin is more efficiently presented to the mouse immune system when targeted to the DEC-205/CD205 receptor on dendritic cells. Ann N Y Acad Sci 1174:6–17
Warger T, Schild H, Rechtsteiner G (2007) Initiation of adaptive immune responses by transcutaneous immunization. Immunol Lett 109:13–20
Weinlich G, Heine M, Stössel H, Zanella M, Stoitzner P, Ortner U, Smolle J, Koch F, Sepp NT, Schuler G, Romani N (1998) Entry into afferent lymphatics and maturation in situ of migrating cutaneous dendritic cells. J Invest Dermatol 110:441–448
Wilson NS, Villadangos JA (2004) Lymphoid organ dendritic cells: beyond the Langerhans cells paradigm. Immunol Cell Biol 82:91–98
Witmer-Pack MD, Valinsky J, Olivier W, Steinman RM (1987) Quantitation of surface antigens on cultured murine epidermal Langerhans cells: rapid and selective increase in the level of surface MHC products. J Invest Dermatol 90:387–394

Yamazaki S, Steinman RM (2009) Dendritic cells as controllers of antigen-specific Foxp3$^+$ regulatory T cells. J Dermatol Sci 54:69–75

Yamazaki S, Dudziak D, Heidkamp GF, Fiorese C, Bonito AJ, Inaba K, Nussenzweig MC, Steinman RM (2008) CD8$^+$ CD205$^+$ splenic dendritic cells are specialized to induce Foxp3$^+$ regulatory T cells. J Immunol 181:6923–6933

Zaba LC, Fuentes-Duculan J, Steinman RM, Krueger JG, Lowes MA (2007) Normal human dermis contains distinct populations of CD11c$^+$BDCA-1$^+$ dendritic cells and CD163$^+$FXIIIA$^+$ macrophages. J Clin Invest 117:2517–2525

Zaba LC, Krueger JG, Lowes MA (2009) Resident and inflammatory dendritic cells in human skin. J Invest Dermatol 129:302–308

Intradermal Rabies Vaccination: The Evolution and Future of Pre- and Post-exposure Prophylaxis

M. J. Warrell

Abstract Inactivated rabies vaccines have been used to pioneer the immunological and economical advantages of intradermal (ID) administration over 35 years. Vaccine shortages or its prohibitive cost stimulated studies of various doses, frequency and sites of injection. An economical regimen for pre-exposure prophylaxis requires one-tenth of an intramuscular dose, but the early popularity of the method has been stifled by pharmaceutical regulations. There has also been reluctance to use multiple-site post-exposure ID regimens, except in a very few Asian counties. A new four-site ID regimen could overcome many of the problems encountered to date. The time is ripe to make dramatic progress towards efficient use of the current excellent vaccines globally, wherever there is a shortage of vaccine or funds.

Contents

M. J. Warrell (✉)
Oxford Vaccine Group, Centre for Clinical Vaccinology & Tropical Medicine,
Churchill Hospital, University of Oxford, Oxford, OX3 7LJ, UK
e-mail: mary.warrell@ndm.ox.ac.uk

Current Topics in Microbiology and Immunology (2012) 351: 139–157
DOI: 10.1007/82_2010_121

Published Online: 26 January 2011

1 Introduction

Prophylaxis against human rabies encephalitis can be 100% effective; no failures of combined pre- and post-exposure treatment have been reported. Therefore, the many thousands of agonising deaths a year are all due to a failure to provide adequate prophylaxis. In developing countries, surveillance is poor or non-existent, especially in most of Africa. The much quoted estimate of 55,270 (90% CI 24,000–93,000) annual human rabies deaths in Asia and Africa is based on assumptions and extrapolation. Probably only 3% of cases are recorded by authorities (Knobel et al. 2005). The dominant reservoir species of this zoonosis is the domestic dog, and dog rabies virus strains are responsible for >99% of human disease (WHO 2007). Worldwide, ten million people are estimated to receive post-exposure prophylaxis annually.

There are seven Lyssavirus genotypes. Genotype 1, rabies, is found in dogs and other terrestrial mammal reservoir species, and in the Americas only, also in bats. Genotypes 2–6 are rabies-related Lyssaviruses whose reservoir hosts are some bats in Europe, Africa and Asia (with the exception of the rare genotype 3, Mokola virus, in rodents in Africa).

The success of prophylaxis is related to the unique pathogenesis of rabies. When the virus is inoculated under the skin during an animal bite, it may infect cells and replicate locally before entering a neuron. The virus hijacks the retrograde axonal transport mechanism, travels up the nerve, replicates, crosses a synapse and progresses thus towards the brain (Schnell et al. 2010; Ugolini 2010). Here intraneuronal replication and viral spread result in encephalitis and inevitable death. Only two patients infected by American bat rabies, one 40 and the other 5 years ago, are reported to have survived rabies encephalitis without severe neurological impairment. Dog virus infection is a more aggressive and intractable disease.

The immunological response which correlates best with protection following rabies challenge in animals is neutralising antibody, which is induced only by the glycoprotein epitopes on the surface of the virion. This association is not perfect, viral nucleoprotein is also immunogenic and cell-mediated immunity is also induced variably by vaccines, but their roles are unknown. In experimental encephalitis, however, the development of a cytotoxic T lymphocyte response correlated with survival (Wiktor et al. 1977). During infection by virulent virus, immune $CD3^{+}$ T cells migrate into the CNS, but are destroyed by apoptosis on contact with infected neurons (Lafon 2005).

There is an opportunity to prevent infection after a bite by killing or neutralising the virus in the wound. Once inside a neuron, the virus is assumed to be protected from immune attack. The first-aid treatment is thorough wound washing with copious soap and water. The lipid in the viral coat is sensitive to detergent. Rapid provision of local neutralising antibody seems to be crucial to survival. Ideally, previous pre-exposure rabies immunisation will have induced circulating antibody and primed T lymphocytes which now respond to an immediate booster dose of rabies vaccine by increasing the titre. Alternatively, in unvaccinated patients, passive immunisation with rabies immunoglobulin (RIG) is injected into and around the wound, because it will take about a week before the primary vaccine course induces antibody.

Since the untreated mortality from proven rabid dog bites is 15–45%, modern post-exposure treatment is remarkably effective. No deaths have been reported in anyone who had pre-exposure vaccination and booster doses after exposure. There are fewer than ten known cases of death despite optimal primary post-exposure treatment started on the day of the bite, in otherwise healthy recipients. Apparent 'failure of treatment' is due to failure to deliver the recommended wound cleaning and active and passive immunisation promptly, or failure of the patients' immune response.

The quality of rabies vaccines has improved slowly over the 120 years since Pasteur's first treatment with desiccated rabbit spinal cord vaccine (Turner 1969). Vaccine homogenates of animal brain contain minute amounts of viral antigen compared with the vast quantity of nervous tissue. However, Semple and Fermi sheep brain vaccines, and also suckling mouse brain vaccine, are still used as daily injections in several countries, although condemned by the WHO. Avian embryo vaccines were an advance, relatively free of neurological reactions, and a purified duck embryo vaccine is now produced in India (after transfer of technology from Switzerland). Higher potency vaccines of tissue culture origin have been used increasingly since the 1970s (Turner 1984). Three of these currently meet the WHO criteria: human diploid cell vaccine (HDCV), purified chick embryo cell vaccine (PCECV) and purified VeRO cell vaccine (PVRV). Other vaccines are made in India, Russia, China and Brazil, but their immunogenicity is uncertain. The standard post-exposure course is five intramuscular (IM) doses over 4 weeks (on days 0, 3, 7, 14 and 28). An alternative shorter four-dose IM regimen has 2 doses on the first day, with single doses on days 7 and 21. The pre-exposure regimen is three doses over 4 weeks (Table 1).

Table 1 ID rabies vaccine regimens compared with standard IM

Vaccine regimen & route	Vaccine administration timeline					Number of visits	Total ampoules
	Day of injection (Number of sites injected)						
Pre-exposure							
IM	0		7		28	3	3
ID 0.1 ml[a]	0		7		28	3	< 1
Post-exposure (+ RIG day 0)							
IM	0	3	7	14	28	5	5
2-site ID	0 **(x2)**	3 **(x2)**	7 **(x2)**		28 **(x2)**	4	< 2
4-site ID[b]	0 **(x4)**		7 **(x2)**		28	3	< 2[c]
Post-exposure if previous vaccine course							
IM	0	3				2	2
ID	0 **(x4)**					1	1 (or < 1)[d]

[a] ID doses are all 0.1 ml/site of injection
[b] ID doses are 0.1 ml/site for PVRV vaccine (0.5 ml/ampoule) or the equivalent dose 0.2 ml per site of injection for PCECV vaccine (1.0 ml/ampoule). See text in Sect. 4.8 for explanation and alternative dose 0.1 ml per site with PCECV
[c] If no sharing of vaccine maximum of three ampoules used
[d] Whole ampoule used, alternatively 0.1 ml/site if sharing 1 ml vaccine. See text in Sect. 5.1 for details
The *red colour* is the main subject of the article, intradermal injections, and the *bold* to differentiate sites of injection from days of treatment.

2 The Beginning of ID Use of Rabies Vaccine

Rabies vaccine was first used ID in 1960 to reduce the amount of potential allergens inoculated during a pre-exposure course of duck embryo vaccine. Three doses of 0.2 ml ID proved immunogenic in 75% of 49 students (Anderson et al. 1960).

2.1 Site of Injection

Injecting duck embryo vaccine ID on the medial surface of the forearm caused more local side effects than inoculating ID over the deltoid, but the forearm injections induced higher antibody titres (Schnurrenberger et al. 1965). Using the same arm for IM injections was more immunogenic than if vaccine was given into alternating arms (Peck and Kohlstaedt 1964). These results may not be applicable to modern potent rabies vaccines because the vaccine tested was a relatively weak antigen. However, in case the site of injection is important, future vaccine trials could record the details, and perhaps investigate immunogenicity at different sites.

2.2 Experiments with Tissue Culture Vaccines ID for Pre-exposure Use

Human diploid cell vaccine, licensed in 1974, was the first tissue culture vaccine to be injected ID for reasons of economy rather than safety by taking advantage of the protective immunological mechanisms which have evolved in the skin. The presence of antigen-presenting dendritic and Langerhans cells at the site of antigen inoculation facilitates transfer to local lymph nodes. T cells are then activated more efficiently and rapidly than after IM inoculation (Nicolas and Guy 2008; Teunissen et al. 2011). One tenth, 0.1 ml, of the dose of HDCV given ID (2 injections a month apart) was as immunogenic as the usual IM dose and induced much higher antibody levels than the then standard duck embryo vaccine (Aoki et al. 1975).

Pre-exposure immunisation aims to induce a prolonged presence of neutralising antibody in 100% of vaccines using the minimum amount of vaccine. A study of 194 volunteers for 3 years showed that higher and more durable antibody titres were induced by 3 doses (days 0, 28 and 56) rather than 2, whether ID or IM. Although the titres were adequate with ID injections, they were higher in the IM groups. The rapid and marked serological response to a booster dose was not influenced by the route of injection of the primary course, although the titres were higher with deep subcutaneous (SC) injection than via the ID route. After boosting, the antibody response began at 48 h and peaked at 8–16 days (Turner et al. 1982). The results of this early study have proved to be the principle features of ID immunisation, borne out by many subsequent reports over 30 years.

To test the immunogenicity of the same dose given ID and IM, a three-dose pre-exposure course of 0.1 ml of vaccine ID was compared with an identical dose IM. Significantly higher titres were induced by the ID route, and all exceeded the WHO minimum level (Fishbein et al. 1987). Similarly a whole dose divided between multiple ID sites was more immunogenic than the same dose IM (Phanuphak et al. 1987; Khawplod et al. 2002b).

2.3 Varying ID Doses and Side Effects

Meanwhile in Germany, between 2 and 4 ID doses of 0.2 ml of HDCV given over 28 days proved immunogenic (vaccine potency only 1.2 IU/ml, half the current minimum of 2.5 IU/ml) (Cox and Schneider 1976). The investigators' concern that ID injection might cause sensitisation proved unfounded. In France, dividing a 0.1 ml ID HDCV dose into two 0.05 ml ID doses gave similar antibody levels. The ID regimens gave good seroconversion but the titres were lower than two SC doses of 1 ml (Ajjan et al. 1980).

Local reactions at ID injection sites were greater during primary than booster inoculation (Nicholson et al. 1978). Studies over 30 years show that the systemic side effects after ID treatment are similar to those of IM doses but that local reactions, usually erythema and irritation, are more frequent.

2.4 The Effects of Incorrect ID Injection Technique

Injecting ID vaccine below the dermis is assumed to impair immunogenicity. When a 0.1 ml ID vaccine dose was erroneously deposited SC, the antibody response was significantly diminished. Although all volunteers seroconverted, not all the SC recipients' results reached 0.5 IU/ml (Bernard et al. 1982). Increasing the SC dose to 0.25 ml was as immunogenic as the 0.1 ml ID route. To investigate the effect of failing to inject the correct amount of vaccine, dilutions of vaccine were given in 0.1 ml doses, both IM and ID, with a full IM dose control. The lowest doses, IM (3% of the full dose) and ID (1% of an IM dose), still induced antibody above the CDC minimum titre (1:5) in all, but some were <0.5 IU/ml. Overall, the dose response curve for the ID route was parallel to, but higher than that for the IM route (Fishbein et al. 1987). The number of subjects in these two studies was about 25 per group, and the potency of the vaccine was 3.8 IU/ml. Phanuphak et al. (1990) simulated erroneous ID injection in two sites and found adequate antibody on day 14, even if one or both injections were SC. The potency of this particular vaccine was high at >10 IU/dose. However, another study compared 0.2 ml of HDCV SC in four sites with the same regimen of 0.1 ml ID per site. The SC gave poor results on day 7 and lower titres throughout (Warrell et al. 1984). The depth of SC injection may be important.

In conclusion: failing to deliver the complete ID dose, or unintended SC or IM injection, could result in lower antibody levels in some cases. For pre-exposure immunisation, this is unlikely to occur with all three inoculations, so the course would still be immunogenic, resulting in an accelerated secondary response to a subsequent post-exposure booster dose. Hence occasional faulty technique is not a cause of concern for 0.1 ml ID pre-exposure prophylaxis.

3 Pre-exposure Immunisation

3.1 The Introduction of ID Pre-exposure Vaccination

At first, the pre-exposure regimens varied in different countries (Roumiantzeff et al. 1988), but three IM doses on days 0, 7 and 28 became accepted as the standard (WHO 1992) (Table 1). The immunogenicity of ID immunisation was proven in several trials in Europe and the USA (Roumiantzeff et al. 1988). In 1984 the WHO first recommended pre-exposure vaccination with an ID dose of 0.1 ml as alternative to IM 1 ml (WHO 1984), and it was recommended for use in the UK (Immunisation against infectious disease 1984). ID treatment was officially recognised as acceptable in the USA in 1982 (CDC 1982). As the vaccine contained no preservative and was not registered as a multi-dose vial, it could not be approved by the FDA, and in 1984 it was recommended for ID use if the whole ampoule was used immediately (CDC 1984). A new packaging containing 1/10th of the IM dose was then sanctioned by the FDA in the USA (Dreesen et al. 1984). However, the 0.1 ml HDCV preparation was expensive to produce, proved uneconomical and was withdrawn.

Peace Corps workers and others immunised in developing counties were found to have lower antibody titres after ID immunisation. A thorough investigation (Bernard et al. 1985) concluded that multiple factors, including the immunosuppressive effect of concomitant chloroquine malaria prophylaxis (Pappaioanou et al. 1986), were responsible. As a result, the CDC ruled that ID immunisation should be completed before departure to a rabies endemic area. Otherwise, and for anyone taking chloroquine, the vaccine should be given IM (CDC 1986). It was considered unnecessary to confirm seroconversion after ID vaccination.

The VeRO cell vaccine, PVRV, was licensed in 1985, with an IM dose of 0.5 ml. The ID dose remained at 0.1 ml for pre-exposure immunisation because it is the smallest volume practicable, although double the amount of antigen is given.

3.2 Current Practice of ID Pre-exposure Rabies Prophylaxis

ID pre-exposure immunisation has now been recommended by the WHO for 25 years.

Serological testing after vaccination is recommended only if immunosuppression is suspected (WHO 2005). Nevertheless, there has been concern over low antibody levels (Lau and Sisson 2002). ELISA serological tests are not considered as accurate as the rapid fluorescent focus inhibition neutralising antibody test, especially at low levels. Checking titres after ID pre-exposure immunisation is, therefore, recommended in some places (Australian Immunisation Handbook 2008; Canada Communicable Disease Report 2005). However, the importance of maintaining a detectable antibody level is unknown. The immune response to booster doses is predictable even if the antibody level was low previously (Turner et al. 1982; Horman et al. 1987; Fishbein et al. 1986). Vaccine is not always available promptly after an exposure, and so a booster dose might be advisable before travel to remote areas. Alternatively serological testing is recommended as another dose is unnecessary if antibody is detectable. There is one report of rabies following pre-exposure prophylaxis with a tissue culture vaccine: that of a Peace Corps worker who received ID immunisation was bitten by a dog in Kenya but had no post-exposure treatment (Bernard et al. 1985). Her death is attributed to failure to give vaccine after exposure.

The ID route is not currently recommended in the USA (Manning et al. 2008) or in the UK (Dept of Health 2006). The main reason is that the vaccines contain no preservative, and so sharing ampoules for ID use does not comply with pharmaceutical regulations for multi-dose vaccines, and is considered 'off label' use in many countries, although ID immunisation may be given on the responsibility of the doctor. There is unsubstantiated concern over the ability of staff to inject ID, but if an ID injection fails to raise a characteristic bleb, another dose can be given immediately at an adjacent site. No problems have been reported by users. Once opened, an ampoule of vaccine can be shared between several people who can be immunised on the same day. A new syringe and needle must be used for each patient. The opened vial is kept in the fridge and discarded after 8 h (WHO 2005).

Pre-exposure immunisation is often considered prohibitively expensive, especially in the USA (Trevejo 2000). About 26% of travellers to rabies endemic areas, who refused vaccination, considered it unaffordable (Altmann et al. 2009).

However, reliance on having post-exposure prophylaxis abroad if exposed to rabies is unwise, as correct treatment was provided locally in only 24% cases (Hatz et al. 1995). Sharing an ampoule within a group reduces the cost and is suitable for use in travel clinics also for families, students, veterinarians, international aid workers, military personnel and most important, for residents of dog rabies endemic areas. Doctors should not be afraid to comply with the WHO guidelines and give vaccine ID to people who would otherwise have none. If there is no time for the complete pre-exposure course, give one or two doses and warn the recipient that they should have full post-exposure prophylaxis if exposed to rabies. The immunisation can be completed or restarted later. Having had any previous vaccine is an immunological advantage if exposed to rabies.

4 Post-exposure Immunisation

4.1 Rabies Tissue Culture Vaccines ID for Post-exposure Prophylaxis

Rabies vaccines are unique because they are usually used in an emergency to induce rapid immunity following exposure to a rabid animal. The criteria required for rabies post-exposure vaccination are, therefore: the speed of antibody induction; to be consistently immunogenic throughout the population; to be easy to use and to be acceptable to patients and staff, and affordable. In Africa the cost of the five-dose post-exposure IM course is US$39, which is prohibitive since half the Sub-Saharan population subsists on less than US$1.25 a day. In Asia, stopping the production of nervous tissue vaccines, usually provided free of charge, has recently increased the need for tissue culture vaccines, for which patients often have to pay. For the past 25 years, attempts have been made to reduce the cost by: decreasing the dose of vaccine; changing the route of injection; the number of sites of application; the timing of the doses and adding adjuvants or immunostimulants.

Multiple-site injection was first suggested by Dr David Tyrrell as emergency prophylaxis for staff caring for two rabies patients in London hospitals, with a limited amount of available vaccine. Four ID injections of 0.1 ml HDCV, one into each limb on day 0, induced detectable rabies neutralising antibody significantly more rapidly (by day 7) than if 0.1 ml of vaccine was given ID as 4 daily doses on days 0, 3, 7 and 14 (Turner et al. 1976). The principle of giving multiple ID doses on the first day was pursued and eight ID 0.1 ml doses were given on a single day anecdotally, including to two people resulting in very much higher antibody levels than the standard IM regimen by day 7 (Nicholson et al. 1979, 1981). Rabbits were protected against viral challenge by four ID doses, at least as effectively as an IM dose of HDCV (Nicholson et al. 1981). For further data on the relationship between ID vaccine dose and immunogenicity see Sect. 4.5.

The initial cell-mediated immune response induced by multiple-site ID HDCV injection was significantly higher than twice the dose by the IM route, according to a lymphocyte transformation test (Ratanavongsiri et al. 1985). Doubling or tripling the initial IM dose of vaccine was explored (Anderson et al. 1981; Suntharasamai et al. 1987a, b), and although the results were encouraging, it was not economical.

4.2 *The Evolution of the First Economical Multi-Site ID Post-exposure Regimen*

The rate and quality of the immune response to nine different economical candidate post-exposure vaccine regimens were compared with the standard regimens of IM HDCV and Semple vaccine (Warrell et al. 1983, 1984). The most rapid, consistently high level of neutralising antibody occurred after a regimen of: a whole ampoule of HDCV divided between eight sites ID on day 0, 0.1 ml ID at four sites on day 7 and 0.1 ml ID at single sites on days 28 and 91. Giving a low dose of antigen risks immunosuppression by concomitant RIG treatment, but adequate antibody was still induced despite an inadvertent double dose of human RIG on day 0 (Warrell et al. 1984). The serological results were still adequate if the first day's dose was changed to only four ID injections (Suntharasamai et al. 1987a), which provides reassurance if the accuracy of the ID injection technique is uncertain. The method uses less than 40% of the vaccine of the IM regimen, and has fewer clinic visits. The eight sites chosen for injection were the deltoid, thigh, suprascapular and lower anterior abdominal wall areas, which all drain to different groups of potentially responsive lymph nodes.

4.3 *Eight-Site ID Regimen*

This eight-site regimen was then tested clinically in 155 patients bitten by proven rabid animals in a randomised comparative trial of the eight-site ID HDCV regimen or with the Semple vaccine used at that time (Warrell et al. 1985). Patients with severe bites also had ERIG. On day 7, 88% of patients given ID HDCV alone had detectable antibody, and in 33% it was >0.5 IU/ml. All in the HDCV groups had antibody >0.5 IU/ml from day 14 to 1 year, and RIG did not significantly suppress the immune response to this reduced dose of antigen. The antibody response to Semple vaccine was much lower. After 2 years no deaths from rabies have been detected amongst the vaccinees. The immunogenicity of the eight-site regimen using PCECV has been confirmed (Suntharasamai et al. 1987a; Madhusudana et al. 2001), including in 32 patients with proven exposure to rabies with or without RIG (Madhusudana et al. 2002). The eight-site regimen meets all the WHO requirements for post-exposure use.

4.4 Two-Site ID Regimen

The new PVRV was licensed with an IM dose of only 0.5 ml, making it unsuitable for use with the eight-site regimen. Hence, in 1990 the Thai Red Cross Institute devised an economical ID regimen for PVRV. Two ID 0.1 ml doses were given over the deltoids on days 0, 3 and 7, with single site ID doses on days 28 and 90. The immunogenicity of this two-site regimen was equivalent to that of the IM 5 dose treatment, and it was chosen for use, despite the fact that double the dose gave higher antibody levels during the crucial early weeks (Phanuphak et al. 1987). In a post-exposure trial, 100 patients bitten by proven rabid animals were given the two-site PVRV regimen with RIG. 19 had severe bites. Serology on only ten patients showed antibody >0.5 IU/ml from day 14 to 1 year, and no rabies deaths occurred (Chutivongse et al. 1990).

The ID dose with PVRV was 0.1 ml, and the equivalent dose with PCECV (1 ml per ampoule) was 0.2 ml/site. The two-site method used the same total amount of vaccine as the eight-site, and the only difference between them is that the large first dose of the eight-site regimen is divided between days 0 and 3 in the two-site regimen, which therefore needs an extra clinic visit. The eight-site method induced higher levels of neutralising antibody than the two-site regimen, from day 7 to a year later (Madhusudana et al. 2001, WHO 2005). These two economical regimens were recommended by the WHO for use where insufficient vaccine was available for the IM regimen (WHO 1997).

Subsequently, half the original dose of PCECV, 0.1 ml per ID site, with the two-site regimen was shown to induce adequate antibody levels (Suntharasamai et al. 1994, Madhusudana et al. 2004). After post-exposure studies (Briggs et al. 2000; Quiambao et al. 2005; Madhusudana et al. 2006) the WHO recommended 0.1 ml as a standard ID dose for either vaccine in 2005. Hence the current two-site regimen with PCECV needs half the amount of antigen than is used for PVRV. The method has been used for several years in parts of Thailand, and also four other Asian countries, where RIG is usually available for severe cases. Unpublished studies gave rise to concern about the immunogenicity of this lower dose two-site regimen, and higher potency PCECV was demanded in Thailand and other countries (Dodet 2007). This should no longer be necessary as an alternative regimen is available. An option was also introduced to omit the day 90 dose and to double the dose on day 28 (WHO 2005, 2007) (Table 1).

4.5 The Relationship Between ID Vaccine Dose and Immunogenicity

To design an economical regimen, the relationship between the amount of vaccine injected and the antibody titre induced is crucial. An increasing antibody response correlated with the number of 0.1 ml ID injections of HDCV (1, 2, 4 or 8 ID doses) given on a single day (Täuber et al. 1986). Diluting PCECV given by a multiple-site ID regimen clearly confirmed that the antibody response rises with the ID antigen dose (Beran et al. 2006). Unfortunately these data failed to reveal an inevitable upper threshold of antigen, above which the antibody levels reach a plateau. Further studies showed that doubling the ID dose of PVRV from approximately half to a whole ampoule of vaccine on days 0 and 3 (Phanuphak et al. 1987) or from one to two ampoules ID on day 0 (Quiambao et al. 2008) gave higher antibody levels on day 7 ($p < 0.0005$, $p < 0.001$, respectively). Another study agreed with the results of Phanuphak, and also showed that two ampoules ID on day 0 showed no immunological advantage over one ampoule on days 0 and 3 (Khawplod et al. 2002b). The same dose IM was less immunogenic in all the studies.

The conclusions are that a whole ampoule on days 0 and 3 gives better results than half that dose and there is no clear further benefit from two ampoules on day 0. Limitations of the data published restrict further interpretation. The minimum antigen threshold giving maximum immunogenicity is at least one ampoule on the first day.

4.6 Problems with ID Post-exposure Vaccine Regimens

The eight-site and the two-site regimens have been recommended by the WHO for 13 years (WHO 1997). They can be economical (Goswami et al. 2005), but their widespread implementation has been hindered by: lack of confidence in low dose regimens against this fatal disease; confusing dosages; the need for more than one patient to be treated the same day; pharmaceutical restrictions over multi-dose vials; the eight-site is inconvenient to use and is not economical with PVRV (0.5 ml per vial) and because they have not been promoted. As a result ID vaccine regimens are used in a few places in Asia, mainly in big clinics, but this approach is practically unknown in Africa. Radical changes are necessary to introduce economical prophylaxis into more counties and especially into rural areas, where most rabies deaths occur.

4.7 Four-Site ID Regimen

The sharing of ampoules of vaccine and number of clinic visits would be reduced by modifying the eight-site regimen to four-site one to give the same antigen dose but in half the number of ID sites, so that it can be used with any vaccine. The four-site ID regimen using PVRV (0.5 ml/ampoule) consists of:

Day 0: 4 × 0.1 ml (approximately) ID injections over the deltoid and thigh.
Day 7: 2 × 0.1 ml ID injections over the deltoid.
Day 28: one dose ID over the deltoid (Table 1).

The timing of this dose may be adjusted to enable economy by sharing vials. For example a clinic might assign just 2 or 3 days a week for the final treatment. This simplified ID regimen was tested in a randomised controlled comparison with the eight-site and the two-site ID regimens and the standard IM regimen. The results demonstrated that the four-site ID regimen is at least as immunogenic as the IM 'gold standard' (Warrell et al. 2008). The method meets the WHO criteria of immunogenicity, and supersedes the eight-site regimen.

Four-site injections of PVRV in this trial used a whole ampoule of vaccine on day 0, but if PCECV (1 ml/ampoule) is used, 0.4 ml is half an ampoule in practice. Ambrozaitis et al. (2006) tested the four-site regimen with these two vaccines, without any comparison with a standard regimen. They found that an ID dose of 0.1 ml/site of both vaccines gave similar antibody levels. They injected deltoid and suprascapular sites, which gives an alternative method which might be helpful in cultures where there is reluctance to expose the thighs.

Quiambao et al. (2008) also confirmed the immunogenicity of the four-site regimen in comparison to the IM and the two-site regimens.

4.8 Practical Aspects of the Four-Site ID Regimen

Only three visits to the clinic are needed with the four-site regimen, on the same days as the routine pre-exposure course (0, 7 and 28), but it uses less vaccine (Table 1). This regimen is economical if two or more patients are treated together, and there still is a saving of vaccine if only one patient is treated (using three vials instead of five doses IM). Any vaccine that is left over can be used as ID pre-exposure vaccination for others, but with a new syringe and needle for each patient, and remaining vaccine must be kept cool and discarded at the end of the day.

With PCECV (1 ml ampoule), a standard 0.1 ml dose per ID site may be suitable for use in clinics treating more than one person on the same day with limited resources. Otherwise and if only one patient is treated on the first day, the dose equivalent to that for PVRV is used: on day 0, a whole 1 ml ampoule is divided between four sites ID over the deltoid and thigh/suprascapular areas. On day 7, two 0.2 ml ID injections over the deltoid, and on day 28 a single 0.2 ml dose ID. Any difficulty in injecting 0.2 ml ID is solved by withdrawing the needle and injecting the remainder in an adjacent area (Chi et al. 2010). This prevents wastage of vaccine on the first day and provides a large immune stimulus immediately, increasing the chance of survival for patients who fail to complete the vaccine course. Accidental SC instead of ID injection should not impair the immunogenicity because a whole ampoule is used and half the ID dose is adequately immunogenic (Ambrozaitis et al. 2006). This gives a wide margin of safety, an essential requirement as it is likely to be used by inexperienced staff especially in developing countries with a high prevalence of HIV infection.

5 Post-exposure Vaccination in Previously Immunised Patients

5.1 A New Single-Day ID Regimen

For those who have already had a complete pre- or post-exposure course of vaccine, no RIG is needed and a shorter course of two IM booster doses of vaccine are given, on days 0 and 3. An alternative single-day treatment is to inject 0.1 ml of vaccine ID at four sites on the deltoid and thigh or suprascapular regions (Table 1). This has proved at least as immunogenic as the IM method (Tantawichien et al. 1999; Khawplod et al. 2002a); it has been used in thousands of patients in Thailand and has been approved by the WHO. In practice using PVRV, the whole (0.5 ml) ampoule of vaccine is divided between 4 ID injections. With PCECV, 0.1 ml × 4 is about half a 1 ml ampoule, giving half the dose. When used in clinics with more than one patient a day, sharing ampoules would be economical, but if only one person is treated, vaccine wastage should be avoided. It is then more practical, and safer in inexperienced hands, to recommend using a whole ampoule of any vaccine divided between four ID sites.

6 The Future?

Inactivated rabies vaccines have been used to pioneer the immunological and economical advantages of ID vaccine administration over 35 years. Recent events have created an opportunity to make dramatic progress towards efficient use of the current excellent vaccines globally, wherever there is a shortage of vaccine or funds.

Changes in pharmaceutical regulations have been precipitated by the hurried registration of 2009 pandemic H1N1 influenza vaccines without any preservative in multi-dose vials. If these rules were applied to rabies vaccines, the avoidable risk of cross-contamination could be rationally balanced against the risk of death from rabies.

6.1 In Developing Countries

Primary vaccination alone may not prevent rabies after severe exposure, but RIG is often not available in many countries in dog rabies enzootic areas, and the patient usually has to bear the cost (Dodet 2006, 2009b). This is unlikely to change even when new rabies monoclonal antibody products are introduced in several years' time, but the need for RIG treatment could be avoided if children were routinely vaccinated. ID pre-exposure vaccination proved immunogenic with a regimen suitable for inclusion in routine immunisation schedules (Vien et al. 2008; Kamoltham et al. 2007), and ID rabies vaccination of school children has begun in the Philippines (Dodet 2009a). This is probably too expensive for widespread use, but it may be economical in areas with a high incidence of potentially rabid dog bites.

The reasons for the dismal uptake of post-exposure ID vaccine regimens in developing counties have been discussed, but the advent of a simplified more practical four-site regimen provides an opportunity to increase confidence in using vaccine ID in the rural areas of Africa and Asia where it is most needed. Co-ordinated activity of professional networks including the Southern and Eastern African Rabies Group, the Africa Rabies Expert Bureau and the Asian Rabies Expert Bureau, provides a means of introducing appropriate improvements in human prophylaxis and dog rabies control.

6.2 In Developed Countries

The importance of economy in rabies vaccine use has resulted from intermittent shortages and the prohibitive cost to governments, patients and to travellers who cannot afford immunisation. A lack of supplies recently caused the CDC temporarily to withhold pre-exposure vaccination in the USA (Bourhy et al. 2009). The reintroduction of pre-exposure ID treatment with current vaccine is being considered (Recuenco et al. 2009) to help overcome future vaccine shortages. In some developed countries ID pre-exposure vaccination may be given on the doctors' responsibility. Since there has been no recorded failure of this treatment if a booster dose is given after exposure to rabies, doctors should not be afraid to implement the WHO guidelines (WHO 1984, 2007) to reduce the costs by sharing vaccine vials, especially for those who would otherwise remain unvaccinated.

Novel devices for delivering antigen ID (Kim et al. 2011) are being evaluated for influenza (Falsey 2010) and other antigens including rabies (Laurent et al. 2010). Although more convenient and less prone to error or contamination, the same amount of antigen has been used as with the usual Mantoux syringe. There has been no comparison of the immunogenicity of the old and new ID injection methods. A microneedle or other delivery system might be useful for the relatively small market of pre-exposure prophylaxis in developed countries, but they are unlikely to be practical in the foreseeable future where rabies vaccine is most needed, as post-exposure prophylaxis in Africa and Asia.

The five-dose post-exposure IM regimen can be reduced to a three dose, four-site ID regimen without contravening any pharmaceutical regulations, although vaccine is wasted. Global rabies prophylaxis in the twenty-first century could become predominantly ID until new vaccines, for example a live genetically engineered virus product (Cenna et al. 2009), prove effective and practicable to implement.

References

Ajjan N, Soulebot JP, Triau R, Biron G (1980) Intradermal immunization with rabies vaccine. Inactivated Wistar strain cultivated in human diploid cells. JAMA 244:2528–2531

Altmann M, Parola P, Delmont J, Brouqui P, Gautret P (2009) Knowledge, attitudes, and practices of French travelers from Marseille regarding rabies risk and prevention. J Travel Med 16:107–111

Ambrozaitis A, Laiskonis A, Balciuniene L, Banzhoff A, Malerczyk C (2006) Rabies post-exposure prophylaxis vaccination with purified chick embryo cell vaccine (PCECV) and purified Vero cell rabies vaccine (PVRV) in a four-site intradermal schedule (4-0-2-0-1-1): an immunogenic, cost-effective and practical regimen. Vaccine 24:4116–4121

Anderson GR, Schnurrenberger PR, Masterson RA, Wentworth FH (1960) Avian embryo rabies immunization I. Duck-embryo vaccine administered intradermally in man. Am J Hyg 71:158–167

Anderson LJ, Baer GM, Smith JS, Winkler WG, Holman RC (1981) Rapid antibody response to human diploid rabies vaccine. Am J Epidemiol 113:270–275

Aoki FY, Tyrrell DA, Hill LE (1975) Immunogenicity and acceptability of a human diploid-cell culture rabies vaccine in volunteers. Lancet 1:660–662

Australian immunisation handbook, 9th edn (2008) Part 3.1 Australian bat lyssavirus infection and rabies. http://www.immunise.health.gov.au/internet/immunise/publishing.nsf/Content/Handbook-lyssavirus. Accessed 13 Jan 2010

Beran J, Honegr K, Banzhoff A, Malerczyk C (2006) How far can the antigen content of tissue culture rabies vaccine be reduced safely? Vaccine 24:2223–2224

Bernard KW, Roberts MA, Sumner J et al (1982) Human diploid cell rabies vaccine. Effectiveness of immunization with small intradermal or subcutaneous doses. JAMA 247:1138–1142

Bernard KW, Fishbein DB, Miller KD et al (1985) Pre-exposure rabies immunization with human diploid cell vaccine: decreased antibody responses in persons immunized in developing countries. Am J Trop Med Hyg 34:633–647

Bourhy H, Goudal M, Mailles A, Sadkowska-Todys M, Dacheux L, Zeller H (2009) Is there a need for anti-rabies vaccine and immunoglobulins rationing in Europe? Euro Surveill 14 (13) pii = 19166

Briggs DJ, Banzhoff A, Nicolay U et al (2000) Antibody response of patients after postexposure rabies vaccination with small intradermal doses of purified chick embryo cell vaccine or purified Vero cell rabies vaccine. Bull World Health Organ 78:693–698

Canada Communicable Disease Report 31, ACS-5, 1 June 2005, An Advisory Committee Statement (ACS), National Advisory Committee on Immunization (NACI). http://www.phac-aspc.gc.ca/publicat/ccdr-rmtc/05vol31/asc-dcc-5/index-eng.php. Accessed 13 Jan 2010

CDC (1982) Recommendation of the Immunization Practices advisory Committee (ACIP). Supplementary statement on pre-exposure rabies prophylaxis by the intradermal route. MMWR Morb Mortal Wkly Rep 31:279–280, 285

CDC (1984) Rabies prevention–United States, 1984. MMWR Morb Mortal Wkly Rep 33:393–402, 407–398

CDC (1986) Rabies prevention: supplementary statement on the preexposure use of human diploid cell rabies vaccine by the intradermal route. MMWR Morb Mortal Wkly Rep 35:767–768

Cenna J, Hunter M, Tan GS et al (2009) Replication-deficient rabies virus-based vaccines are safe and immunogenic in mice and nonhuman primates. J Infect Dis 200:1251–1260

Chi RC, Rock MT, Neuzil KM (2010) Immunogenicity and safety of intradermal influenza vaccination in healthy older adults. Clin Infect Dis 50:1331–1338

Chutivongse S, Wilde H, Supich C, Baer GM, Fishbein DB (1990) Postexposure prophylaxis for rabies with antiserum and intradermal vaccination. Lancet 335:896–898

Cox JH, Schneider LG (1976) Prophylactic immunization of humans against rabies by intradermal inoculation of human diploid cell culture vaccine. J Clin Microbiol 3:96–101
Department of Health (2006) Immunisation against infectious disease 2006—The green book. Chapter 27 Rabies 329–342. Stationary Office, London. http://www.dh.gov.uk/prod_consum_dh/groups/dh_digitalassets/documents/digitalasset/dh_110418.pdf. Accessed 13 Jan 2010
Dodet B (2006) Preventing the incurable: Asian rabies experts advocate rabies control. Vaccine 24:3045–3049
Dodet B (2007) Advocating rabies control in Asia. Vaccine 25:4123–4124
Dodet B (2009a) Report of the fifth AREB meeting Ho Chi Minh City, Vietnam, 17–20 November 2008. Vaccine 27:2403–2407
Dodet B (2009b) The fight against rabies in Africa: from recognition to action. Vaccine 27:5027–5032
Dreesen DW, Brown WJ, Kemp DT, Brown J, Reid FL, Baer GM (1984) Pre-exposure rabies prophylaxis: efficacy of a new packaging and delivery system for intradermal administration of human diploid cell vaccine. Vaccine 2:185–188
Falsey AR (2010) New emerging technologies and the intradermal route: the novel way to immunize against influenza. Vaccine 28(Suppl 4):D24–D32
Fishbein DB, Bernard KW, Miller KD et al (1986) The early kinetics of the neutralizing antibody response after booster immunizations with human diploid cell rabies vaccine. Am J Trop Med Hyg 35:663–670
Fishbein DB, Pacer RE, Holmes DF, Ley AB, Yager P, Tong TC (1987) Rabies preexposure prophylaxis with human diploid cell rabies vaccine: a dose-response study. J Infect Dis 156:50–55
Goswami A, Plun-Favreau J, Nicoloyannis N, Sampath G, Siddiqui MN, Zinsou JA (2005) The real cost of rabies post-exposure treatments. Vaccine 23:2970–2976
Hatz CF, Bidaux JM, Eichenberger K, Mikulics U, Junghanss T (1995) Circumstances and management of 72 animal bites among long-term residents in the tropics. Vaccine 13: 811–815
Horman JT, Rullan JV, Myers RA, Bond JO, Israel E, Joseph JM (1987) Antibody response after a two-year intradermal booster of rabies human diploid cell vaccine. J Am Vet Med Assoc 191:185–187
Joint Committee on Vaccination and Immunisation (1984) Chapter 17 Rabies. In: Immunisation against infectious disease. HMSO, London, p 105.
Kamoltham T, Thinyounyong W, Phongchamnaphai P et al (2007) Pre-exposure rabies vaccination using purified chick embryo cell rabies vaccine intradermally is immunogenic and safe. J Pediatr 151:173–177
Khawplod P, Benjavongkulchai M, Limusanno S, Chareonwai S, Kaewchompoo W, Tantawichien T et al (2002a) Four-site intradermal postexposure boosters in previously rabies vaccinated subjects. J Travel Med 9:153–155
Khawplod P, Wilde H, Tepsumethanon S et al (2002b) Prospective immunogenicity study of multiple intradermal injections of rabies vaccine in an effort to obtain an early immune response without the use of immunoglobulin. Clin Infect Dis 35:1562–1565
Kim YC, Jarrahian C, Zehrung D, Mitragotri S, Prausnitz MR (2011) Delivery systems for intradermal vaccination. Curr Top Microbiol Immunol 351:77–112
Knobel DL, Cleaveland S, Coleman PG et al (2005) Re-evaluating the burden of rabies in Africa and Asia. Bull World Health Organ 83:360–368
Lafon M (2005) Modulation of the immune response in the nervous system by rabies virus. Curr Top Microbiol Immunol 289:239–258
Lau C, Sisson J (2002) The effectiveness of intradermal pre-exposure rabies vaccination in an Australian travel medicine clinic. J Travel Med 9:285–288
Laurent PE, Bourhy H, Fantino M, Alchas P, Mikszta JA (2010) Safety and efficacy of novel dermal and epidermal microneedle delivery systems for rabies vaccination in healthy adults. Vaccine 28:5850–5856

Madhusudana SN, Anand NP, Shamsundar R (2001) Evaluation of two intradermal vaccination regimens using purified chick embryo cell vaccine for post-exposure prophylaxis of rabies. Natl Med J India 14:145–147

Madhusudana SN, Anand NP, Shamsundar R (2002) Economical multi-site intradermal regimen with purified chick embryo cell vaccine (Rabipur) prevents rabies in people bitten by confirmed rabid animals. Int J Infect Dis 6:210–214

Madhusudana SN, Sanjay TV, Mahendra BJ, Suja MS (2004) Simulated post-exposure rabies vaccination with purified chick embryo cell vaccine using a modified Thai Red Cross regimen. Int J Infect Dis 8:175–179

Madhusudana SN, Sanjay TV, Mahendra BJ et al (2006) Comparison of safety and immunogenicity of purified chick embryo cell rabies vaccine (PCECV) and purified vero cell rabies vaccine (PVRV) using the Thai Red Cross intradermal regimen at a dose of 0.1 ML. Hum Vaccin 2:200–204

Manning SE, Rupprecht CE, Fishbein D, Hanlon CA, Lumlertdacha B, Guerra M, Meltzer MI, Dhankhar P, Vaidya SA, Jenkins SR, Sun B, Hull HF (2008) Human rabies prevention—United States, 2008: recommendations of the Advisory Committee on Immunization Practices. MMWR Recomm Rep 57:1–28

Nicholson KG, Turner GS, Aoki FY (1978) Immunization with a human diploid cell strain of rabies virus vaccine: two-year results. J Infect Dis 137:783–788

Nicholson KG, Cole PJ, Turner GS, Harrison P (1979) Immune responses of humans to a human diploid cell strain of rabies virus vaccine: lymphocyte transformation, production of virus-neutralizing antibody, and induction of interferon. J Infect Dis 140:176–182

Nicholson KG, Prestage H, Cole PJ, Turner GS, Bauer SP (1981) Multisite intradermal antirabies vaccination. Immune responses in man and protection of rabbits against death from street virus by postexposure administration of human diploid-cell-strain rabies vaccine. Lancet 2:915–918

Nicolas JF, Guy B (2008) Intradermal, epidermal and transcutaneous vaccination: from immunology to clinical practice. Expert Rev Vaccines 7:1201–1214

Pappaioanou M, Fishbein DB, Dreesen DW et al (1986) Antibody response to preexposure human diploid-cell rabies vaccine given concurrently with chloroquine. N Engl J Med 314:280–284

Peck FB Jr, Kohlstaedt KC (1964) Pre-exposure rabies prophylaxis problems and procedures. Ind Med Surg 33:17–21

Phanuphak P, Khawplod P, Sirivichayakul S et al (1987) Humoral and cell-mediated immune responses to various economical regimens of purified Vero cell rabies vaccine. Asian Pac J Allergy Immunol 5:33–37

Phanuphak P, Khaoplod P, Benjavongkulchai M, Chutivongse S, Wilde H (1990) What happens if intradermal injections of rabies vaccine are partially or entirely injected subcutaneously? Bull World Health Organ 68:83–85

Quiambao BP, Dimaano EM, Ambas C et al (2005) Reducing the cost of post-exposure rabies prophylaxis: efficacy of 0.1 ml PCEC rabies vaccine administered intradermally using the Thai Red Cross post-exposure regimen in patients severely exposed to laboratory-confirmed rabid animals. Vaccine 23:1709–1714

Quiambao BP, Gepanayao C, Bermal N et al (2008) Immunogenicity and safety of three intradermal anti-rabies vaccination regimens using purified vero cell rabies vaccine. APCRI J 10:15–19

Ratanavongsiri J, Sriwanthana B, Ubol S, Phanuphak P (1985) Cell-mediated immune response following intracutaneous immunisation with human diploid cell rabies vaccine. Asian Pac J Allergy Immunol 3:187–190

Recuenco S, Warnock E, Urazova O et al (2009) Intradermal administration of PCEC rabies vaccine: preliminary results of a human clinical trial in the USA. Abstract at international conference on Rabies in the Americas (RITA), October 19th to 23, Quebec City

Roumiantzeff M, Ajjan N, Vincent-Falquet JC (1988) Experience with preexposure rabies vaccination. Rev Infect Dis 10(Suppl 4):S751–S757

Schnell MJ, McGettigan JP, Wirblich C, Papaneri A (2010) The cell biology of rabies virus: using stealth to reach the brain. Nat Rev Microbiol 8:51–61

Schnurrenberger PR, Bashe WJ, Helwig JH (1965) Avian embryo rabies immunization. 3. Optimal site and timing of intradermal inoculations in pre-exposure regimens. Am J Epidemiol 81:146–149

Suntharasamai P, Warrell MJ, Viravan C et al (1987a) Purified chick embryo cell rabies vaccine: economical multisite intradermal regimen for post-exposure prophylaxis. Epidemiol Infect 99:755–765

Suntharasamai P, Warrell MJ, Warrell DA et al (1987b) Early antibody responses to rabies post-exposure vaccine regimens. Am J Trop Med Hyg 36:160–165

Suntharasamai P, Chaiprasithikul P, Wasi C, Supanaranond W, Auewarakul P, Chanthavanich P, Supapochana A, Areeraksa S, Chittamas S, Jittapalapongsa S et al (1994) A simplified and economical intradermal regimen of purified chick embryo cell rabies vaccine for postexposure prophylaxis. Vaccine 12:508–512

Tantawichien T, Benjavongkulchai M, Limsuwan K et al (1999) Antibody response after a four-site intradermal booster vaccination with cell-culture rabies vaccine. Clin Infect Dis 28:1100–1103

Täuber MG, Putzi R, Fuchs P, Wyler R, Luthy R (1986) High rate of insufficient antibody titers after single-day immunization with human diploid-cell-strain vaccine against rabies. Klin Wochenschr 64:518–521

Teunissen MBM, Haniffa M, Collin MP (2011) Insight into the immunobiology of human skin and functional specialization of skin dendritic cell subsets to innovate intradermal vaccination design. Curr Top Microbiol Immunol 351:25–76

Trevejo RT (2000) Rabies preexposure vaccination among veterinarians and at-risk staff. J Am Vet Med Assoc 217:1647–1650

Turner GS (1969) Rabies vaccines. Br Med Bull 25:136–142

Turner GS (1984) Trends and advances in the approach to the problems of rabies: a review of recent progress. Abst Hyg Commun Dis 59:R1–R12

Turner GS, Aoki FY, Nicholson KG, Tyrrell DA, Hill LE (1976) Human diploid cell strain rabies vaccine. Rapid prophylactic immunisation of volunteers with small doses. Lancet 1:1379–1381

Turner GS, Nicholson KG, Tyrrell DA, Aoki FY (1982) Evaluation of a human diploid cell strain rabies vaccine: final report of a three year study of pre-exposure immunization. J Hyg (Lond) 89:101–110

Ugolini G (2010) Advances in viral transneuronal tracing. J Neurosci Methods 194:2–20

Vien NC, Feroldi E, Lang J (2008) Long-term anti-rabies antibody persistence following intramuscular or low-dose intradermal vaccination of young Vietnamese children. Trans R Soc Trop Med Hyg 102:294–296

Warrell MJ, Warrell DA, Suntharasamai P et al (1983) An economical regimen of human diploid cell strain anti-rabies vaccine for post-exposure prophylaxis. Lancet 2:301–304

Warrell MJ, Suntharasamai P, Nicholson KG et al (1984) Multi-site intradermal and multi-site subcutaneous rabies vaccination: improved economical regimens. Lancet 1:874–876

Warrell MJ, Nicholson KG, Warrell DA et al (1985) Economical multiple-site intradermal immunisation with human diploid-cell-strain vaccine is effective for post-exposure rabies prophylaxis. Lancet 1:1059–1062

Warrell MJ, Riddell A, Yu LM et al (2008) A simplified 4-site economical intradermal post-exposure rabies vaccine regimen: a randomised controlled comparison with standard methods. PLoS Negl Trop Dis 2:e224

WHO (1984) WHO Expert Committee on Rabies. Seventh report. Technical report series 709. World Health Organization, Geneva

WHO (1992) WHO Expert Committee on rabies. Eighth report. Technical report series 824. World Health Organization, Geneva

WHO (1997) WHO recommendations on rabies post-exposure treatment and the correct technique of intradermal immunization against rabies. WHO/EMC/ZOO.96.6. http://whqlibdoc.who.int/hq/1996/WHO_EMC_ZOO_96.6.pdf. Accessed 13 Jan 2010

WHO (2005) World Health Organization Expert Consultation on rabies. WHO technical report series 931 first report. http://www.wpro.who.int/NR/rdonlyres/B1ED8443-0993-408C-BF09-D1D06A6E1B45/0/FINALTEXTWHOTechnicalReportSeries090605.pdf. Accessed 13 Jan 2010

WHO (2007) Rabies vaccines. WHO position paper. Wkly Epidemiol Rec 82:425–435. http://www.who.int/wer/2007/wer8249_50.pdf. Accessed 13 Jan 2010

Wiktor TJ, Doherty PC, Koprowski H (1977) Suppression of cell-mediated immunity by street rabies virus. J Exp Med 145:1617–1622

Intradermal Vaccination to Protect Against Yellow Fever and Influenza

A. H. E. Roukens, L. B. S. Gelinck and L. G. Visser

Abstract The viral infections yellow fever and influenza can lead to large epidemics, which may deplete limited vaccine supplies. The intradermal vaccination route of yellow fever and influenza vaccines has received renewed attention, because it allows dose reduction without loss of efficacy. In this chapter, we review these two vaccines, the history of vaccine development, correlates of protection, immune response to vaccination and current knowledge concerning intradermal vaccination, including the immunological background, both in healthy subjects and immunocompromized individuals.

Contents

A. H. E. Roukens · L. G. Visser (✉)
Department of Infectious Diseases, Suite C5-P, Leiden University Medical Centre, Albinusdreef 2, 2333 ZA Leiden, The Netherlands
e-mail: l.g.visser@lumc.nl

L. B. S. Gelinck
Department of Internal Medicine, Medisch Centrum Haaglanden, P.O. Box 432, 2501 CK, The Hague, The Netherlands

Current Topics in Microbiology and Immunology (2012) 351: 159–179
DOI: 10.1007/82_2011_124

Published Online: 17 March 2011

1 Introduction

Intradermal (ID) vaccination has recently entered the main arena for several commercially available vaccines. The driving force behind ID vaccination with reduced vaccine doses are cost reduction and increased coverage of vaccination programs despite limited vaccine supplies. In addition, the proven immunological superiority has sparked the development of easy to use ID vaccination devices. Still many practical obstacles to ID vaccination remain.

In this review, we discuss two different viral infections, yellow fever and influenza. The history of vaccine development and the current state of affairs concerning ID vaccination, including the immunological background, both in healthy subjects and immunocompromized individuals are discussed for these two viruses.

2 Clinical Consequences of Infection

2.1 *Yellow Fever*

The yellow fever virus is a small (40–60 nm) positive-sense, single-stranded RNA virus, belonging to the flavivirus family, which also include viruses such as Dengue virus, West Nile virus, Japanese encephalitis virus and Tick Borne Encephalitis virus. The genome of the yellow fever virus consists of a single open reading frame which encodes three structural proteins (capsid, premembrane, and envelope proteins), and eight non-structural proteins which are involved in the replication of the virus (Monath 2008a).

Infection with yellow fever virus causes yellow fever, a mosquito-borne hemorrhagic fever that occurs mostly in sub-Saharan Africa (90% of cases worldwide) and tropical regions of South America. Approximately 200,000 cases of yellow fever occur annually (Monath 2008a). It is a major public health threat to hundreds of millions of people living in endemic regions, and for millions of travelers to yellow fever endemic areas (WHO 2003). Infection with yellow fever virus can give rise to a wide spectrum of clinical manifestations, from subclinical infection in 75% of those infected, to a life-threatening disease with multi-organ failure, jaundice, and hemorrhage. The classical illness is characterized by three stages. The first stage is marked by non-specific symptoms such as malaise, fever, headache, myalgia, anorexia, and nausea. After 3 to 4 days, a period of remission occurs that can last up to 48 h. Many patients recover at this stage, but 25% enter the intoxication phase that is characterized by hepatic, renal and myocardial dysfunction, and hemorrhage. Fifty percent of those who enter the intoxication phase die (Monath 2008a). Antivirals such as ribavirin, and immune modulators such as interferon alpha, are effective when administered within 2 days after yellow fever infection (when symptoms are indistinguishable from many other viral infections), but ineffective when given after the infection is established (Monath 2008b), rendering vaccination the only real protection against the disease.

2.2 *Influenza*

Influenza viruses belong to the family of Orthomyxoviridae. These enveloped viruses have a spherical or filamentous form (80–120 nm) and contain a segmented genome of negative-sense single-stranded RNA. Three distinct influenza types are recognized: influenza A, influenza B, and influenza C virus. Influenza A viruses are subtyped according to their major surface antigens: hemagglutinin (H) and neuraminidase (N). Although at least 16 different H and 9N antigens have been found (of which most exclusively in birds), only few H–N combinations have been found to efficiently infect humans. Influenza A/H3N2, A/H1N1 and influenza B have been the dominant viruses infecting the human population during the last decades. Smaller, more contained, epidemics with influenza A/H5N1 and A/H7N7 have occurred (Treanor 2009).

Influenza viruses display a high degree of gradual adaptation by antigenic alterations over time. Furthermore, they have a more efficient global spread than any other known infectious agent. For these reasons official influenza nomenclature also includes place of initial isolation, strain designation and year of isolation. In moderate climates, influenza activity typically peaks during the winter months. Influenza viruses escape existing immunity of the human population by (minor) antigenic changes called antigenic drift. Typically some cross-reactive immunity against these viruses exists that helps to contain the extent of the epidemic. When larger antigenic adaptations occur (antigenic shift) the entire human population may become susceptible to such a virus, possibly leading to a pandemic. The 2009 influenza A/H1N1 strain was a new antigen for the younger population but not for the elderly who had been infected with the 1918 influenza A/H1N1 virus or related viruses. This pre-existing immunity has dampened the impact of the influenza pandemic for those who are classically the most vulnerable to this virus (Kelly and Grant 2009).

The clinical manifestations of influenza range from asymptomatic to a severe disease with pneumonia, myocarditis, or encephalitis. Typical manifestations of influenza are a sudden onset of (high) fever with chills and malaise (including headache and myalgia), mostly accompanied by respiratory symptoms of the upper airways. The disease typically has a self-limiting character, with fever subsiding after 3–5 days. Morbidity and mortality are higher in the elderly, in cardiovascular or pulmonary compromized patients, and in those with impaired immunity. Annually, influenza is a major cause of morbidity and mortality, and has major economical consequences through missed working days. Several anti-viral drugs are available for influenza. Antiviral treatment should be initiated promptly in order to affect the course of the disease. Especially in immuno-compromized patients, who fail to clear the virus, resistance associated with treatment failure has been documented. Resistant strains can cause epidemics. In the US, over 90% of all tested circulating influenza A/H1N1 strains were oseltamivir resistant; the subsequent 2009 influenza A/H1N1 strain was innately amantadin resistant (Centers for Disease Control and Prevention (CDC) 2009).

3 History of Vaccination

3.1 Yellow Fever Vaccine Development

In the 1920s, the yellow fever virus was isolated by English-American researchers from a Ghanaian patient, called Asibi, who suffered from yellow fever. The virus was inoculated into a monkey to use as a model for yellow fever infection (Stokes et al. 2001). Concurrently, French researchers isolated the virus from a patient in Dakar. This virus was used to develop a mouse model of yellow fever infection, which was employed to demonstrate protection against yellow fever infection by serum antibodies. In the following years, both research groups attenuated the wild-type yellow fever virus with the aim of inducing protective immunity in humans, without causing disease. The French researchers developed the French Neurotropic Virus (FNV), derived from the Dakar-strain (Sellards 1931). After intramuscular inoculation, FNV induced severe neurological symptoms, but these were diminished after vaccine delivery by scarification. The English-American group propagated the Asibi-strain on mouse embryo tissue. To abate the neurotropism that was observed with the attenuated Dakar-strain, the Asibi-virus was passaged on mouse embryo tissue stripped of nervous tissue. In the later and final stages, the virus was attenuated by repeated passage on chicken embryo tissue, of which the nervous tissue had been removed, and after 227 and 229 passages, this led to the development of an immunogenic and safe Yellow Fever-17D (YF-17D) vaccine strain (Theiler and Smith 1937).

The FNV and YF-17D strains were used concurrently for immunization against yellow fever, until in 1965, when a vaccination campaign in Senegal with FNV resulted in an epidemic of vaccine-related encephalitis in children mostly between 2 and 11 years (children <2 years were excluded from vaccination) (Mar et al. 1967). After the restriction of vaccinating with FNV under the age of 14, the French vaccine lost its popularity and production was discontinued in 1980. Since then, YF-17D has been the only available vaccine strain for yellow fever vaccination. Two different

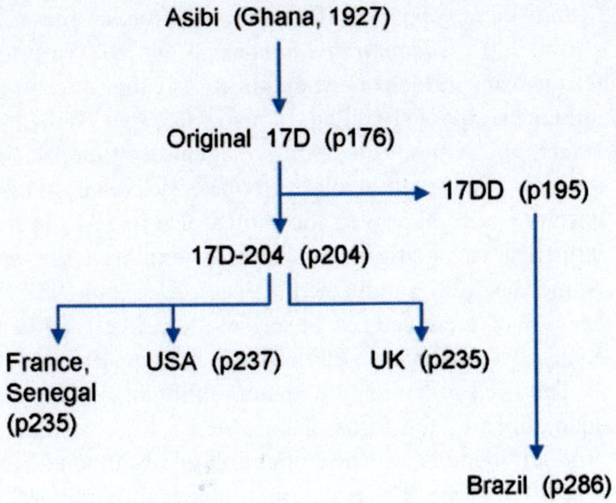

Fig. 1 Derivation and passage histories of yellow fever vaccines according to the WHO. p = number of passages. China, Colombia, Switzerland and Russia produce small quantities of the vaccine. Figure is adapted from Marianneau et al. (2001)

substrains derived from the 17D yellow fever strain, called 17DD and 17D-204, are used for the manufacturing of yellow fever vaccines today (Fig. 1). The 17DD substrain is used in Brazil and the 17D-204 substrain in all other countries where yellow fever vaccine is manufactured (Monath 2005).

3.2 *Yellow Fever Vaccine: Correlates of Protection*

Protection against yellow fever is determined by the development of neutralizing antibodies (NA). A protective antibody titer is defined as a log 0.7 (=80%) reduction of viral infectivity by minimally diluted (1:10) serum of the vaccinee, measured by the plaque reduction neutralization test. This assay measures the reduction of cell clusters (plaques) of cells infected by YF-17D in the presence of serum containing NA. A log 0.7 plaque reduction has been shown to correlate to protection in monkeys, when challenged with 10^3 mouse lethal dose$_{50}$ administered subcutaneously 20 weeks after vaccination (Mason et al. 1973). The plaque reduction neutralization test is considered the most sensitive and specific test to measure yellow fever NA (Niedrig et al. 1999). Recently, the role of cellular immunity in yellow fever vaccination has been investigated. Although these studies provide a very interesting insight into the development of the response against the yellow fever vaccine, the NA titer has historically proved useful as a correlate of protection, since no reports on yellow fever infection have been published in individuals with protective NA titers.

3.3 *Influenza Vaccine Development*

Although influenza epidemics have been recognized since the sixteenth century, influenza virus was first isolated in 1933 by Wilson Smith and colleagues

(Smith et al. 1933). Before the isolation of the virus, the disease was faultily attributed to *Haemophilus influenzae*, which was often isolated from patients suffering from influenza. Attempts to use this micro-organism to vaccinate against influenza, obviously failed. In his 1933 paper, Wilson Smith also refuted the role of *Haemophilus* spp. as a causative agent of influenza (in ferrets). The recognition of the viral etiology immediately boosted vaccination research. Commercial influenza vaccines were approved for clinical use in 1945 in the United States. The earliest influenza vaccination trials already explored the possibility of ID vaccination. Numerous studies published between 1947 and 1958 explore this vaccination route, because of a reduced risk of serious side effects, while saving antigen and achieving equal post-vaccination titers (Appleby et al. 1951; McCarroll and Kilbourne 1958).

The need to annually update the influenza vaccine, in response to the antigenic adaptations of the virus, has created a highly efficient vaccine development and production industry. The epidemiology of influenza viruses is constantly monitored across the globe. The isolation of a new antigenic influenza A/H1N1 variant by the US Centers for Disease Control and Prevention in April of 2009, led to the cloning and distribution of an appropriate vaccine strain within 30 days. The typical vaccine strain is a construct of gene segments encoding for the hemagglutinin, neuraminidase, and a polymerase from a current strain combined with the remaining genes taken from a 1934 'backbone' influenza virus. Several vaccine manufacturers then started the process of mass production, in which embryonated eggs are inoculated to grow these viruses in larger amounts, so that clinical studies could be conducted in July 2009. The first results of these studies were published in September, less than 6 months after isolation of this new strain (Greenberg et al. 2009).

The classical influenza vaccine is a split or subunit vaccine, which only contains the immunogenic antigens (primarily the hemaglutinin, but also the neuramidase). For several decades, the development of live-attenuated influenza viruses has been investigated. Similar to the live-attenuated yellow fever vaccine virus, these live vaccine strains have to be attenuated so that they will still generate immunity, without causing fever or disease and without the risk of transmission or reversion to the wild type virus. Several techniques of attenuation of these influenza strains have been tested. The currently registered live-attenuated influenza virus strains have been attenuated by cold adaptation.

3.4 Influenza Vaccine: Correlates of Protection

Inactivated vaccines contain a controlled minimal amount of haemagglutin per strain (usually 15 μg), and also contain other antigens. Virus strain-specific antibodies directed against the major viral surface glycoproteins are the main outcome of vaccination with inactivated viruses. The most commonly used test to assess the immunogenicity of influenza vaccination is the haemagglutination inhibition (HI) assay. This test relies on the ability of the virus specific antibodies to inhibit haemagglutination caused by the viral haemagglutin. This test correlates well with other quantitative measurements that determine neutralizing antibodies. HI titers are correlated with clinical protection against influenza in healthy adults. On the basis of data derived from 12 publications concerning healthy adults, it was estimated that a median HI titer of 28 protected 50% of the vaccinees against the virus (Beyer et al. 2004; de Jong et al. 2003; Plotkin 2008). A titer of $\geq$40 is usually considered to be protective. The primary outcome of vaccination trials is mostly determined by the geometric mean titer of anti-influenza antibodies. The large differences in post-vaccination geometric mean titers, between different strains (within one year and over longer periods) make this outcome measurement less suitable to compare results from different studies over time. Other outcome measurements are derived from the antibody titer. The protection rate (the percentage of a population with a post-vaccination titer $\geq$40) is considered to be a clinically relevant outcome, although this percentage is influenced by the proportion that already had a titer >40 before vaccination. Other vaccination outcomes, such as the response rate, try to correct for this effect by including a response criterion (such as a fourfold titer increase). In clinical practice, protection rate, response rate, and other outcomes are clearly correlated.

Cold-adapted, live-attenuated influenza viruses have been shown to be effective especially in children; adults show relatively poor serological response measured by HI, although there was good clinical protection. This is suggestive of a different route of immunological protection when live adapted viruses are used. Local mucosal immunity and cellular responses might even represent more relevant outcomes of vaccination than serum anti-influenza antibody titers. Subunit vaccines only transiently enhance cytotoxic T lymphocyte responses (McMichael et al. 1981).

4 Immune Response Against Yellow Fever Vaccine and Influenza Vaccine

4.1 Response Against Yellow Fever Vaccine in Immunocompetent Persons

The YF-17D vaccine virus strain induces a viraemia that can be detected in 50% of vaccinees and generally occurs from day 3 to day 7 with a peak on the fifth day after vaccination (Monath 2005). After local replication, that probably occurs in cells of the innate immune system, such as dendritic cells and macrophages of the skin or subcutaneous tissue, the virus is carried to the draining lymph nodes, from where it reaches other organs via the bloodstream and lymphatic system. NA have been found to recognize epitopes on the envelope protein that is essential for virus entry into the cell (Gould et al. 1986; Pincus et al. 1992). By opsonising the virus shortly after infection, NA could hamper viral replication by blocking cell entry. Ten days after vaccination, 95% of vaccinees showed protective NA levels, and after 30 days, 99% are protected. NA declined gradually with time after vaccination (Niedrig et al. 1999), but have been shown to circulate in vivo up to 30–35 years after a single vaccination (Poland, Bull World Health Organ, 1981). Among revaccinated healthy subjects, the vaccine boosted NA levels (Roukens et al. 2008), indicating a good memory response; although some have reported that the height of pre-existing NA may inversely affect the height of the booster response (Hepburn et al. 2006).

Until recently, the cellular immune response after YF-17D vaccination was a black box. The reason why it was hardly investigated is probably the fact that the vaccine is very effective and that the correlate of protection by NA is sufficient in daily practice. With the development of new research techniques and increased interest in the mechanism of this effective vaccine response, interesting results concerning the cellular immune response against YF-17D have been published recently. The peak of proliferation of natural killer cells was demonstrated on day 7 after vaccination, and T cell proliferation ($CD4^+$ and $CD8^+$) was most profound 14 days after vaccination. In addition, yellow fever vaccination induces a robust memory response shown by highly proliferative $CD4^+$ and $CD8^+$ T cells that were drawn from vaccinees 60–90 days after vaccination (Akondy et al. 2009; Gaucher et al. 2008). A mixed $CD4^+$ T helper cell type 1 (Th1) and T helper cell type 2 (Th2) response was found, measured by proliferation and cytokine production, with a variable Th1/Th2 balance per individual (Gaucher et al. 2008). The development of a mixed Th1 and Th2 response had been suggested previously, since YF-17D activates multiple Toll-like receptors (TLRs), including TLRs 2, 7, 8, and 9, that induce diverse types of adaptive immune responses (Querec et al. 2006).

4.2 Response Against Yellow Fever Vaccine in Immunocompromized Persons

The yellow fever vaccine virus is a live-attenuated virus that replicates after inoculation, in order to induce a protective immune response. Immunocompromized persons have always been excluded from vaccination because of the risk of inducing unrestricted replication of the vaccine virus and thereby causing a yellow fever-like illness. Serious adverse events following YF-17D vaccination, known as yellow fever-associated viscerotropic or neurotropic disease (YEL-AVD or YEL-AND), could result from such an unrestricted viral replication due to the failing immune response to YF-17D. YEL-AVD has been reported more frequently after primary yellow fever vaccination in individuals older than 60 years of age, although young and apparently immunocompetent individuals have also been reported to develop these serious adverse events. In general, the immune response to vaccines can be impaired in elderly (Weinberger et al. 2008), and this may subsequently increase the susceptibility to acquire infectious diseases. In the case of yellow fever vaccination, the development of YEL-AVD or YEL-AND by vaccination is a more important concern than an impaired response to the vaccine. Although the early humoral immune response is be hampered in the elderly (Roukens, unpublished results), NA titers are comparable to that of younger vaccinees at 30 days post-vaccination (Monath et al. 2005).

The fact that impaired immunity can indeed be a risk factor for YEL-AVD is shown by case reports of this fatal condition in immunocompromized persons. For example, a human immunodeficiency virus (HIV) infected patient with a CD4 cell count of 108 cells/mm^3, who died shortly after yellow fever vaccination (Kengsakul et al. 2002), and the development of YEL-AVD in patients who underwent thymectomy prior to vaccination (Barwick 2004). Recently, a retrospective study of HIV infected patients with a mean CD4 cell count of 537 cells/mm^3 at the time of vaccination, included six patients with a CD4 cell count <200 cells/mm^3 who did not develop serious adverse events following YF vaccination. A significantly larger proportion of first-time vaccinated HIV-infected patients (19%) did not show a protective neutralizing antibody (NA) response in reaction to vaccination, compared to non-infected controls, in whom 3% of the individuals did not show seroprotection. Out of all the HIV-infected participants, 83% developed protective NA titers in the first year after vaccination, compared to 93% of the controls. HIV-infected patients had significantly lower NA than non-infected individuals, both within the first year after vaccination and thereafter. The CD4 cell count was found to be a predictor of the development of the NA titer (Veit et al. 2009). Of the six participants with a CD4 cell count <200 cells/mm^3, two did not develop a protective NA titer. None of these six patients developed serious adverse events following yellow fever vaccination.

The response against yellow fever vaccination in patients who take immunosuppressive medication (e.g. transplant recipients, patients with rheumatoid arthritis or inflammatory bowel disease) has not been investigated. However, immune suppression by cyclophosphamide in hamsters showed 50% mortality due to neurological disease after YF-17D vaccination compared to no mortality in the mock-treated animals (Mateo et al. 2007). In the daily practice, this means that severely immunocompromized individuals (HIV infected with CD4 cell counts <200/ml; patients using immunosuppressive medication, because of solid organ transplantation, rheumatologic or inflammatory bowel disease; patients with a history of thymectomy) are advised to avoid endemic and transitional areas of yellow fever. Mildly immunocompromized, including elderly, are vaccinated if they visit yellow fever endemic or transitional regions, and advised to use anti-mosquito bite protection if traveling to low-risk regions (Roukens and Visser 2008). Recent research by Gaspard et al. showed that the subcutaneous injection of inactivated YF-17D into mice induced an immune response that protected against intracerebral inoculation of a lethal dose of YF-17D immune response, although with lower NA titers than live-attenuated vaccine (Gaspar et al. 2008). ID injection of inactivated YF-17D is not potentially harmful to immunocompromized persons, and should be investigated in order to induce a better response.

4.3 Response against Influenza Vaccine in Immunocompetent Persons

In healthy adults, peak antibody levels reach values of 2–10 times the protection threshold (≥40), giving rise to post-vaccination protection rates that are generally >90%. Anti-influenza titers wane rather rapidly, leaving the majority with a HI titer of <40 one year after vaccination. Clinical protection from illness however has been shown to persist for several years after vaccination in a decreasing proportion of the vaccinated population. Waning titers and drifting antigens do however necessitate annual vaccination (Russell et al. 2008).

Additional determinants of the immune response are amongst others, age and previous exposure. Overall the antibody response diminishes with increasing age. The absolute number of na (CD4 and CD45RA positive) T cells is inversely correlated with age. The decreasing numbers of na T cells secondary to a diminishing thymus size are the result of a physiological aging process and affect the immune response in the elderly (Bains et al. 2009; Lynch et al. 2009). This explains also why the immune recovery after starting combined anti-retroviral therapy in HIV-infected individuals is better at a younger age (Cohen Stuart et al. 2002; Douek et al. 1998). Many other factors have been described that might be correlated with this so-called immunosenescence (Pfister and Savino 2008). Age effects should be reported in every influenza vaccination study.

Previous exposure to the vaccine antigen is also relevant in all vaccination trials. Pre-vaccination titers are generally higher in patients who have been vaccinated before. Furthermore, relatively high anti-influenza titers may persist for a long time after developing influenza, even if the disease course was mild and not recognized as ‘flu’ by the individual. We found that up to 70% of the healthy previously unvaccinated controls had antibodies against the influenza A/H3N2 vaccine strain. Previous influenza vaccination or previous exposure to the virus can act as an important confounding factor in determining vaccination outcomes and should be addressed in every influenza vaccination study. In some, but not all studies, we found lower post-vaccination titers in subjects with a history of previous vaccination, even when that vaccine antigen was identical to the one administered the year before. This counter intuitive outcome has been described before and was named ‘the Hoskins’ paradox’ after the author of several influenza vaccination studies in the early 1970s (Beyer et al. 1998; Hoskins et al. 1979; Smith et al. 1999). Two processes might play a role in the paradoxal lower post-vaccination titers in previously vaccinated subjects: (1) neutralization of vaccine antigen (or the forming of immune complexes) by circulating antibodies and (2) a phenomenon know as the ‘original antigenic sin’: a related antigen (drift variant) will boost the response to the original antigen, instead of to the newly administered antigen, if there is enough resemblance.

Gender has been reported in some vaccination studies as a relevant factor for which adjustment was necessary. Both male and female gender have been correlated with better outcomes in different studies, however in influenza vaccination trials gender does not seem to play an important role (Overton et al. 2007; de Vries-Sluijs et al. 2008). Many other factors have been implied as variables that influence the outcome upon vaccination: among them the site of vaccine administration (e.g. deltoid vs. gluteal muscle), body weight and smoking (Chlíbek et al. 2007; Mackenzie and Fimmel 1978).

4.4 *Response against Influenza Vaccine in Immunocompromized Persons*

Influenza vaccination can be applied as a tool to measure the severity of the immunodeficiency by determining the height of post-vaccination titers in several patient groups with different forms of immunodeficiency, using a similar vaccination protocol. We could find a clear hierarchy between different groups (Gelinck et al. 2009). In patients infected with HIV, there is a correlation between post-vaccination geometric mean titers and the number of $CD4^+$ T lymphocytes. Individuals with a CD4 count below $200/mm^3$ clearly show impaired serological responses. Patients on successful suppressive anti-retroviral therapy still show impaired responses, although the percentage with a protective titer 4 weeks after vaccination is not dramatically lower than in healthy volunteers. The efficacy of influenza vaccination in HIV-infected individuals has been confirmed in placebo-controlled trials (Madhi and al 2009; Tasker et al. 1999).

Most groups of immunocompromized patients (solid organ transplant patients; patients treated with immunosuppressive agents such as anti-TNF-α or methotrexate because of auto-immune diseases; haemodialysis patients) show clear trends towards an impaired response upon influenza vaccination in antibody response, cellular response and even in clinical protection (Kunisaki and Janoff 2009). Post-vaccination antibody titers upon influenza vaccination are clearly lower in haematological stem cell transplantation patients and patients treated with anti-CD20 (rituximab). Rituximab depletes $CD20^+$ B cells which are the progenitors of antibody-producing plasma cells, and thus inhibits the final common pathway of both T cell-dependent and -independent humoral immune responses (van Assen et al. 2010; Gelinck et al. 2007; van der Kolk et al. 2002; Oren et al. 2008; Takata et al. 2009). This B cell depletion typically lasts more than 6 months.

5 Increased Vaccine Coverage by Reduced-Dose Intradermal Vaccination

5.1 *Intradermal Administration of Yellow Fever Vaccine*

ID vaccination is a recently rediscovered possibility of dose reduction through augmented immune stimulation and has received much attention from vaccinologists

(Glenn and Kenney 2006; Lambert and Laurent 2008; Nicolas and Guy 2008). By reducing the vaccine dose needed for immunization, costs per vaccine dose decrease and vaccine stockpiles last longer, possibly leading to higher vaccine coverage. ID administration of reduced amounts of both yellow fever and influenza vaccines—1/5th of the yellow fever vaccine or 1/5th of the influenza vaccine—elicited protective immune responses (Belshe et al. 2004; Gelinck et al. 2009; Kenney et al. 2004). We have shown that in case of yellow fever, the reduced dose injected ID is non-inferior to the subcutaneous dose, but we have not demonstrated the superiority of ID immunization per se since no comparison was made between ID and conventional immunization route of the reduced vaccine dose (Roukens et al. 2008).

In support of the superiority of the ID route, Cubas et al. recently showed that ID injection of virus-like particles (VLPs) of simian-HIV in mice induced enhanced immune responses compared to intramuscular, intraperitoneal, and subcutaneous inoculation routes with the same dose. By optical imaging, the trafficking of the VLPs after immunization was directly visualized, thereby showing that ID immunization led to the highest level of lymph node involvement for the longest period of time, which correlated with the strongest humoral and cellular immune responses (Cubas et al. 2009). These findings should now be investigated with respect to other antigenic formulations. The immune response following ID immunization is depicted in Fig. 2. In response to the injected antigen, with or without adjuvant, immature dendritic cells (DCs) residing at the site of vaccination (Langerhans cells or dermal DCs) undergo a maturation process that is characterized by expression of costimulatory molecules and inflammatory cytokines (Pulendran and Ahmed 2006). With respect to yellow fever, the in vivo sites of replication of YF-17D have been determined in cynomolgus macaques (Monath 2005). After subcutaneous inoculation, small amounts of 17D virus were found in the skin at the site of inoculation, in the draining lymph nodes and mesenteric lymph nodes at the peak of viraemia (day 3 for these primates). By day 7, liver, spleen, bone marrow, thymus, and adrenal glands were found to harbor YF-17D. The spleen and lymph nodes remained positive for the virus up to 14 days after inoculation, and by day 46 the virus was undetectable. These data indicate that the attenuated vaccine virus has a tissue tropism similar to that of wild-type YF, and that the initial process of immune activation occurs between the site of inoculation and the draining lymph nodes, similar to inactivated vaccine antigens. In support of the hypothesis of the response being initiated at the site of inoculation, recent data showed that YF-17D replicates in DCs and is then rapidly processed (Palmer et al. 2007). The predilection of YF-17D for DCs of the skin would not be unexpected, given the natural route of infection via mosquito bites.

5.2 *Intradermal Administration of Influenza Vaccine*

ID influenza vaccination received most attention in times of vaccine shortage caused by pandemics (e.g. the 1957 influenza A/H2N2 pandemic) or in case of

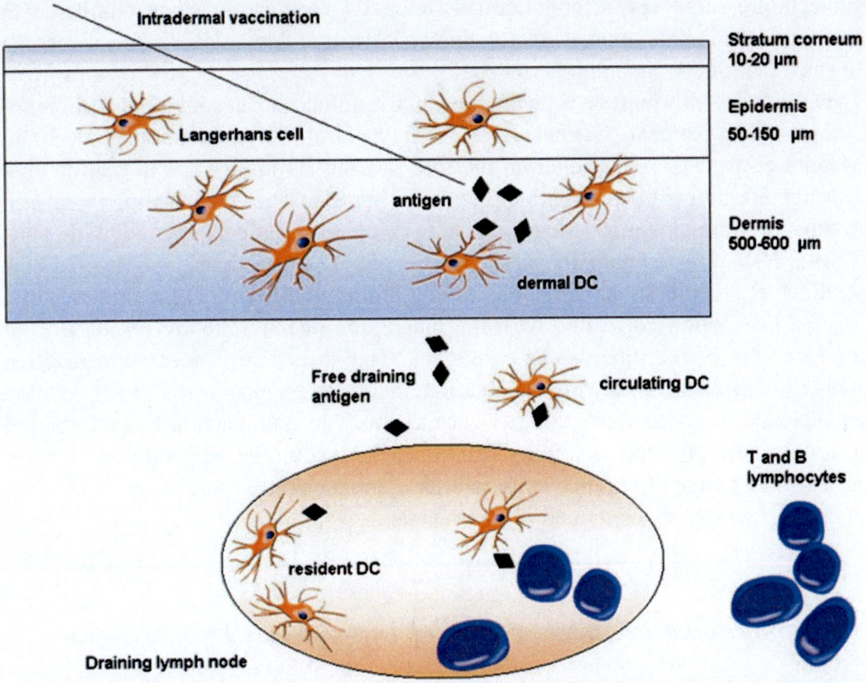

Fig. 2 Schematic representation of ID immunization and subsequent initiation of adaptive immune response. Figure is based on a figure by Nicolas and Guy (2008). DC = dendritic cell

manufacturing problems such as in 1973 and 2004 (Belshe et al. 2004; Kenney et al. 2004). These studies concentrated on the immune responses of healthy subjects (Kenney et al. 2004). These studies show that it is feasible to use reduced dose ID influenza vaccination, as compared to routine intramuscular vaccination, with similar outcomes in the parameters reported in these studies. Several studies confirm the true immunological superiority of a reduced influenza vaccine dose administered ID versus an equal dose administered intramuscular in risk groups such as the elderly (Arnou et al. 2009; Holland et al. 2008). This serves as proof of a more efficient immune response upon ID vaccine delivery. Besides the immunologic benefit of ID vaccination, there is an obvious economic advantage in saving up to 80% of vaccine required for protection, allowing for full vaccination coverage even in times of vaccine shortages (MIV Study Group 2005; Roukens et al. 2008).

There are however also some inherent practical disadvantages to ID vaccination, especially relevant in mass vaccination campaigns, such as the annual influenza vaccination campaigns or in the response to a pandemic influenza outbreak. The vaccination technique itself is more difficult and time consuming than intramuscular vaccination. Recently developed ID vaccination devices will bring an end to these practical complications. Furthermore, local side effects in healthy subjects are more severe and frequent upon ID vaccination when compared to intramuscular vaccination, a factor known to negatively impact vaccine uptake (Ryan et al. 2006; Smedley et al. 2007).

Only little information is available on ID influenza vaccination in immunocompromized patients (Gelinck et al. 2009; Jo et al. 2009; Khanlou et al. 2006; Manuel et al. 2007). We reported on dose sparing ID influenza vaccination as a feasible alternative for the routine practice of intramuscular vaccination in several groups of immunocompromized subjects, including patients treated with anti-TNF-α, HIV-infected patients and hematopoietic stem cell transplantation patients (Gelinck et al. 2009). An interesting finding of this study was that the presence of a local skin reaction correlated with the magnitude of the antibody response to at least one out of the three vaccine antigens. The absence of a local skin reaction within the first 48 h following vaccination, identified patients who did not develop an adequate response at day 28 after vaccination. The skin reaction was interpreted as a delayed-type hypersensitivity reaction, which could be directed at either one of the three hemagglutinin or neuraminidase antigens or even at traces of chicken egg or preservatives contained in the vaccine.

5.3 *Immunological Background of Intradermal Immunization*

Both primary and secondary immune responses take place in lymphoid tissue and the physiology of this response upon vaccination is reasonably well described in healthy subjects (Siegrist 2008). B cell activation upon antigen binding will upregulate CCR7, a molecule that will drive antigen-specific B cells to the outer T-cell zone of lymphoid tissues. Antigen-specific B cells are captured and retained by follicular dendritic cells that, in cooperation with follicular T cells, facilitate massive clonal proliferation. The class switch from IgM to IgG, IgA or IgE secreting plasma cells and affinity maturation will take place in the germinal centers that are formed upon this proliferation. In a high turnover state the B cell with the highest affinity for the vaccine antigen will bind that antigen from the follicular dendritic cells, and undergo subsequent T cell help for proliferation. Cells with lower affinity antigen binding will not survive this process. This process, also known as the somatic hypermutation process, drives the response towards the most specific antibody producing cells. In healthy subjects, the forming of a germinal center reaction takes about 2 weeks, negative feedback starts within 3–6 weeks, thus peak IgG levels can be found 4–6 weeks after primary vaccination.

Until today, the precise role of distinct DC subsets such as Langerhans cells, dermal DCs, and plasmacytoid DCs in the immunology of ID immunization remains largely unknown. Besides, the involvement of skin resident DCs in the initial antigen–antigen-presenting cell contact, circulating DC precursors can be recruited into the dermis upon ID vaccination with a soluble protein, via enhanced expression of chemokine receptor/ligand CCR6/CCL20 (Le Borgne et al. 2006).

After the uptake and processing of antigens, the maturing DCs migrate to the T cell rich areas of the draining lymph nodes, where they express as a mature phenotype (Pulendran and Ahmed 2006).

The role of migratory DCs in the induction of $CD8^+$ T cell responses upon viral inoculation in the skin with different viruses is not uniform, as shown by the following mouse experiments. For example, in response to Herpes Simplex virus migratory DCs merely ferry viral antigens to the lymph node and immediately transfer the Herpes Simplex virus-antigens to $CD8^+$ DCs residing in the lymph node for cross-presentation (Allan et al. 2006). In contrast, He et al. (2006) showed that migratory skin DCs did directly present lentivirus derived ovalbumin (OVA) to lymph node $CD8^+$ T cells, without cross-presentation to lymph node resident DCs (Hepburn et al. 2006). Nonetheless, Allan et al. demonstrated that inhibition of migration of skin DCs, impaired the cytotoxic T lymphocyte response in the induction of immunity against Herpes Simplex virus (Allan et al. 2006), thereby implicating the importance of migratory skin DCs. Besides the trafficking of antigens through migrating DCs, recent research has highlighted the additional role of direct lymphatic drainage of free soluble antigen within hours after inoculation. This free antigen flows through afferent lymphatics into the subcapsular sinuses of the draining lymph node and is taken up and processed by lymph node resident DCs. After 24 h, a second antigen wave is delivered to the lymph node by influx of dermal DCs (not Langerhans cells) (Itano et al. 2003). Even though the lymph node resident DCs were responsible for the initial T cell activation, the DCs that acquired antigen at the injection site and migrated to the lymph node were needed to sustain the expression of the IL-2 receptor on the T cells.

Several hypotheses have been postulated to explain the relative success of ID vaccination. Firstly, a more direct antigen–antigen-presenting cell contact could lead to a smaller 'loss' of antigen in subcutaneous tissue or blood circulation where possibly less antigen-presenting cells are present. This hypothesis is particularly attractive in the case of live-attenuated viruses, which need to replicate intracellularly in order to induce a potent immune response. For soluble protein antigens, direct flow via the afferent lymphatic vessels could also contribute to the response (Itano et al. 2003; Pape et al. 2007). Interestingly, it has been shown recently that locally activated mast cells can, via enhanced DC migration, augment the immune response to several vaccine antigens, such as protein antigens and vaccinia, a live viral antigen (McLachlan et al. 2008). We described the protective antibody response to YF-17D in chicken egg allergic individuals who received the reduced dose yellow fever vaccine ID and developed strong local urticarial reactions (Roukens et al. 2009). In the presence of this hypersensitivity reaction, these individuals developed sufficient neutralizing antibodies. Unfortunately, whether their antibody response was enhanced compared to non-allergic individuals could not be verified, as their response could not be measured at set time points.

Secondly, ID immunization can trigger the activation and migration of dermal DCs, thereby amplifying the immune response (Itano et al. 2003). In contrast, intramuscular immunization enhances, via the bloodstream, the activation of plasmacytoid DCs which enter the lymph node via high endothelial venules, similar to B and T cells (Liu 2005). Plasmacytoid DCs are activated through TLR7 and TLR9 signaling, leading to type-1 IFN secretion. Their functional capacity in terms of vaccination (i.e. antigen presentation and T cell priming) remains to be investigated.

Finally, suggested by the findings of Cubas et al. (2009) the greater number of lymph nodes engaged upon ID immunization might be attributed to the lymphatic structure in the intradermal zone. In the skin, lymphatic vessels form two plexuses (Skobe and Detmar 2000). The superficial plexus contain branches that drain vertically into larger lymphatic vessels located in the lower dermis and the superficial zone of the subcutaneous tissue. These deep lymphatic vessels contain numerous valves through which antigen can be taken up. In addition, the limited space in the dermis and relatively large volume inoculated, could affect the permeability of the lymph vessels and thereby increase antigen uptake (Nicolas and Guy 2008). This argument of the volume of inoculation influencing the immune response has been suggested by Fox et al. (1943) and should be considered when designing new trials studying the ID immunization route.

The growing interest in ID immunization by vaccinologists has led to the development of many different technologies to accurately administer vaccine doses into the dermis. These techniques include fine-gauge needles and microneedle arrays, as well as various types of needle-free devices such as jet injectors and patches. Novel technologies for ID delivery may simplify the logistics of vaccine administration, avoid the dangers of needles and overcome other drawbacks facilitating vaccination mass campaigns (Glenn and Kenney 2006; Lambert and Laurent 2008; Nicolas and Guy 2008).

6 State-of the-Art: Future Perspectives

Antivirals have no value in the combat against yellow fever, and only a limited value in the combat against influenza epidemics, due to the rapid emergence and efficient spread of resistant strains. The unpredictable nature of influenza epidemiology calls for flexible vaccination policies. The global monitoring of influenza viruses, even before they enter the human reservoir, might be the most relevant action in containing viral spread. It might give health authorities a head start to prevent pandemic spread, even when the antigenic characteristics of a virus have altered enough to escape from pre-existing immunity. Using cell lines instead of embryonated eggs, will certainly help in making influenza vaccine production more flexible. In the production of yellow fever vaccine, an alternative to the production on embryonated chicken eggs is necessary to increase vaccine dose availability. Until then vaccine shortage is prone, and ID vaccination provides a relative solution to this shortage.

The two goals that will drive vaccination campaigns are the protection of those most vulnerable for morbidity and mortality and the interruption of spread by vaccination of transmission chains in nursery homes and (pre-)schools.

Vaccines with a higher immunogenicity have an added value for the elderly and immunocompromized hosts, who tend to have worse responses as compared to younger healthy controls. ID vaccination has been proved to be a feasible approach in times of vaccine shortage, especially for those with compromized immunity.

References

Akondy RS, Monson ND, Miller JD et al (2009) The yellow fever virus vaccine induces a broad and polyfunctional human memory CD8+ T cell response. J Immunol 183:7919–7930

Allan RS, Waithman J, Bedoui S et al (2006) Migratory dendritic cells transfer antigen to a lymph node-resident dendritic cell population for efficient CTL priming. Immunity 25:153–162

Appleby JC, Himmelweit F, Stuart-Harris CH (1951) Immunisation with influenza virus A vaccines, comparison of intradermal and subcutaneous routes. Lancet 1:1384–1387

Arnou R, Icardi G, De Decker M, Ambrozaitis A, Kazek MP, Weber F, Van Damme P (2009) Intradermal influenza vaccine for older adults: a randomized controlled multicenter phase III study. Vaccine 27:7304–7312

Bains I, Antia R, Callard R, Yates AJ (2009) Quantifying the development of the peripheral naive CD4+ T-cell pool in humans. Blood 113:5480–5487

Barwick R (2004) History of thymoma and yellow fever vaccination. Lancet 364:936

Belshe RB, Newman FK, Cannon J et al (2004) Serum antibody responses after intradermal vaccination against influenza. N Engl J Med 351:2286–2294

Beyer WE, de Bruijn IA, Palache AM, Westendorp RG, Osterhaus AD (1998) The plea against annual influenza vaccination? 'The Hoskins' Paradox' revisited. Vaccine 16:1929–1932

Beyer WE, Palache AM, Luchters G, Nauta J, Osterhaus AD (2004) Seroprotection rate, mean fold increase, seroconversion rate: which parameter adequately expresses seroresponse to influenza vaccination? Virus Res 103:125–132

Centers for Disease Control and Prevention (CDC) (2009) Pandemic influenza A (H1N1) virus infections—Chicago, Illinois, April–July 2009. MMWR Morb Mortal Wkly Rep 58(33):913–918

Chlíbek R, Smetana J, Sindelár R, Cecetková B, Prymula R, Kohl I (2007) Immunogenicity of vaccines against viral hepatitis A and B in the population above 40 years of age—impact of risk factors. Epidemiol Mikrobiol Imunol 56:119–128

Cohen Stuart J, Hamann D, Borleffs J, Roos M, Miedema F, Boucher C, de Boer R (2002) Reconstitution of naive T cells during antiretroviral treatment of HIV-infected adults is dependent on age. AIDS 16:2263–2266

Cubas R, Zhang S, Kwon S et al (2009) Virus-like particle (VLP) lymphatic trafficking and immune response generation after immunization by different routes. J Immunother 32: 118–128

de Jong JC, Palache AM, Beyer WE, Rimmelzwaan GF, Boon AC, Osterhaus AD (2003) Haemagglutination-inhibiting antibody to influenza virus. Dev Biol 115:63–73

de Vries-Sluijs TE, Hansen BE, van Doornum GJ, Springeling T, Evertsz NM, de Man RA, van der Ende ME (2008) A prospective open study of the efficacy of high-dose recombinant hepatitis B rechallenge vaccination in HIV-infected patients. J Infect Dis 197:292–294

Douek DC, McFarland RD, Keiser PH et al (1998) Changes in thymic function with age and during the treatment of HIV infection. Nature 396:690–695

Fox JP, Luty Kossobudski S, Fonseca da Cunha J (1943) Field studies on the immune response to 17D yellow fever virus. Relation to virus substrain, dose and route of inoculation. Am J Hyg 38:113–138

Gaspar LP, Mendes YS, Yamamura AM et al (2008) Pressure-inactivated yellow fever 17DD virus: implications for vaccine development. J Virol Methods 150:57–62

Gaucher D, Therrien R, Kettaf N et al (2008) Yellow fever vaccine induces integrated multilineage and polyfunctional immune responses. J Exp Med 205:3119–3131

Gelinck LBS, Teng YKO, Rimmelzwaan GF, Van den Bemt BJF, Kroon FP, Van Laar JM (2007) Poor serological responses upon influenza vaccination in patients with rheumatoid arthritis treated with rituximab. Ann Rheum Dis 66:1402–1403

Gelinck LB, van den Bemt BJ, Marijt WA, van der Bijl AE, Visser LG, Cats HA, Rimmelzwaan GF, Kroon FP (2009) Intradermal influenza vaccination in immunocompromized patients is immunogenic and feasible. Vaccine 27:2469–2474

Glenn GM, Kenney RT (2006) Mass vaccination: solutions in the skin. Curr Top Microbiol Immunol 304:247–268

Gould EA, Buckley A, Barrett ADT, Cammack N (1986) Neutralizing (54 K) and nonneutralizing (54 K and 48 K) monoclonal antibodies against structural and non-structural yellow fever virus proteins confer immunity in mice. J Gen Virol 67:591–595

Greenberg ME, Lai MH, Hartel GF et al (2009) Response to a monovalent 2009 influenza A (H1N1) vaccine. N Engl J Med 361:2405–2413

He Y, Zhang J, Donahue C, Falo LD Jr (2006) Skin-derived dendritic cells induce potent CD8(+) T cell immunity in recombinant lentivector-mediated genetic immunization. Immunity 24:643–656

Hepburn MJ, Kortepeter MG, Pittman PR, Boudreau EF, Mangiafico JA, Buck PA, Norris SL, Anderson EL (2006) Neutralizing antibody response to booster vaccination with the 17d yellow fever vaccine. Vaccine 24:2843–2849

Holland D, Booy R, De Looze F, Eizenberg P, McDonald J, Karrasch J, McKeirnan M, Salem H, Mills G, Reid J, Weber F, Saville M (2008) Intradermal influenza vaccine administered using a new microinjection system produces superior immunogenicity in elderly adults: a randomized controlled trial. J Infect Dis 198:650–658

Hoskins TW, Davies JR, Smith AJ, Miller CL, Allchin A (1979) Assessment of inactivated influenza-A vaccine after three outbreaks of influenza A at Christ's Hospital. Lancet 1:33–35

Itano AA, McSorley SJ, Reinhardt RL, Ehst BD, Ingulli E, Rudensky AY et al (2003) Distinct dendritic cell populations sequentially present antigen to CD4 T cells and stimulate different aspects of cell-mediated immunity. Immunity 19:47–57

Jo YM, Song JY, Hwang IS, Lee J, Oh SC, Kim JS, Kim SR, Kim WJ, Cheong HJ (2009) Dose sparing strategy with intradermal influenza vaccination in patients with solid cancer. J Med Virol 81:722–727

Kelly H, Grant K (2009) Interim analysis of pandemic influenza (H1N1) 2009 in Australia: surveillance trends, age of infection and effectiveness of seasonal vaccination. Euro Surveill 14. pii: 19288

Kengsakul K, Sathirapongsasuti K, Punyagupta S (2002) Fatal myeloencephalitis following yellow fever vaccination in a case with HIV infection. J Med Assoc Thai 85:131–134

Kenney RT, Frech SA, Muenz LR, Villar CP, Glenn GM (2004) Dose sparing with intradermal injection of influenza vaccine. N Engl J Med 351:2295–2301

Khanlou H, Sanchez S, Babaie M, Chien C, Hamwi G, Ricaurte JC et al (2006) The safety and efficacy of dose-sparing intradermal administration of influenza vaccine in human immunodeficiency virus-positive patients. Arch Intern Med 166:1417

Kunisaki KM, Janoff EN (2009) Influenza in immunosuppressed populations: a review of infection frequency, morbidity, mortality, and vaccine responses. Lancet Infect Dis 9:493–504

Lambert PH, Laurent PR (2008) Intradermal vaccine delivery: Will new delivery systems transform vaccine administration? Vaccine 26:3197–3208

Le Borgne M, Etchart N, Goubier A et al (2006) Dendritic cells rapidly recruited into epithelial tissues via CCR6/CCL20 are responsible for CD8+ T cell crosspriming in vivo. Immunity 24:191–201

Liu YJ (2005) IPC: professional type 1 interferon-producing cells and plasmacytoid dendritic cell precursors. Annu Rev Immunol 23:275–306

Lynch HE, Goldberg GL, Chidgey A, Van den Brink MR, Boyd R, Sempowski GD (2009) Thymic involution and immune reconstitution. Trends Immunol 30:366–373

Mackenzie JS, Fimmel PJ (1978) The effect of ABO blood groups on the incidence of epidemic influenza and on the response to live attenuated and detergent split influenza virus vaccines. J Hyg (Lond) 80:21–30

Macroepidemiology of Influenza Vaccination (MIV) Study Group (2005) The macro-epidemiology of influenza vaccination in 56 countries, 1997–2003. Vaccine 23:5133–5143

Madhi S et al. (2009) Efficacy of influenza vaccine in HIV-infected (HIV+) adults: a double-blind, placebo randomised controlled trial in South Africa. In: 5th IAS conference on HIV pathogenesis, treatment and prevention. 19–22 July 2009, Cape Town. Late breaker poster LBPEB04. http://www.ias2009.org/pag/Abstracts.aspx?AID=3805

Manuel O, Humar A, Chen MH et al (2007) Immunogenicity and safety of an intradermal boosting strategy for vaccination against influenza in lung transplant recipients. Am J Transplant 11:2567–2572

Mar ID, Niang I, Guicheney A, Berne C, Collomb H, Rey M, Satgé P (1967) Encephalitis following anti-yellow fever vaccination (from 248 cases observed at Dakar in 1965). Ann Pediatr (Paris) 143:181–191

Marianneau P, George-Courbot M, Deubel V (2001) Rarity of adverse effects after 17D yellow-fever vaccination. Lancet 358:84–85

Mason RA, Tauraso NM, Spertzel RO, Ginn RK (1973) Yellow fever vaccine: direct challenge of monkeys given graded doses of 17D vaccine. Appl Microbiol 25:539–544

Mateo RI, Xiao SY, Travassos da Rosa AP, Lei H, Guzman H, Lu L, Tesh RB (2007) Yellow fever 17-D vaccine is neurotropic and produces encephalitis in immunosuppressed hamster. Am J Trop Med Hyg 77:919–924

McCarroll JR, Kilbourne ED (1958) Immunization with Asian-strain influenza vaccine, equivalence of the subcutaneous and intradermal routes. NEJM 259:618–621

McLachlan JB, Shelburne CP, Hart JP et al (2008) Mast cell activators: a new class of highly effective vaccine adjuvants. Nat Med 14:536–541

McMichael AJ, Gotch F, Cullen P, Askonas B, Webster RG (1981) The human cytotoxic T cell response to influenza A vaccination. Clin Exp Immunol 43:276–284

Monath TP (2005) Yellow fever vaccine. Expert Rev Vaccines 4:553–574

Monath TP (2008a) Yellow fever. In: Plotkin SA, Orenstein WA, Paul A (eds) Vaccines, 5th ed. Saunders Elsevier, Philadelphia, p 959

Monath TP (2008b) Treatment of yellow fever. Antiviral Res 78:116–124

Monath TP, Cetron MS, McCarthy K et al (2005) Yellow fever 17D vaccine safety and immunogenicity in the elderly. Hum Vaccin 1:207–214

Nicolas JF, Guy B (2008) Intradermal, epidermal and transcutaneous vaccination: from immunology to clinical practice. Expert Rev Vaccines 7:1201–1214

Niedrig M, Lademann M, Emmerich P, Lafrenz M (1999) Assessment of IgG antibodies against yellow fever firus after vaccination with 17D by different assays: neutralization test, haemagglutination inhibition test, immunofluorescence assay and ELISA. Trop Med Int Health 12:867–871

Oren S, Mandelboim M, Braun-Moscovici et al (2008) Vaccination against influenza in patients with rheumatoid arthritis: the effect of rituximab on the humoral response. Ann Rheum Dis 67:937–941

World Health Organisation (2003) Yellow fever vaccine. WHO position paper, Wkly Epidemiol Rec 40:349–359

Overton ET, Nurutdinova D, Sungkanuparph S, Seyfried W, Groger RK, Powderly WG (2007) Predictors of immunity after hepatitis A vaccination in HIV-infected persons. J Viral Hepat 14:189–193

Palmer DR, Fernandez S, Bisbing J et al (2007) Restricted replication and lysosomal trafficking of yellow fever 17D vaccine virus in human dendritic cells. J Gen Virol 88:148–156

Pape KA, Catron DM, Itano AA, Jenkins MK (2007) The humoral immune response is initiated in lymph nodes by B cells that acquire soluble antigen directly in the follicles. Immunity 26:491–502

Pfister G, Savino W (2008) Can the immune system still be efficient in the elderly? An immunological and immunoendocrine therapeutic perspective. Neuroimmunomodulation 15:351–364

Pincus S, Mason PW, Konishi E, Fonseca BA, Shope RE, Rice CM, Paoletti E (1992) Recombinant vaccinia virus producing the prM and E proteins of yellow fever virus protects mice from lethal yellow fever virus encephalitis. Virology 187:290–297

Plotkin SA (2008) Correlates of vaccine-induced immunity. Clin Infect Dis 47:401–409

Pulendran B, Ahmed R (2006) Translating innate immunity into immunological memory: implications for vaccine development. Cell 124:849–863

Querec T, Bennouna S, Alkan S, Laouar Y, Gorden K, Flavell R, Akira S, Ahmed R, Pulendran B (2006) Yellow fever vaccine YF-17D activates multiple dendritic cell subsets via TLR2, 7, 8, and 9 to stimulate polyvalent immunity. J Exp Med 203:413–424

Roukens AH, Visser LG (2008) Yellow fever vaccine: past, present and future. Expert Opin Biol Ther 8:1787–1795

Roukens AH, Vossen AC, Bredenbeek PJ, van Dissel JT, Visser LG (2008) Intradermally administered Yellow Fever vaccine at reduced dose induces a protective immune response: a randomized controlled non-inferiority trial. PLoS ONE 3:e1993

Roukens AH, Vossen AC, van Dissel JT, Visser LG (2009) Reduced intradermal test dose of yellow fever induces protective immunity in individuals with egg allergy. Vaccine 27:2408–2409

Russell CA, Jones TC, Barr IG et al (2008) The global circulation of seasonal influenza A (H3N2) viruses. Science 320:340–346

Ryan J, Zoellner Y, Gradl B, Palache B, Medema J (2006) Establishing the health and economic impact of influenza vaccination within the European Union 25 countries. Vaccine 24:6812–6822

Sellards AW (1931) The behaviour of the virus of yellow fever in monkeys and mice. Proc Natl Acad Sci U S A 17:339–343

Siegrist CA (2008) Vaccine immunology. In: Plotkin S, Orenstein W, Offit P (eds) Vaccines, 5th edn. Saunders Elsevier, Philadelphia

Skobe M, Detmar M (2000) Structure, function, and molecular control of the skin lymphatic system. J Investig Dermatol Symp Proc 5:14–19

Smedley J, Poole J, Waclawski E et al (2007) Influenza immunisation: attitudes and beliefs of UK healthcare workers. Occup Environ Med 64:223–227

Smith W, Andrews C, Laidlaw P (1933) A virus obtained from influenza patients. Lancet 2:66–68

Smith DJ, Forrest S, Ackley DH, Perelson AS (1999) Variable efficacy of repeated annual influenza vaccination. Proc Natl Acad Sci U S A 96:14001–14006

Stokes A, Bauer JH, Hudson NP (2001) The transmission of yellow fever to *Macacus rhesus*. Rev Med Virol 11:141–148

Takata T, Suzumiya J, Ishikawa T, Takamatsu Y, Ikematsu H, Tamura K (2009) Attenuated antibody reaction for the primary antigen but not for the recall antigen of influenza vaccination in patients with non-Hodgkin B-cell lymphoma after the administration of rituximab-CHOP. J Clin Exp Hematol 49:9–13

Tasker SA, Treanor JJ, Paxton WB, Wallace MR (1999) Efficacy of influenza vaccination in HIV-infected persons: a randomised, double-blind, placebo-controlled trial. Ann Intern Med 131:430–433

Theiler M, Smith HH (1937) The use of yellow fever virus modified by in vitro cultivation for human immunization. J Exp Med 65:787–800

Treanor JJ (2009) Influenza viruses, including avian influenza and swine influenza. In: Mandell GL, Bennett JE, Dolin R (eds) Mandell, Douglas, and Bennett's principles and practice of infectious diseases, 7th edn. Elsevier, Philadelphia

van Assen S, Holvast A, Benne CA et al (2010) Humoral responses after influenza vaccination are severely reduced in patients with rheumatoid arthritis treated with rituximab. Arthritis Rheum 62:75–81 van der Kolk LE, Baars JW, Prins MH, van Oers MH (2002) Rituximab treatment results in impaired secondary humoral immune responsiveness. Blood 100:2257–2259

Veit O, Niedrig M, Chapius-Taillard C, Cavassini M, Mossdorf E, Schmid P, Bae HG, Litzba N, Staub T, Hatz C, Furrer H, Swiss HIV Cohort Study (2009) Immunogenicity and safety of yellow fever vaccination for 102 HIV-infected patients. Clin Infect Dis 48:659–666

Weinberger B, Herndler-Brandstetter D, Schwanninger A, Weiskopf D, Grubeck-Loebenstein B (2008) Biology of immune responses to vaccines in elderly persons. Clin Infect Dis 46:1078–1084

The Dermis as a Portal for Dendritic Cell-Targeted Immunotherapy of Cutaneous Melanoma

D. Oosterhoff, B. J. R. Sluijter, B. N. Hangalapura and T. D. de Gruijl

Abstract Complete surgical excision at an early stage remains the only curative treatment for cutaneous melanoma with few available adjuvant therapy options. Nevertheless, melanoma is a relatively immunogenic tumor type and particularly amenable to immunotherapeutic approaches. A dense network of cutaneous dendritic cells (DC) may account for the reported efficacy of vaccination through the skin and provide an attractive target for the immunotherapy of melanoma. Several phenotypically distinct DC subsets are discernable in the skin, among others, epidermal Langerhans cells and dermal DC. Upon appropriate activation both subsets can efficiently migrate to melanoma-draining lymph nodes (LN) to prime T cell-mediated responses. Unfortunately, from an early stage, melanoma development is characterized by strong immune suppression, facilitating unchecked tumor growth and spread. Particularly the primary tumor site and the first-line tumor-draining LN, the so-called sentinel LN, bear the brunt of this melanoma-induced immune suppression—and these are exactly the sites where anti-melanoma effector T cell responses should be primed by DC in order to prevent early metastasis. Through local immunopotentiation or through DC-targeted vaccination, the dermis may be utilized as a portal to activate DC and kick-start or boost effective T cell-mediated anti-melanoma immunity, even in the face of this immune suppression.

D. Oosterhoff · B. N. Hangalapura · T. D. de Gruijl (✉)
Department of Medical Oncology, VU University Medical Center,
De Boelelaan 1117, 1081 HV, Amsterdam, The Netherlands
e-mail: td.degruijl@vumc.nl

B. J. R. Sluijter
Department of Surgical Oncology, VU University Medical Center,
De Boelelaan 1117, 1081 HV, Amsterdam, The Netherlands

Current Topics in Microbiology and Immunology (2012) 351: 181–220
DOI: 10.1007/82_2011_136

Published Online: 18 June 2011

Contents

1 Introduction

Malignant and invasive growth of melanocytes, which are normally located in the basal layer of the epidermis, is termed melanoma cutis or cutaneous melanoma. Although it represents only 4% of all diagnosed cases of skin cancer, melanoma of the skin is one of the most aggressive types of cancer with a high invasive and metastasizing potential. As yet, the only curative treatment option remains excision of the primary tumor at early stages of the disease, before it penetrates into the dermis where it can access lymphatic and blood vessels for metastatic spread. The classification of the different stages of melanoma by the American Joint Committee on Cancer is provided in Box 1 (Balch et al. 2001, 2009b; Cecchi et al. 2007; Starz and Balda 2007). Once metastases are present, therapeutic options are limited and most patients do not survive for more than 6 months after being diagnosed with advanced disease. Although cutaneous melanoma is not sensitive to traditional chemo- and radiotherapy, it is highly immunogenic. Case reports of spontaneous regressions have been documented and are suggestive of immune-mediated tumor rejection. In addition, melanoma-specific T cells can be found early on in the blood and tumor-draining lymph nodes (TDLN) of most patients (Banchereau et al. 2001; Romero et al. 1998, 2006). This knowledge has led to extensive research of immunotherapeutic approaches aimed at controlling local melanoma growth and eliminating distant metastasis. The immunomodulatory drugs IL-2 and IFN-α have both been FDA approved for the treatment of melanoma patients. However, treatment will only follow after diagnosis of local or distant metastases, although Stage II melanoma (Box 1) is already considered to be of intermediate risk for local recurrence or distant metastasis. Adjuvant therapy could be of value to these patients since 5-year survival rates for Stages IIA–IIC range from 53 to 80% (Balch et al. 2009b). The same applies to patients with Stage III melanoma: these tumors spread to regional lymph nodes (LN) without evidence of distant metastasis (Box 1). Even with treatment, Stage III disease is considered to be of intermediate to high-risk for local recurrence or distant metastasis and 5-year survival rates for Stage IIIC drop as low as 27% (Balch et al. 2001). Clearly, patients in early stages of melanoma might benefit from adjuvant immunotherapy, aiming to control tumor growth and spread at the primary tumor site and the TDLN. Possible treatment approaches for these patients are local immunomodulation or vaccination. Local management of the disease has the advantage that it is less likely to cause severe systemic side effects. Moreover, there is evidence that local immune activation may lead to systemic immune protection (Molenkamp et al. 2008; Ridolfi et al. 2001). The dermis provides an ideal portal for the delivery of immunopotentiating agents or vaccines. It contains a variety of different immune effector cell populations and provides ready access to skin-draining LN through a network of afferent lymphatic vessels. By boosting local innate and adaptive immune responses in the dermis, the growth and local spread of melanoma may be contained in the early stages of its development. Dendritic cells (DC) are the central initiators and orchestrators of the immune response with a unique ability to prime and skew T cell responses (Banchereau et al. 2000). During their activation they receive environmental input that determines their cytokine release patterns, which in turn direct the type of T cell responses that are elicited (Macagno et al. 2007). They are prime candidates to target with local immunomodulation. Here, we will discuss how developing melanomas influence their microenvironment to effectively suppress the local immune system and we will propose ways in which DC or T cells in the dermis and draining LN may be targeted and modulated to overcome this immune suppression in aid of melanoma immunotherapy.

Box 1: Staging of Melanoma Cutis According to the American Joint Committee on Cancer and Eligibility for Immunopotentiation in the Adjuvant Setting

Stage 0 melanoma: When the epidermis, but not the underlying dermis is tumor involved, this is called Stage 0 melanoma or melanoma in situ. There is no invasion of surrounding tissues, lymph nodes, or distant sites. After radical excision Stage 0 is considered very low risk for disease recurrence, or for tumor spread to lymph nodes or distant sites. Five-year survival is >97%.

Stage I melanoma: Stage I melanomas are tumors with a Breslow thickness of $\leq$ 2.0 mm without ulceration or $\leq$ 1.0 mm with ulceration, that have not spread to nearby lymph nodes or distant sites. Timely resection of these lesions results in low risk for recurrence and metastasis. Ten year survival rates for Stage IA–IB range from 85 to 99%.

Stage II melanoma: Stage II melanomas are tumors with a Breslow thickness of ≥2.0 mm without ulceration or ≥1.0 mm with ulceration that have not spread to nearby lymph nodes or distant sites. Even with treatment, Stage II disease is considered to be intermediate risk for local recurrence or distant metastasis: 16% develop a recurrence, which is associated with a significant decrease in survival. Five-year survival rates for Stages IIA–IIC are 53–80%.

Stage III melanoma: Stage III melanomas are tumors that have spread to regional lymph nodes without evidence of distant metastasis. With treatment, Stage III disease is considered to be intermediate to high-risk for local recurrence or distant metastasis. The 5-year survival rates for Stages IIIA–IIIC range from 40 to 78%.

Stage IV melanoma: Stage IV melanomas are associated with metastasis to distant sites in the body. Five-year survival rates range from 10 to 28% depending on the anatomical location of the metastases; median survival after the onset of distant metastases is usually only 6–9 months.

NB: Patients with Stages I–III melanoma might benefit from adjuvant local immunopotentiation. (*Source* Balch et al. 2001, 2009b)

2 The Challenges of Generating Anti-Melanoma Immunity

In cutaneous melanoma, skin-resident DC take up and transport melanoma-associated antigens (MAA) to TDLN (Banchereau et al. 2000; Toriyama et al. 1993). The relatively large number of identified MAA underlines the immunogenicity of this tumor. Different types of MAA are discerned, among others cancer/testis antigens (e.g. MAGE, NY-ESO, and PRAME) and melanocyte differentiation antigens (e.g. tyrosinase, tyrosinase-related proteins-1 and -2 (TRP-1/-2), MART-1/Melan-A, and gp100) (Dranoff 2009). In order to activate T cells specifically recognizing these MAA, the skin-emigrated DC need to become activated, i.e. express high levels of co-stimulatory molecules as well as appropriate chemokine receptors to migrate to the paracortical T cell areas of the TDLN (Macagno et al. 2007). In the T cell areas of the TDLN the MAA-presenting DC bind and specifically activate recirculating naïve and memory T-helper (Th) cells and cytotoxic T lymphocytes (CTL) (Schoenberger et al. 1998). Activated effector CTL leave the LN via efferent vessels and home to tumor sites in order to eradicate melanoma cells. Although tumor-infiltrating lymphocytes (TIL) specifically recognizing MAA can be readily found in primary tumors, TDLN, and metastases, they obviously cannot prevent ultimate melanoma growth and spread (Romero et al. 2006). Nevertheless, important clinical studies, in which autologous TIL were adoptively transferred to advanced melanoma patients, have clearly demonstrated the powerful intrinsic ability of these TIL to eliminate bulky melanoma metastases (reviewed by Rosenberg and Dudley 2009). In order for this approach to be effective, the TIL need to be extricated from the immunosuppressive tumor environment and expanded in vitro. Moreover, patients receive lymphodepleting chemotherapy to eliminate suppressor cells and other effector cells that may compete for growth factors with the adoptively transferred TIL, prior to infusion of billions of expanded TIL. By eliminating the suppressive microenvironment of the tumor and systemically "resetting" the immune system of the patient through lymphodepleting chemotherapy, adoptive T cell transfer has proven effective, achieving objective regression of melanoma metastases in up to 70% of treated patients (Rosenberg and Dudley 2009). These studies serve as an impressive demonstration of the immune system's capacity to eradicate melanoma tumors. One of the challenges in the adjuvant setting, where distant metastases have not yet developed, is to curb the melanoma's immunosuppressive traits and kick-start a protective anti-tumor immune response in order to prevent metastatic spread. Central to the premise of local immunopotentiation in melanoma is the enhancement or restoration of anti-tumor DC and T cell functions in the tumor and its draining LN, even in the face of immunosuppressive conditions imposed by the tumor (Cochran et al. 2006; Molenkamp et al. 2006; Rabinovich et al. 2007). The elimination of these suppressive conditions is also a prerequisite for any MAA-based vaccine to be effective.

3 The Immune Microenvironment and Dendritic Cell Subsets of the Skin

As the first and main physical barrier between the body and the outside world, the skin can be regarded as the largest immune organ of the body. It consists of a large number of epidermis- and dermis-resident immune effector cells that under steady state conditions maintain homeostasis and tolerance, but in case of infection or inflammation can prime specific immune responses (Nestle and Nickoloff 2007). Besides DC, skin-resident leukocytes include macrophages, T cells, NKT cells, mast cells, and granulocytes (review by Nestle et al. 2009). Moreover, non-immune cells in the epidermis and dermis, such as keratinocytes and fibroblasts, should not be regarded as immunologically inactive. Keratinocytes express a wide range of Toll-like receptors (TLR) and can sense microbial infection through binding of TLR-ligands (Lebre et al. 2007). Upon their TLR-mediated activation keratinocytes release protective antimicrobial peptides, but also a variety of cytokines (among others IL-1, -6, -10, -18, and TNF-α) that in turn can activate DC and condition dermal fibroblasts to secrete chemokines that attract DC and further recruit immune effector cells (Ouwehand et al. 2008, 2010). Besides microbial recognition, keratinocytes are also endowed with the ability to sense tissue damage and stress (e.g. induced by toxins, irritants, ultraviolet radiation, or tumor growth) through so-called nucleotide-binding domain, leucin-rich repeat (NLR) containing proteins, linking to the inflammasome complex and inducing the cleavage of IL-1β and/or IL-18 from their pro-cytokines. This will start a cascade of events, resulting in immune activation (Nestle et al. 2009).

Besides this crosstalk between immune and non-immune cells in support of immune surveillance, the dermis also contains a dense network of blood and lymph vessels, facilitating both the rapid recruitment of immune effector cells from blood and ready access to skin-draining LN, where adaptive B and T cell responses can be primed or boosted (Mathers and Larregina 2006). These features have made the skin a favored site for delivery of vaccines and immunomodulatory agents (Mikszta and Laurent 2008; Stoitzner et al. 2010b). Vaccination through the skin has been shown to result in effective anti-tumor immunity (Mikszta and Laurent 2008; Mitsui et al. 2010; Stoitzner et al. 2008). Particularly for melanoma, being a skin-derived tumor, skin-based immunization approaches may be very effective (Stoitzner et al. 2010a). This is in part attributable to the fact that effector-memory T cells primed in skin-draining LN efficiently and preferentially home to the skin through the expression of skin-homing molecules such as cutaneous lymphocyte-associated antigen (CLA). This is a process referred to as imprinting and involves skin-derived DC (Edele et al. 2008; Mora et al. 2005).

A dense network of readily accessible and differentially specialized DC subsets lines the skin and upon any sign of danger can rapidly initiate immune activation. Nevertheless, which of the thus-far identified subsets should be targeted for optimal CTL induction remains unclear. Indeed, all DC subsets may be targetable for potentiation of the anti-melanoma immune response (Sparber et al. 2010). Figure 1 shows a FACS dot plot of human skin explant-emigrated CD11c^{+} myeloid cells stained for CD1a and CD14. This plot illustrates the diversity of DC subsets in the human skin environment; at least five populations can be discerned: (1) CD1a^{hi}CD14^{-} Langerhans cells (LC) that also express the C-type lectin Langerin at their cell surface and are mature based on CD83 expression; (2) CD1a^{+}CD14^{-} dermal DC (DDC) that do not express surface Langerin or DC-SIGN but are mature (i.e. express CD83) and can express intracellular DC-SIGN upon IL-4 modulation (Fig. 2); (3) CD1a^{+}CD14^{+} DDC that over time can convert into (4) CD1a^{-}CD14^{+} DDC; and (5) CD1a^{-}CD14^{-} DDC, a fraction of which can express DC-SIGN at their surface (de Gruijl et al. 2006). It is important to realize that in many cases it is not absolutely clear if these are actual distinct subsets, or merely DC from the same subset with different phenotypes, dictated by micro-environmental factors. Study of this matter is ongoing, but complicated by the extremely low numbers in which DC are present in vivo. Moreover, care should be taken in extrapolation to the human situation of murine findings, since a variety of murine DC subsets in skin, LN, and spleen have been identified, but the equivalents have not (yet) been found in humans (Romani et al. 2010). Below, a brief

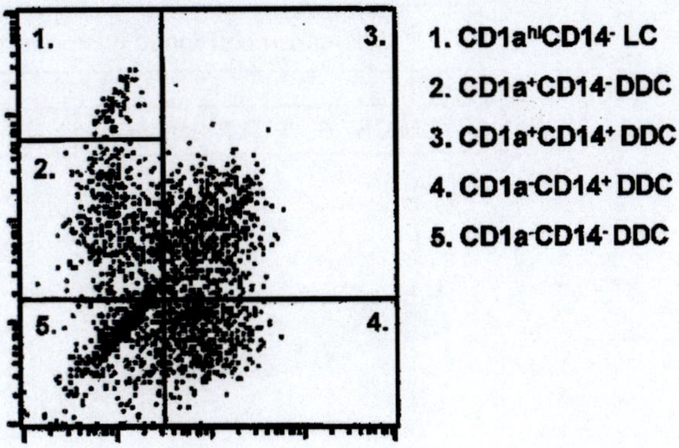

Fig. 1 Human skin-emigrating dendritic cell subsets. CD1a (*vertical axis*)/CD14 (*horizontal axis*) phenotype of 2-day migrated CD11c^{hi} conventional DC from cultured human skin explants, according to our earlier described methods (de Gruijl et al. 2006)

overview is given of DC and other antigen-presenting cell subsets in skin and skin-draining LN. Of note, all these subsets can be targeted by intradermal (ID) delivery of immunomodulatory agents or vaccines.

3.1 Langerhans Cells

LC are the DC of the epidermis and were the first DC to be described. In the steady state LC are derived from precursor cells residing in the skin, whereas under inflammatory conditions they can also develop from monocytes recruited from the blood (Geissmann et al. 2010; Merad et al. 2008). They express high levels of CD1a and Langerin at their cell surface, as well as the epithelial adhesion molecule EpCAM. There is evidence to suggest that upon their activation and migration to LN, LC preferentially bind and activate T cells (Klechevsky et al. 2009). In keeping with this, LC-like cells generated from monocytes or CD34^{+} precursors were shown to be superior CTL activators (Klechevsky et al. 2008, 2009). As cell-mediated immunity is generally believed to be crucial in tumor eradication, it may therefore be beneficial to specifically target LC and their precursors for tumor immunotherapy. However, in contrast with these claims, our own studies with human skin-emigrated LC and DDC have shown DDC to be even more efficient CTL primers than LC ex vivo (Santegoets et al. 2008a). In conclusion, both subsets remain viable targets for melanoma immunotherapy strategies.

While DDC may easily be targeted through ID injection, LC targeting usually involves transcutaneous approaches (Stoitzner et al. 2008, 2010a, b). However, there are ways to attract LC to the dermis, where they can also be targeted for immunization purposes. Moreover, a recent study showed that ID injected antibodies were able to pass the basal membrane and bind LC in the epidermis (Flacher et al. 2010), suggesting that even ID delivery of large proteins can result in targeting of epidermal LC.

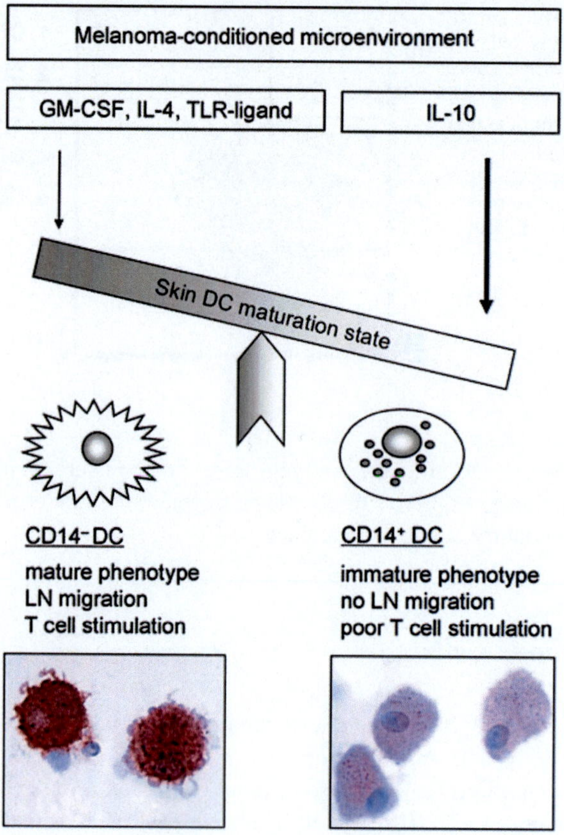

Fig. 2 The balance between dendritic cell maturation-inducing factors (TLR-ligands, cytokines) and IL-10 in the dermal microenvironment of invading melanomas will determine the phenotypic activation state and functionality of skin-emigrating DC. IL-10 induces a phenotypic switch in migrating DC from a mature T cell-stimulatory to an immature macrophage-like phenotype, resulting in possible immunological silence. DC-activating cytokines and TLR-ligands can induce a stable DC maturation that is resistant to the suppressive effects of IL-10 (de Gruijl et al. 2006). Photographic inserts: human skin-explant emigrated DC stained for DC-SIGN, 7 days after start of explant culture. Explants were ID injected on day 0 with 100 ng GM-CSF and 1000 IU IL-4 (*left panel*) or 10 ng IL-10 (*right panel*); magnification 400×

3.2 *CD1a*$^+$ *Dermal Dendritic Cells*

In contrast to LC, CD1a$^+$ DDC do not express Langerin and only intermediate to low levels of CD1a. Instead, DDC can express an alternative set of lectins, including the mannose receptor (MR) and DC-SIGN, as well as Factor XIIIa (Mathers and Larregina 2006). The differential expression pattern of antigen-capture receptors between LC and DDC should enable the specific targeting of each subset for vaccination purposes. DDC have been shown to produce IL-10 and to be able to direct the generation of type-2 humoral responses, vital to the initiation of humoral immunity (Mathers and Larregina 2006; Sen et al. 2010). However, the T cell skewing abilities of interstitial DC/DDC are not fixed, but rather dictated by a balance of factors in the microenvironment, their number, and activation state, resulting in differential Th1, Th2, or Th17 profiles (Mathers and Larregina 2006; Mathers et al. 2009; Morelli et al. 2005). The ability to modulate this balance may be of crucial importance for successful immunotherapy of cancer.

Recently, Langerin$^+$ and CD103$^+$ DDC were identified in murine studies as a major migratory DC subset from skin with the ability to cross-present proteins from the skin environment (Bedoui et al. 2009; Farrand et al. 2009; Ginhoux et al. 2007). It has been suggested that CD1a$^+$ DDC may be the human equivalent of this subset (Klechevsky et al. 2009), but evidence to back up this claim is lacking. We have performed a genome-wide transcriptional profiling analysis of freshly isolated human CD1a$^+$ DDC versus LC and found DDC to express a far wider range of adhesion and co-stimulatory molecules, chemokines, and cytokines (and at higher levels), pointing to a putatively superior migratory and T cell stimulatory ability over LC (Santegoets et al. 2008b). Indeed, our own comparative ex vivo study of the ability of these subsets to prime CD8$^+$ effector T cells against a MART-1 epitope, are in keeping with these transcriptional analyses (Santegoets et al. 2008a).

3.3 *CD14$^+$ Dermal Dendritic Cells and Dermal Macrophages*

Several reports have pointed to the existence of another CD1a$^-$CD14$^+$ DDC subset in human skin under steady state conditions with an immature macrophage-like phenotype and lacking T cell priming ability (Fig. 1) (Angel et al. 2007; de Gruijl et al. 2006; Klechevsky et al. 2008, 2009; Nestle and Nickoloff 2007; Zaba et al. 2009). Our own unpublished studies have shown that they are the most prevalent DDC subset migrating from full-thickness skin explants taken from skin overlying breast tumors (in contrast to healthy skin where CD1a$^+$ DDC are the most frequent subset among migrating DDC, Lindenberg et al. manuscript in preparation). These CD14$^+$ DC appeared immunologically silent (i.e. lacking co-stimulatory signals and the LN-homing chemokine receptor CCR7) and were further characterized by expression of the C-type lectin BDCA3 (de Gruijl et al. 2006).

Besides CD14$^+$ DDC, also CD14$^+$ resident macrophages were found in the steady state dermis. These macrophages were strongly positive for the macrophage markers CD68 and CD163 (Zaba et al. 2007), but surprisingly have also been reported to express the DC-associated C-type lectin DC-SIGN (Ochoa et al. 2008). CD14$^+$ dermal macrophages can be discerned from CD14$^+$ DDC through their lack of CD1b or CD1c (Zaba et al. 2007, 2009). While, like CD14$^+$ DDC, dermal macrophages display a poor ability to induce T cell proliferation, they may nevertheless contribute to T cell activation through their release of inflammatory cytokines (Zaba et al. 2007).

3.4 Plasmacytoid Dendritic Cells

In contrast to the above described peripheral conventional DC (cDC) subsets, immature plasmacytoid DC (pDC) with a plasma cell-like appearance and a more lymphoid phenotype, preferentially seed LN straight from the blood through L-selectin-mediated homing (Yoneyama et al. 2004). In the steady state they reside in LN rather than in skin, constantly screening the surroundings for signs of infection. However, under pathological or inflammatory conditions (e.g. psoriasis) pDC may also be recruited from the blood to the reticular dermis, likely in a CXCR3-mediated fashion (Asselin-Paturel et al. 2005; Skrzeczynska-Moncznik et al. 2009). Differential TLR expression (Jarrossay et al. 2001) or specific expression of C-type lectins [e.g. BDCA2 or DCIR (Dzionek et al. 2001; Fanning et al. 2006; Meyer-Wentrup et al. 2008; Riboldi et al. 2009)] may allow for the specific targeting of pDC for immunotherapy. However, caution is warranted as DCIR or BDCA2 engagement can interfere in the pDC's cytotoxic and stimulatory abilities, possibly resulting in tumor escape and/or tolerisation. To avoid this, pDC targeting through specific C-type lectins may have to be combined with activating stimuli.

3.5 Dendritic Cell Subsets in Skin-Draining LN

As ID delivered substances will also rapidly diffuse to skin-draining LN, DC subsets residing in these LN may be directly modulated and/or targeted. In contrast to mice, very little is known about cDC subsets present in human LN that drain the skin. From our own melanoma sentinel LN (SLN) studies we can discern at least three different cDC populations, besides a pDC population (Molenkamp et al. 2007; Vuylsteke et al. 2004).

1. $CD1a^+$ DC: These DC express high levels of co-stimulatory molecules, CD83, and CCR7. ID administration of granulocyte–macrophage colony-stimulating factor (GM-CSF) leads to further upregulation of their co-stimulatory machinery and CD83 and to increased numbers of these DC in the paracortical LN areas (Vuylsteke et al. 2004). A high and significant correlation was found between densities of $CD1a^+$ DC in the papillary dermis and matching SLN, strongly suggesting the $CD1a^+$ DC subset in the SLN to derive from dermis-emigrating $CD1a^+$ LC and/or DDC (Molenkamp et al. 2005, 2007). Frequencies of these mature $CD1a^+$ DC in the SLN also correlated significantly with

melanoma-specific CD8$^+$ effector T cells, indicative of the validity of this DC subset for tumor vaccine targeting (Vuylsteke et al. 2006).

2. CD11c^{hi}CD14$^-$ DC: These DC do not express CD1a, but do express CD83 and co-stimulatory molecules on their surface, albeit at lower levels than the CD1a$^+$ DC (Molenkamp et al. 2007). We found the frequencies of this DC subset to be up-regulated in melanoma SLN upon CpG administration (Molenkamp et al. 2007). The most likely explanation for this is the recruitment and/or differentiation of LN-resident or blood-derived monocytes or other DC precursors under the influence of pDC-derived IFN-α. The functional abilities of this novel subset remain to be established, although expression of TRAIL on their surface suggests a direct cytolytic ability. Expression of the C-type lectin BDCA3/CD141 on at least part of these DC (Sluijter et al., submitted) suggests that the BDCA3$^+$ cDC subset in peripheral blood may be their direct precursor, but this remains to be established. Interestingly, a recent genome-wide transcriptional profiling study suggested BDCA3$^+$ DC to be the human equivalent of the CD8α^+ DC subset in murine spleen, which is known to be the subset with cross-priming and powerful CTL priming abilities (Robbins et al. 2008). Indeed, recent in vitro studies provided evidence for the cross-priming abilities of human BDCA3$^+$ DC and thus confirmed this hypothesis (Bachem et al. 2010; Crozat et al. 2010; Jongbloed et al. 2010; Poulin et al. 2010).
3. CD11c^{hi}CD14$^+$ DC: Although at least part of these cells most likely represent monocytes or macrophages, low CD83 expression on a subpopulation seems to suggest a semi-mature DC phenotype (Sluijter et al. submitted). These might derive from migratory CD14$^+$ DDC, but this is not consistent with our observations from skin explant studies that migratory CD14$^+$ DDC are immature and do not express CD83 (de Gruijl et al. 2006). Thus, their origins and function for the moment remain obscure.

   Both DC-SIGN and Langerin expression is apparent by immunohistochemistry on DC-like cells in the LN paracortex (Engering et al. 2004; Geissmann et al. 2002). However, neither DC-SIGN nor Langerin surface expression is discernable by flow cytometry on any of the above listed cDC subsets, leaving their relation to skin subsets obscure for the moment. Of note, the strongest expression of DC-SIGN is found in marginal zone and sinus macrophages (Granelli-Piperno et al. 2005 and own unpublished observation), leaving its relevance for selective DC targeting in doubt.
4. BDCA2/CD303$^+$CD123$^+$ pDC: In the steady state pDC reside in LN in low numbers (which rise in melanoma-draining LN) and can bind microbial products through receptors such as TLR9 (Gerlini et al. 2007, 2010). TLR9 binds bacterial DNA-derived unmethylated CpG oligodinucleotide-containing motifs and activates pDC, which then release IFN-α. In turn IFN-α can boost CTL and NK cell responses (Liu et al. 2008; Salio et al. 2003) as well as promote the differentiation and maturation of bystander cDC and their precursors (Gursel et al. 2002; Molenkamp et al. 2007). In addition, pDC can also directly (cross-) present MAA-derived epitopes and thus prime melanoma-specific CTL (Liu et al. 2008; Mouries et al. 2008; Villadangos and Young 2008).

4 Subverting the Immune Response: Melanoma-Induced Dendritic Cell Suppression

The very reason that melanoma is such an attractive target for immunotherapy, i.e. its intrinsically high immunogenicity, is most likely also why it is a powerful immunosuppressive tumor type and refractory to conventional tumor vaccination approaches. In order to survive the host immune response and enable tumor outgrowth and spread, it had to develop ingenious ways through which to subvert and escape the anti-tumor immune response (Mellor and Munn 2008). The main challenge for tumor immunotherapists is to identify these suppressive mechanisms and devise novel strategies to overcome them.

An obvious target of this tumor-induced immunosuppression is the central immune orchestrator, the DC. Hampered DC differentiation and activation has been reported in many tumors and decreased tumor infiltration by mature DC is generally recognized as a poor prognostic factor (Ishigami et al. 2010; Iwamoto et al. 2003; Ladanyi et al. 2007). Immature DC with ready access to MAA, derived from primary or metastatic tumor sites, can induce specific tolerance through inappropriate or abortive T cell activation (Hawiger et al. 2001; Jonuleit et al. 2001). Indeed, immature cDC isolated from melanoma metastases were reported to induce T cell tolerance (Enk et al. 1997; Gerlini et al. 2004), while cDC in TDLN were similarly reported to display immature characteristics (Cochran et al. 2001, 2006; Huang et al. 2000). cDC development and activation can both be frustrated by inhibitory factors commonly associated with melanoma, such as VEGF, TGF-β, IL-10, or gangliosides (Cochran et al. 2006; Enk et al. 1997; Gerlini et al. 2004; Peguet-Navarro et al. 2003). Over the past years it has become clear that many of these tumor-derived suppressive factors exert their suppressive effects on cDC through activation (i.e. phosphorylation) of signal transducer and activator of transcription-3 (STAT3) (Yu et al. 2009). STAT3 activation during later stages of DC development may block DC differentiation and instead favor the development of macrophages and immature myeloid-derived suppressor cells. Rather than by mature DC, tumors will be infiltrated by alternatively activated, tumor-associated macrophages, and myeloid-derived suppressor cells, which release immunosuppressive arginase, inducible nitric-oxide synthase, reactive oxygen species, and TGF-β (Nagaraj et al. 2009; Yu et al. 2009).

pDC also infiltrate melanomas and their draining LN (Gerlini et al. 2007, 2010; Vermi et al. 2003) and are recruited by stromal cell-derived factor-1 (SDF-1/CXCL12) and CCL20, both of which are expressed by melanomas (Mohty et al. 2004; Salio et al. 2003; Zou et al. 2001). Tumor-associated pDC have been shown to induce immunosuppressive IL-10-producing T cells (Zou et al. 2001), to express low levels of TLR9 and to harbor a diminished capacity for IFN-α production (Hartmann et al. 2003). Moreover, although virtually absent from normal LN, indoleamine 2,3-dioxygenase (IDO)-expressing pDC were found in abundant numbers in melanoma TDLN (Gerlini et al. 2007; Lee et al. 2003; Vermi et al. 2003). IDO is a tryptophan-catabolizing enzyme, which can induce tryptophan depletion from the tumor-conditioned micro-environment, which in turn hampers T cell proliferation and reduces specific T cell responses in vivo (Munn and Mellor 2007). A high content of IDO$^+$ pDC in TDLN from patients with early stage melanoma (without detectable metastases) correlated significantly with reduced overall survival (Munn et al. 2004a; Munn and Mellor 2007). Suppressive CD4$^+$CD25^{hi}FoxP3$^+$ regulatory T cells (Tregs) are found at increased frequencies in the blood, tumors, and TDLN of melanoma patients (Cesana et al. 2006; Tuve et al. 2007) and have been reported to enhance IDO expression by DC through a CTL antigen-4 (CTLA-4)-dependent mechanism (Munn et al. 2004b). Excessive IDO expression in turn leads to abortive effector T cell activation and facilitates the further recruitment and activation of Tregs (Brody et al. 2009; Sharma et al. 2007, 2009), which in melanoma LN metastases was shown to be associated with decreased survival (Brody et al. 2009). These activated Tregs express high levels of CTLA-4 and may thus perpetuate this vicious cycle by in turn enhancing IDO expression by DC (Munn and Mellor 2006).

The degree of immunosuppression in TDLN was found to be directly related to their distance from the primary tumor (Cochran et al. 2006), indicating the causative agents to be tumor-derived. The first LN to directly drain the primary tumor, the SLN, is a preferential site of early lymph-borne metastasis (Bostick et al. 1999; Gershenwald et al. 1999; Statius Muller et al. 2000) and shows the most pronounced immunosuppression, even at the earliest stages of melanoma development (Cochran et al. 2001, 2006): the density of activated cDC in the paracortical T cell areas of SLN is often reduced and most cDC present in melanoma SLN lack dendritic morphology and display lower expression levels of co-stimulatory molecules as compared to cDC in more downstream draining LN (Cochran et al. 2001; Essner and Kojima 2002). These profoundly suppressive conditions imposed by tumors have led to the concept to consider the TDLN as an immune-privileged site (Munn and Mellor 2006). Local immunomodulation aimed at potentiating DC and T cell functions at the site of the primary melanoma and its draining LN (and the SLN in particular), may therefore offer a valuable therapy option in the adjuvant setting to prevent both local and systemic metastases.

5 Dendritic Cell Suppression in the Skin: Lessons from Human Skin Explant Studies

As primary melanomas grow and invade the dermis, immunosuppressive factors will condition the dermis to become permissive for tumor growth. To study the effects of tumor-induced suppression we have injected various melanoma-associated suppressive cytokines into the dermis of healthy human skin ex vivo and studied their effects on skin-emigrating DC. To this end 6-mm diameter explants were taken from the ID injection spots and cultured for 2 days while floating in medium with the epidermal side up. Emigrating DC were collected over the next 2 days and immediately analysed or cultured for an additional 5 days in the explant-conditioned medium. Of all the tested suppressive factors, we only observed suppressive effects for IL-10 (de Gruijl et al. 2006). Dermal conditioning by IL-10 resulted in a shift from mature $CD83^+CD1a^+$ cDC to immature $CD83^-CD14^+$ DC with more macrophage-like qualities. During the additional 5 day culture period, virtually all $CD1a^+$ DC converted to $CD14^+$ cells, passing through a $CD1a^+CD14^+$ stage (Fig. 1). Interestingly, $CD1a^+CD14^-$ and $CD1a^+CD14^+$ DC, as well as $CD1a^-CD14^+$ cells, are commonly found in the afferent lymph from normal human skin (Brand et al. 1999). The observed post-migrational phenotypic switch also occurred in medium-injected control explants, but was accelerated and reinforced by IL-10 (de Gruijl et al. 2006). Importantly, it was preventable by co-injection of the DC-activating cytokines GM-CSF and/or IL-4. Experiments with separated epidermal and dermal sheets showed these events to occur both in LC and DDC, but for full conversion to a $CD14^+$ macrophage-like state to occur, the dermis microenvironment was required. Our own recent observations suggest a role for dermal fibroblasts in this process (Ouwehand et al. submitted). IL-10-conditioned skin DC acquired a macrophage-like granular appearance and lost expression of CD83, CD1a, Langerin, and DC-SIGN, while GM-CSF/IL-4-conditioned skin DC maintained their dendritic morphology and phenotype (Fig. 2). Further, IL-10-conditioned DC display up-regulated expression of the macrophage markers CD14 and CD68, down-regulated expression of maturation and co-stimulatory markers, lacked expression of the LN-homing receptor CCR7, were unable to prime allogeneic T cells, and secreted higher levels of IL-10 (de Gruijl et al. 2006). IL-10 is secreted in the epidermis by melanocytes and possibly keratinocytes in response to environmental stress (Enk and Katz 1992; Nickoloff et al. 1994; Rivas and Ullrich 1992; Teunissen et al. 1997) and in the dermis by activated macrophages (Chung et al. 2007; Randow et al. 1995). The CD1a-to-CD14 switch, observed upon migration of LC and DDC in the absence of strong maturation-inducing signals, could thus be a mechanism to maintain tolerance in the face of tissue damage and avoid the induction of collateral autoimmunity.

In conclusion, the post-migrational CD1a-to-CD14 conversion of dermis-emigrating DC may serve to maintain immunological ignorance under steady state conditions, but reinforced by melanoma-secreted IL-10, it will interfere with the generation of effective anti-tumor immunity. Indeed, high IL-10 levels in melanoma metastases have been linked to a disturbed DC phenotype with high levels of CD14 (Gerlini et al. 2004). So, immunopotentiation of the melanoma-infiltrated dermis might result in normalized DC activation supporting the induction of protective immunity (Fig. 2). Two approaches can be applied, both targeting the microenvironment of the dermis and its draining LN: (1) local immunopotentiation of DC and T cell functions, and (2) DC-targeted vaccination. Ultimately, both approaches may be combined for an immunostimulatory therapy that can be generally applied to all patients as off-the-shelf formulations. Both approaches will be discussed in the following paragraphs.

6 Local Immunopotentiation of the Primary Melanoma Site and the Skin-Draining LN

By ID delivery of immunostimulatory agents, both the primary melanoma site and TDLN may be conditioned to permit re-activation of primed melanoma-specific $CD8^+$ T cells. A staggering 20 billion T cells are estimated to be present in normal, healthy skin (Nestle et al. 2009). Many of these are effector-memory T cells that can persist locally for years and provide rapid protection upon rechallenge (Clark 2010). Thus, previously primed tumor-specific effector T cells at primary melanoma site and in the draining LN may be re-activated by immune modulation, even without further antigenic exposure. We have indeed found evidence for this in SLN upon ID administration of GM-CSF or CpG (Molenkamp et al. 2008; Vuylsteke et al. 2006). Such local immune modulation strategies may afford local and systemic T cell-mediated control of metastatic outgrowth and prove of considerable value as adjuvant therapy. Lymphatic mapping and selective SLN excision is a minimally invasive procedure, which allows for the identification of patients at risk of LN metastasis who should undergo a full therapeutic LN dissection. The SLN procedure in melanoma has proven a useful prognostic tool for the assessment of melanoma relapse and mortality risk (Morton et al. 2008). In addition, the routine SLN procedure, as carried out in early stage melanoma patients, provides an ideal platform to test options for local pre-operative strengthening of SLN immune effector functions, i.e. through ID applied immunostimulatory compounds around the primary tumor excision site.

Growing knowledge of the complexity of DC maturation, migration, and T cell activation, as well as of immune escape mechanisms employed by tumors, has led to the identification of a substantial number of druggable targets to influence these processes in favor of generating anti-tumor immunity. Recently, a panel of experts composed a ranked list of immune response modifiers that should be made available for expedited clinical development (Cheever 2008). These include DC activators and growth factors, vaccine adjuvants, T cell stimulators and growth factors, immune-checkpoint inhibitors and neutralizing agents for suppressive cells, cytokines, and enzymes. There is consensus that only combinations of agents from these different classes of modifiers will ultimately yield optimal anti-tumor efficacy. Examples of these immune modulatory therapeutic agents that show promise for local immunopotentiation and that have either already entered or are about to enter the clinical testing phase, will be discussed below.

6.1 Dendritic Cell-Stimulatory Cytokines

Cytokines employed in (experimental) melanoma therapies target either DC (GM-CSF and IFN-α), effector T cells or NK cells (IL-2 and IFN-α), in an attempt to harness anti-tumor immune responses. Below, a brief overview is given of clinical experience with the administration of the DC-modulatory cytokines GM-CSF and IFN-α and how they may be applied locally in aid of anti-tumor immunity.

Granulocyte–macrophage colony-stimulating factor: GM-CSF stimulates proliferation and differentiation of progenitor cells of myeloid lineages, among others, neutrophilic and eosinophilic granulocytes and monocytes. Additionally, GM-CSF has immunological effects on macrophages, fibroblasts, and DC. It was found to promote the proliferation, survival, maturation, and migration of DC and its precursors, to induce their cytokine production, to up-regulate MHC class II and co-stimulatory molecules, all of which are vital to the induction of a T cell response. As a result, GM-CSF has become a prime candidate for use in immunotherapeutic strategies (Waller 2007). Vectors carrying the GM-CSF gene have been used to transduce tumor cells and DC for adoptive transfer, but have also been directly injected in vivo (Dranoff 2003). All these approaches resulted in effective T cell-mediated anti-tumor immunity in murine models (Dranoff 2003; Kass et al. 2001; Sun et al. 2002). In clinical studies with melanoma patients, evidence has been found for enhanced anti-tumor T cell responses and increased autoimmunity in the form of vitiligo upon systemic administration of GM-CSF, but clinical responses have usually been modest with some reports of stabilized disease.

Local administration of low-dose GM-CSF may prove effective without unwanted side effects. Indeed, local release of GM-CSF has been reported to result in enhanced recruitment of activated DC to draining LN in a murine model (Kass et al. 2001) and GM-CSF has been used as an adjuvant in tumor-vaccination protocols (Clive et al. 2010). These features make GM-CSF a good candidate to test its local immunomodulatory effects on melanoma in a clinical setting. In a first pilot study, 16 melanoma patients with advanced disease received intralesional GM-CSF followed by subcutaneous IL-2 injections (Ridolfi et al. 2001). Partial responses ($n = 2$), minimal responses ($n = 2$), and stable disease ($n = 9$) were observed. Interestingly, responses were also observed in non-treated lesions, indicative of the enhancement of systemic immunity. A likely explanation for this may be the induction or re-activation of melanoma-specific T cells through the activation of DC at the tumor site or in the tumor-draining LN. Indeed, this was also observed in a small single-blinded phase II study, carried out by us, in which 12 Stage I melanoma patients were included to receive four daily ID injections of GM-CSF (at 3 μg/kg) or saline around the primary tumor excision site (Vuylsteke et al. 2004, 2006). On the day of the last GM-CSF administration, the patients underwent an SLN excision procedure. We have developed a method whereby the SLN can be sampled for live immune effector cells without interference in subsequent diagnostic procedures (Vuylsteke et al. 2002). We employed this technique to monitor the phenotype of DC in the SLN through flow cytometry and to assess the frequency and functionality of $CD8^+$ T cells responding to specific melanoma-derived peptides in an IFN-γ Elispot assay. The GM-CSF-receiving patients showed a significant increase in the number and maturation state of $CD1a^+$ cDC, which was associated with a more robust melanoma-specific $CD8^+$ T cell response in the SLN, as compared to saline injected patients. Of note, melanoma-specific T cell rates correlated directly to mature $CD83^{+}CD1a^{+}$ DC frequencies in the SLN, confirming the importance of properly activated DC in the induction of an anti-melanoma immune response. These data are in keeping with findings by Lee et al. who showed that peritumoral administration of GM-CSF resulted in a type-1 cytokine profile consistent with enhanced cell-mediated immunity (Lee et al. 2005).

Recently, GM-CSF has received some bad press. Filipazzi et al. (2007) reported increased frequencies of a $CD14^{+}HLA\text{-}DR^{lo}$ subset of myeloid-derived suppressor cells in Stage IV melanoma patients upon subcutaneous vaccination with an HSP-peptide complex combined with GM-CSF. In addition, two groups separately reported that repeated administration of GM-CSF, added as adjuvant to peptide or tumor cell-based vaccines, to Stage II–IV melanoma patients over a prolonged period of time, resulted in lower anti-vaccine T cell responses (Slingluff et al. 2009) and decreased overall survival rates (Faries et al. 2009). A mouse study accompanying these two reports suggested that these findings might be attributable to GM-CSF-induced increases in Treg rates and/or activation status (Lacelle et al. 2009). Indeed, GM-CSF was previously shown to lead to the production by antigen-presenting cells of milk fat globule EGF 8, which attenuated the vaccination efficacy of GM-CSF-transduced melanoma cells through induction of Tregs in a mouse model (Jinushi et al. 2007). The latter mouse studies thus provide a rationale for combining GM-CSF administration with strategies aimed at eliminating Tregs or other T cell-mediated suppressive mechanisms (e.g. anti-CD25-conjugated toxins or anti-CTLA-4) (Eggermont 2009). Single low-dose administration of GM-CSF acting in a strictly localized fashion may not have the detrimental effects described in the above discussed papers, but this remains to be established.

Interferon-α: IFN-α has anti-angiogenic, cytotoxic, and cytostatic effects on tumors and also stimulates T and NK cells. Systemic administration of IFN-α has been extensively evaluated in (adjuvant) therapy trials with melanoma patients (Ascierto and Kirkwood 2008; Pfeffer et al. 1998). Meta-analyses of randomized trials on the adjuvant treatment with IFN-α in Stages II and III melanoma patients showed increased recurrence-free, but not overall survival for IFN-α treatment (Ascierto and Kirkwood 2008). Current and planned trials with IFN-α are now aimed at identification of subgroups of Stages II/III melanoma patients that will benefit most from treatment.

Emerging evidence on the immunological effects of IFN-α argues in favor of exploring its use as a local immunomodulator (Glaspy et al. 2009). Gogas et al. (2006) described an association between improved recurrence-free and overall survival and serological and clinical autoimmune parameters in melanoma patients receiving high-dose IFN-α. This is reminiscent of observations for other immunomodulators, e.g. anti-CTLA-4, where such autoimmune events correlate with anti-tumor responses. This observation remains to be confirmed by other studies (Bouwhuis et al. 2009), but raises the possibility that IFN-α exerts its anti-tumor effects, at least in part, through immunopotentiation. Wang et al. observed decreased activation (i.e. phosphorylation) of the signaling protein STAT3 in SLN upon administration of high-dose IFN-α to Stage IIIB melanoma patients. Decreased levels of phosphorylated STAT3 (pSTAT3) and increases in pSTAT1/pSTAT3 ratios following high-dose IFN-α treatment suggest its efficacy in suppressing melanoma-induced immune suppression (Wang et al. 2007), in which STAT3 activation has been identified as a key regulator (Yu et al. 2009). In addition, IFN-α-exposed monocytes quickly differentiate into mature $CD83^{+}CD14^{+}$ antigen-presenting cells with the ability to boost memory T cells (Gerlini et al. 2008); this characteristic may contribute to an anti-melanoma response through re-activation of in vivo primed anti-tumor CTL. Combined, these findings indicate that local conditioning of melanoma tumors and their draining LN by IFN-α may well contribute to reversal of immunosuppression and thus to immune potentiation of the anti-tumor immune response.

6.2 TLR-Ligands

TLR expressed on DC or assessory cells constitute attractive targets for immunopotentiation. So far, ten TLR have been identified in humans each able to detect their own class of pathogen-derived molecules. For example, TLR1, -2, and -4 are present on the cell surface and can bind bacterial glycoproteins and endotoxins, while TLR3, -7, -8, and -9 are intracellular receptors that bind viral or bacterial RNA or DNA (Palm and Medzhitov 2009). Of note, LC and DDC express a distinct TLR-expression pattern (van der Aar et al. 2007). With the exception of TLR3, all TLR elicit a response via MyD88 signaling, eventually leading to nuclear translocation of NF-κB and transcriptional activation of pro-inflammatory mediators (Palm and Medzhitov 2009). Ample evidence from an ever growing number of mouse studies shows that TLR-ligands are instrumental in inducing pro-inflammatory cytokine release from antigen-presenting cells in support of long-term effector T cell-mediated immunity (Palm and Medzhitov 2009). This characteristic has also sparked interest for their implementation in anti-tumor immunotherapies, alone or in combination with vaccines or other immune modulators. Below, a brief outline is given of experience with clinically explored options in the local treatment of melanoma.

Imiquimod and Resiquimod: TLR7 and -8 agonists (i.e. ssRNA analogues) have shown powerful anti-tumor effects in preclinical studies, mainly through induction of the release of type-1 skewing immune mediators, but also through the induction of DC with direct anti-tumor activity (Schon and Schon 2008). Imiquimod (formulated as Aldara cream for topical application) is a synthetic agonist for TLR7 and -8. It has been FDA approved for treatment of basal cell carcinoma (BCC), actinic keratosis, and human papillomavirus-induced warts. TLR7 is present on cDC, pDC, and B cells (Hornung et al. 2002; Mancuso et al. 2009). Triggering of TLR7 leads to the release of high amounts of IFN-α, and also of TNF-α and IL-1, -6, -8 and -12 (Hornung et al. 2002; Stanley 2002). These cytokines in turn activate cDC, monocytes and macrophages, NK, Th1 cells, and CTL (Hornung et al. 2002;

Wenzel et al. 2008). This activation of a type-1 cell-mediated immunity is consistent with the anti-viral properties of imiquimod and also suggests anti-tumor efficacy.

Two groups reported 100% clearance of Stage 0 (i.e. epidermal) melanoma lesions with imiquimod (Ray et al. 2005; Wolf et al. 2005, 2007). Biopsies before, during, and after treatment revealed an increase in Th cells and granzyme-B^+ CTL in the affected area during treatment (Wolf et al. 2007). Two other papers also described the use of imiquimod for the treatment of (sub)cutaneous metastases of melanoma with promising results (Bong et al. 2002; Green et al. 2007), i.e. histopathologically confirmed reductions of in-transit metastases after imiquimod application only and a restored Th1/Th2 balance upon additional intralesional IL-2 injections (Green et al. 2008). Overall, a clinical response rate of 50.5% was seen, with 91% of the complete regressions appearing in patients with cutaneous lesions. Of note, pre-conditioning of cutaneous vaccination sites with imiquimod was well tolerated and resulted in the efficient induction of both humoral and cell-mediated immune responses against an NY-ESO-based vaccine in Stages II/III melanoma patients (Adams et al. 2008). These results clearly warrant the further development of imiquimod as the local immunomodulator and adjuvant constituent of cutaneously applied melanoma vaccines.

R848 (or resiquimod), a TLR7 and -8 agonist, topically applied in combination with subcutaneous administration of ovalbumin, was reported to generate robust antigen-specific CTL with anti-melanoma activity (Chang et al. 2009). Interestingly, R848 also induced TRAIL-mediated tumor-cytolytic activity of pDC (Chaperot et al. 2006). An ID delivered gp100/MAGE-A3 melanoma vaccine with or without an R848-based adjuvant is about to enter clinical testing and should provide further insight into the clinical efficacy of R848 (Anon 2010).

CpG oligodeoxynucleotides: Adjuvants based on bacterial unmethylated CpG dinucleotide sequences have strong immunogenic properties (Krieg 2002). All classes of CpG oligodeoxynucleotides (CpG ODN) bind to TLR9 (Krieg 2001, 2002) leading to DC and B cell activation and maturation and subsequent Th1-skewing of cytokine production (IL-12, IFN-α) resulting in both antigen-specific memory and na $CD8^+$ T cell induction (Jakob et al. 1998; Krieg 2008; Warren et al. 2000). Interestingly, CpG-mediated TLR9 activation was shown to be attenuated by STAT3 activation, leading to immune suppression (Kortylewski et al. 2009a). This was prevented by conjugating CpG ODN to STAT3 siRNA prior to delivery (Kortylewski et al. 2009b). These findings argue in favor of combining CpG ODN with newly developed small-molecule JAK2/STAT3 inhibitors (Hedvat et al. 2009).

PF-3512676, formerly known as CpG 7909, is a B-type CpG ODN that has been tested extensively in humans. It has a strong effect on the activation of B cells, but a modest effect on IFN-α production by pDC, in contrast to A- and C-class ODN, which strongly induce IFN-α secretion (Krieg 2001). In a phase II study conducted by us, 23 Stages I/II melanoma patients received one ID injection of either 8 mg PF-3512676 or saline. Patients receiving PF-3512676 showed a clear enhancement of both pDC and $CD1a^+$ cDC maturation and activation in the

SLN by flow-cytometric analyses (Molenkamp et al. 2007). Also, a significant decrease in Treg frequencies and significantly higher CD8$^+$ T cell response rates to MAA-derived epitopes in blood and the SLN were detected (Molenkamp et al. 2008). Moreover, a significant and direct correlation was found between pDC activation in the SLN (by CD86 and CD40 expression levels) and the aggregate increase in frequencies of MAA peptide-reactive CD8$^+$ T cells in post-treatment peripheral blood. This indicates a direct role for the locally CpG-modulated pDC in the SLN in the generation of the observed systemic anti-melanoma CD8$^+$ T cell response. In the same trial we observed infiltrates of activated cDC, pDC, and T cells in the dermis upon ID injection of CpG (van den Hout et al. manuscript in preparation). This was also recently reported for combined GM-CSF and CpG administration (Haining et al. 2008) and hints at a possible utility of local CpG ODN administration to recruit lymphocytic effector infiltrates to tumor sites. In keeping with this notion, in another Phase I trial the effects were studied of intralesional treatment with PF-3512676 in five patients with Basal Cell Carcinoma (BCC) and five patients with (sub)cutaneous melanoma metastases (Hofmann et al. 2008). Patients received doses of up to 10 mg intralesional CpG every 14 days. Two complete regressions were observed (in one BCC and one melanoma patient) and four partial regressions in BCC patients. Moderate to abundant cellular infiltrates of lymphocytes were found post-treatment in most biopsies.

Systemic and prolonged administration of PF-3512676 has been studied in combination with chemotherapy in large randomized Phase III trials in patients with non-small cell lung cancer. A few years back these trials were prematurely terminated due to disappointing clinical results in interim analyses (Schmidt 2007). This caused a major setback in the development of CpG ODN as anticancer therapeutics, although it offered the possibility to re-evaluate the most viable opportunities for clinical application of CpG ODN, such as local administration, possibly combined with other TLR-ligands and/or viral or tumor vaccines (Krieg 2008). The above described clinical studies in melanoma patients demonstrate that local CpG-mediated activation of the immune system can lead to a systemically detectable anti-tumor response with the possibility of recognition and elimination of metastatic tumor cells by circulating T cells.

6.3 Immunomodulatory Antibodies

Various antibodies targeting tumor-associated markers are now part of the oncologist's arsenal of therapeutics and many more are in clinical development, some of which have entered the clinical testing phase. A few examples with possible relevance to local immunopotentiation are discussed below.

Anti-CD40: In numerous preclinical studies CD40-mediated activation of DC was identified as a key event in the generation of long-term CTL-mediated immunity (Koschella et al. 2004; Melief et al. 2002; Rieger and Kipps 2003; Schoenberger et al. 1998; Toka et al. 2005). CD40 stimulation also results in the reversal of T cell tolerance (Ichikawa et al. 2002), renders DC resistant to the suppressive effects of IL-10 (Haenssle et al. 2008), and releases them from the control of Tregs (Serra et al. 2003). Findings from a Phase I trial of a single systemic administration of the anti-CD40 monoclonal antibody CP-870,893 (Vonderheide et al. 2007) established the maximum-tolerated dose at 0.2 mg/kg. Most side effects were attributable to a transient cytokine release syndrome on the day of administration. Encouragingly, four patients with melanoma (i.e. 27% of enrolled melanoma patients) showed objective partial responses, demonstrating the possible utility of CP-870,893 in the immunotherapy of melanoma. The application of agonistic anti-CD40 may also lead to immunopotentiation of TDLN. In a recent paper CP-870,893 was shown to induce DC maturation in vitro and to enhance anti-tumor reactivity in autologous co-cultures of tumor cells and TDLN suspensions ex vivo (Hunter et al. 2007). By local administration of CP-870,893, powerful activation of DC subsets may thus be achieved in the melanoma SLN, releasing them from immunosuppressive conditions.

Anti-CTLA-4 and anti-PD-1: Besides suppression at the DC level, suppression of T cell reactivity is another possible obstacle in the effective triggering of an anti-melanoma immune response. The CTLA-4 and programmed death-1 (PD-1) receptors represent crucial checkpoints in the control of T cell reactivity (Zang and Allison 2007). CTLA-4 is expressed on activated T cells and binds to CD80 and CD86 on DC with higher avidity than its competitor ligand CD28. In contrast to CD28, CTLA-4 provides inhibitory signals to the T cell and blocks activating signals originating from CD28 to CD86/CD80 interactions. The importance of this negative feedback loop is evidenced by the observation that CTLA-4-deficient mice die by 3–4 weeks of age from lymphoproliferative disease with lymphocytic infiltration in multiple organs (Waterhouse et al. 1995). CTLA-4 blockade also breaks through inhibitory feedback loops in tumor-specific T cells and may lead to preferential expansion of high-avidity effector CTL (Egen et al. 2002). Besides these processes at the intrinsic effector T cell level, it has also been suggested that CTLA-4 blockade might abrogate suppressive functions of Tregs (Munn and Mellor 2006).

Pre-clinical and clinical studies have clearly indicated enhanced anti-tumor efficacy upon blocking of CTLA-4 and strongly support further implementation of anti-CTLA-4 in immunotherapeutic approaches to the treatment of melanoma (Egen et al. 2002; Hodi et al. 2003; Phan et al. 2003). Clinical responses and prolonged survival have been observed upon systemic treatment of melanoma patients with the anti-CTLA-4 monoclonal antibodies ipilimumab or tremelimumab (Hodi et al. 2010; Kirkwood et al. 2010; Sarnaik and Weber 2009). Clinical responses coincided with Th17-associated autoimmune-breakthrough events (ABE) that could generally be controlled with immunosuppressive drugs (without interfering with the anti-tumor response), but that in some cases were quite severe (Sarnaik and Weber 2009). The close correlation observed between these ABE and clinical anti-tumor efficacy in patients with advanced melanoma (Attia et al. 2005; Phan et al. 2003) raises the question whether the anti-tumor effects may be achievable without collateral autoimmunity. In all these trials anti-CTLA-4 was administered systemically at high-dose levels (3–10 mg/kg) over long periods of time (monthly for up to 6 months). A single local administration of anti-CTLA-4 aimed at conditioning of the primary melanoma site and the SLN in an adjuvant setting should allow for the use of relatively low anti-CTLA-4 dosages without excess risk of autoimmune effects. Indeed, even upon systemic administration of high doses, autoimmune effects were mostly observed upon repeated administration (Attia et al. 2005; Sarnaik and Weber 2009). In support of localized low-dose application of anti-CTLA-4, Simmons et al. recently reported favorable results obtained in the B16 melanoma model with vaccination with GM-CSF- and anti-CTLA-4-secreting tumor cells. Equivalent anti-tumor activity to systemic administration of high-dose anti-CTLA-4 was observed at significantly lower anti-CTLA-4 serum levels and with serological evidence of reduced systemic autoimmunity (Simmons et al. 2008). In a similar vein, Tuve et al. showed that tumor-localized expression of anti-CTLA-4 resulted in significantly delayed tumor outgrowth, mediated by $CD8^+$ effector cells (Tuve et al. 2007). Of note, anti-CTLA-4 treatment has been reported to be more effective when combined with booster vaccinations than with primary vaccinations (Gregor et al. 2004). This may be explained by up-regulation of CTLA-4 upon activation of T cells and its absence from naïve, unstimulated T cells (Egen et al. 2002). Since the MAA-specific $CD8^+$ T cells detected in our previous SLN trials most likely represent re-activated T cells that were previously primed in vivo (Molenkamp et al. 2008; Vuylsteke et al. 2006), anti-CTLA-4 may prove particularly effective in releasing any anti-CTLA-4-mediated inhibitory effects on these T cells.

PD-1, like CTLA-4, forms a checkpoint for T cell activation. It becomes up-regulated upon T cell activation and binds B7-H1 (PD-L1) and B7-DC (PD-L2) (Chen 2004). Upon binding of PD-1, T cells become inactivated and enter a reversible state of anergy (Barber et al. 2006; Freeman et al. 2000). PD-1 knock-out mice developed autoimmune glomerulonephritis and arthritis (Barber et al. 2006; Keir et al. 2008). PD-1 has been implicated in clonal exhaustion of T cells and high levels of PD-1 are found on tumor-infiltrating T cells and on chronically stimulated T cells (Barber et al. 2006; Chen 2004). Its ligand B7-H1 is often expressed on tumors and may thus interfere with activation of tumor-infiltrating T cells (Ghebeh et al. 2006; Iwai et al. 2002; Ohigashi et al. 2005). In a melanoma mouse model anti-PD-1 was shown to enhance the anti-tumor efficacy of a cell-based vaccine (Li et al. 2009). PD-1 blockade was also shown to facilitate the expansion and eliminate the suppression of MAA-specific CTL, possibly through inhibition of Treg activity (Fourcade et al. 2009; Wang et al. 2009). A first Phase 1 clinical trial has been conducted to study the effects of intravenous anti-PD-1 (MDX-1106) administration in 39 patients, including nine melanoma patients (Brahmer et al. 2010). Results were encouraging with signs of clinical anti-tumor efficacy, $CD8^+$ T cell infiltration at tumor sites and relatively mild autoimmune symptoms. This first clinical trial has now opened the possibility to also test anti-PD-1 as a locally applied immunostimulant.

7 Dendritic Cell-Targeted Vaccines in the Skin Microenvironment

Numerous clinical trials are underway studying the effect of DC-based vaccination with specific MAA. A common strategy is the ex vivo generation of autologous DC from blood-derived DC precursors, which are then loaded with MAA proteins or MAA-derived peptides, carrying known CTL and/or Th epitopes, and subsequently re-administered to the patient. Alternatively, MAA-encoding genes can be transferred to DC. A genetic MAA vaccine provides a long-lived continuous source of antigen and will lead to relatively protracted presentation of MAA by the transduced DC. In addition, endogenous MAA expression resulting from gene transfer ensures access to the MHC class I processing pathway for subsequent activation of specific CTL. With the wide array of molecular recombinant techniques at our disposal and a rapidly growing knowledge of DC biology, it has now become possible to genetically modify vaccines to specifically target them to DC in vivo and at the same time achieve DC activation. Direct in vivo administration of vectors carrying the genetic code of MAA may present a more attractive and standardized alternative to classic DC-based melanoma vaccination, obviating the need for costly, time-consuming, and laborious approaches involving the generation and loading of autologous DC ex vivo.

Vaccines based on the targeting and triggering of tissue-resident DC should be designed in such a way that they exploit the natural physiological processes that facilitate DC activation, migration, LN-homing, and subsequent T cell activation. The presence of different DC subsets in skin allows for the targeting of a range of DC subsets that have been demonstrated to hold potent immunostimulatory capacities, facilitating both $CD4^+$ and $CD8^+$ T cell responses. In mouse studies, in vivo immunotargeting of protein antigens to DC-restricted markers, such as CD11c, CLEC9A, or DEC-205, was shown to induce immune responses (Bonifaz et al. 2004; Mahnke et al. 2005; Sancho et al. 2008; van Broekhoven et al. 2004). However, targeting of a model antigen to the DEC-205 receptor on murine DC led to specific T cell unresponsiveness within 7 days after immunization. This unresponsiveness was only overcome after the co-injection of a CD40 agonistic antibody (Bonifaz et al. 2002). Similarly, CD11c- or DEC-205-targeted cancer vaccines were only effective when DC-activating reagents such as anti-CD40 or TLR-ligands were co-administered (Johnson et al. 2008; Mahnke et al. 2005; Wei et al. 2009).

The choice of molecules to target for DC-specific gene transfer is closely related to the subset, the maturation state, and the anatomical location of the DC in question. The different skin DC subsets are targetable through different surface molecules. The most attractive targets should be only expressed on DC, be rapidly internalized upon binding, and induce DC maturation and migration upon binding, to allow for optimal CTL activation. Pattern recognition receptors (like TLR) and antigen-capture receptors (like C-type lectins) are attractive targets, because it is their natural function to internalize antigens and mediate their routing to antigen-processing pathways in order to start a T cell response. In addition, their differential expression on the LC and DDC subsets may allow for subset-specific targeting; e.g. Langerin on LC and MR, DEC205, and DC-SIGN on DDC (Teunissen et al. 2011).

Depending on their size ID injected vaccine vehicles will either remain ("get stuck") in the dermis (>100 nm, e.g. liposomes) or rapidly drain to the LN (<50 nm, e.g. nanoparticles) (Combadiere and Mahe 2008). This will clearly be a determining factor in what DC subsets will be targeted and should therefore be taken into account. With our current knowledge it is hard to oversee all the consequences of targeting specific skin-associated DC subsets. However, a common trait of any DC-targeted vaccine formulation should be that the targeted DC become properly activated in order to kick-start a T cell-mediated immune response. Based on our current knowledge, $CD1a^+$ DDC (and their $CD1a^+$ equivalents in skin-draining LN) may be the most attractive subsets for vaccine targeting purposes because of their high intrinsic activation state, T cell activation capacity, and easy accessibility (de Gruijl et al. 2002; Santegoets et al. 2008a; Sparber et al. 2010).

8 CD40-Targeted Adenovirus: a Dendritic Cell-Targeting Vaccine Delivered to the Dermis

The use of viral vectors for gene delivery to DC has some major advantages (de Gruijl et al. 2004). (1) Many viruses exhibit a natural tropism for DC (e.g. lentiviruses) that may be utilized for DC-targeted vaccination; (2) viruses have a natural ability to infect target cells and to be efficiently endocytosed by DC; (3) viruses have developed mechanisms to efficiently transfer their genetic cargo to the host cytoplasm and/or nucleus in order to take over the host replication and/or transcription machinery and ensure high-level expression of the transgenes they carry. These characteristics make viruses extremely attractive vaccine vehicles. Non-viral vehicles (e.g. liposomes and nanoparticles) often need to be chemically altered and optimized to achieve the above listed advantageous traits for DC-targeted vaccination that viruses naturally possess (Altin and Parish 2006; Reddy et al. 2006; Tacken et al. 2007). One of the most commonly used gene transfer vectors for DC is the adenovirus (Ad). Advantages of replication-deficient Ad over other delivery vehicles are that Ad can efficiently infect both dividing and non-dividing cells at high efficiencies, so that they can be produced at high titers and are safe, as they do not integrate into the host cell genome (de Gruijl et al. 2004; Timares et al. 2004). Various studies have demonstrated that adenoviral transduction of DC in vitro results in high expression of the tumor antigen and efficient activation of immune responses directed to the tumor upon injection of the transduced DC (de Gruijl et al. 2004; Timares et al. 2004). Unfortunately, direct ID administration of Ad as a vaccine is hampered by the fact that DC exhibit

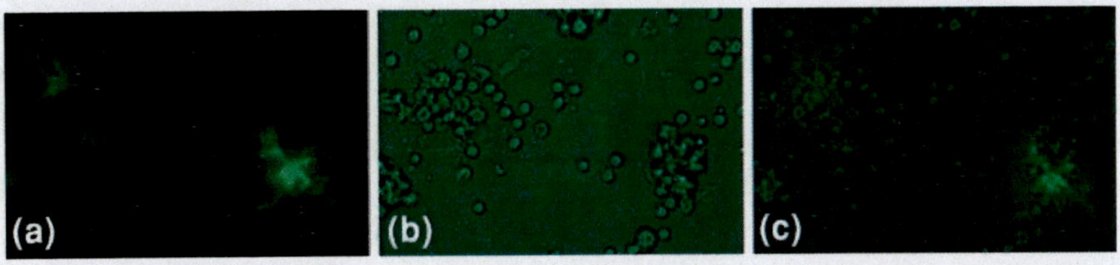

Fig. 3 Melanoma-draining lymph node suspensions were incubated with CD40-targeted adenoviruses encoding enhanced *green fluorescent protein* for 24 h and then examined under a fluorescence microscope. Photographs show **a** transduction of DC and **b** their binding of lymphocytes: a sign of their activated state. Photographs taken with **a** dark field microscopy, **b** conventional microscopy and **c** an overlay of both; magnification 400×

limited expression levels of the Ad-docking receptor coxsackie and adenovirus receptor (CAR), whereas CAR is abundantly expressed on other residential cell types in the dermis, e.g. on fibroblasts (de Gruijl et al. 2004). A logical approach to circumvent inefficient CAR-mediated Ad5 transduction of DC in vivo is redirecting Ad5 entry (i.e. retargeting) via alternative cell surface molecules abundantly expressed on DC (Timares et al. 2004).

We previously reported the successful retargeting of Ad vectors to DC through CD40, resulting in enhanced and selective transduction and simultaneous maturation induction both of in vitro generated monocyte-derived DC and of human skin DC in situ (Brandao et al. 2003; de Gruijl et al. 2002; Hangalapura et al. 2010; Tillman et al. 1999). This CD40-mediated retargeting was achieved either through the use of bispecific conjugates, binding and neutralizing the Ad fiber knob on the one hand and agonistically binding CD40 on the other, or through genetic incorporation of the active TNF-like domain of CD40L into the Ad viral knob (Brandao et al. 2003; de Gruijl et al. 2002; Korokhov et al. 2005; Tillman et al. 1999). In the skin environment, high expression levels of CD40 are mainly restricted to DDC or migrating LC in the dermis (de Gruijl et al. 2002). Migrated DC in a human skin explant model were shown to be transduced at a higher efficiency, to express higher levels of the transgene, display enhanced phenotypic maturation, and maintain the ability to specifically activate CTL over longer periods of time, after ID transduction by CD40-targeted Ad rather than untargeted Ad (de Gruijl et al. 2002). CD40-targeted Ad vectors thus appear to ensure both DC-specific transduction and appropriate DC activation in the context of the skin microenvironment for the effective subsequent priming of anti-tumor immunity. Besides transduction of mature cDC in the dermis, CD40-retargeted Ad vectors can also selectively transduce DC in cutaneous melanoma-draining LN suspensions (Fig. 3) (Hangalapura et al. 2010). This may well be very relevant as the size of Ad vectors (±80 nm) will also allow for their direct lymphatic drainage to skin-draining LN and in situ transduction of DC subsets residing in the LN. CD40-Ad-transduced DC vaccines were shown to afford superior $CD8^+$ T cell-dependent tumor protection in murine tumor models (Kim et al. 2010; Tillman et al. 2000) and ID injection of CD40-targeted Ad resulted in a Th1-skewed immune response in an infectious mouse model (Huang et al. 2008). Similarly, stronger T cell and IgG2 antibody responses (indicative of Th1 skewing) were observed against the tumor antigen CEA upon ID delivery of a CD40-targeted Ad vaccine in a canine model (Thacker et al. 2009). We recently reported that CD40-targeting of Ad5/MART-1 results in enhanced induction of high-avidity CTL, both from human peripheral blood mononuclear cells and in melanoma SLN (Hangalapura et al. 2010). In addition, we have now obtained evidence that ID delivered and CD40-retargeted Ad-gp100 can slow melanoma growth in the B16 mouse model in a therapeutic setting (Hangalapura et al. submitted). There is thus abundant in vitro and in vivo evidence for the enhanced efficacy of ID delivered Ad vaccines encoding full-length MAA genes when they are targeted to CD40 on DC in skin and skin-draining LN. We now aim to translate this approach to the clinic. The envisioned methodology entails local recruitment of a dense and activated LC and DDC infiltrate in the dermis (e.g. through ID injection of GM-CSF) and ID delivery of a CD40-targeted and MAA encoding Ad vector.

9 Summary and Conclusions

There is urgent need for an effective adjuvant therapy for melanoma. Before distant metastasis occurs, local immunopotentiation of the primary tumor site and its draining LN may be a valid strategy to (re-)establish local immune control. Novel and powerful immunomodulatory agents with proven clinical activity and/or efficacy are becoming available to combat melanoma-imposed immune suppression on both DC and T cells. The dermis provides an ideal site for delivery of these compounds. A network of DDC and effector-memory T cells in the dermis are available for re-activation and subsequent generation of an effector immune response. Moreover, the dermis provides ready access to draining LN, where the respective memory and naïve T cell responses can be further boosted or primed. Such approaches may be combined with DC-targeted vaccines, delivered to the dermis, for further MAA-specific T cell activation. Prior conditioning of the ID vaccination site can be employed to activate and mobilize both DDC and LC. Combined targeting of both subsets, provided that appropriate maturation-inducing signals are applied, will ensure a broad immune reactivity involving both the cellular and the humoral arm of the adaptive immune system. CD40-targeted Ad vectors may provide a very useful tool to achieve this. Moreover, the employed Ad vectors can be modified to encode immunomodulatory sequences besides the targeted MAA, e.g. short hairpin RNA (e.g. for STAT3 or IDO) or single-chain Fv fragments (e.g. anti-CD40 or anti-CTLA-4). Exciting new developments in the treatment of melanoma include the use of targeted therapeutics to modulate aberrantly activated signaling cascades in melanoma, e.g. in patients carrying activating b-raf mutations (Smalley 2010). As many of these signaling cascades also affect immune functions, it will be interesting to see how these new therapeutics influence the patient's immune status and how they may be combined with immunotherapeutic approaches. Importantly, the dermis-targeted and localized immunomodulatory strategies discussed in this paper may not only provide protection against local tumor spread but the activated effector T cells can also recirculate and home to distant metastatic sites. Thus, also patients in later stages of melanoma may experience benefit from these approaches. It now seems of utmost importance to establish the most optimal combinations of immunotherapeutic agents. Rather than testing the clinical efficacy of monotherapies in large-scale Phase III trials, it might be more prudent to first study combination therapies in multiple small-scale and carefully designed Phase II trials with biological readouts. This would allow for the more rational design of multi-targeted therapies with a better chance of attaining improved clinical efficacy in randomized Phase III trials.

References

Adams S, O'Neill DW, Nonaka D, Hardin E, Chiriboga L, Siu K, Cruz CM, Angiulli A, Angiulli F, Ritter E, Holman RM, Shapiro RL, Berman RS, Berner N, Shao Y, Manches O, Pan L, Venhaus RR, Hoffman EW, Jungbluth A, Gnjatic S, Old L, Pavlick AC, Bhardwaj N (2008) Immunization of malignant melanoma patients with full-length NY-ESO-1 protein using TLR7 agonist imiquimod as vaccine adjuvant. J Immunol 181:776–784

Anon (2010) http://clinicaltrials.gov/ct2/show/NCT00960752

Altin JG, Parish CR (2006) Liposomal vaccines-targeting the delivery of antigen. Methods 40:39–52

Angel CE, Lala A, Chen CJ, Edgar SG, Ostrovsky LL, Dunbar PR (2007) CD14+ antigen-presenting cells in human dermis are less mature than their CD1a+ counterparts. Int Immunol 19:1271–1279

Ascierto PA, Kirkwood JM (2008) Adjuvant therapy of melanoma with interferon: lessons of the past decade. J Transl Med 6:62

Asselin-Paturel C, Brizard G, Chemin K, Boonstra A, O'Garra A, Vicari A, Trinchieri G (2005) Type I interferon dependence of plasmacytoid dendritic cell activation and migration. J Exp Med 201:1157–1167

Attia P, Phan GQ, Maker AV, Robinson MR, Quezado MM, Yang JC, Sherry RM, Topalian SL, Kammula US, Royal RE, Restifo NP, Haworth LR, Levy C, Mavroukakis SA, Nichol G, Yellin MJ, Rosenberg SA (2005) Autoimmunity correlates with tumor regression in patients with metastatic melanoma treated with anti-cytotoxic T lymphocyte antigen-4. J Clin Oncol 23:6043–6053

Bachem A, Guttler S, Hartung E, Ebstein F, Schaefer M, Tannert A, Salama A, Movassaghi K, Opitz C, Mages HW, Henn V, Kloetzel PM, Gurka S, Kroczek RA (2010) Superior antigen cross-presentation and XCR1 expression define human CD11c+ CD141+ cells as homologues of mouse CD8+ dendritic cells. J Exp Med 207:1273–1281

Balch CM, Buzaid AC, Soong SJ, Atkins MB, Cascinelli N, Coit DG, Fleming ID, Gershenwald JE, Houghton A, Kirkwood JM, McMasters KM, Mihm MF, Morton DL, Reintgen DS, Ross MI, Sober A, Thompson JA, Thompson JF (2001) Final version of the American Joint Committee on Cancer staging system for cutaneous melanoma. J Clin Oncol 19:3635–3648

Balch CM, Gershenwald JE, Soong SJ, Thompson JF, Atkins MB, Byrd DR, Buzaid AC, Cochran AJ, Coit DG, Ding S, Eggermont AM, Flaherty KT, Gimotty PA, Kirkwood JM, McMasters KM, Mihm MC, Jr., Morton DL, Ross MI, Sober AJ, Sondak VK (2009a) Final version of 2009 AJCC melanoma staging and classification. J Clin Oncol 27:6199–6206

Balch CM, Gershenwald JE, Soong SJ, Thompson JF, Atkins MB, Byrd DR, Buzaid AC, Cochran AJ, Coit DG, Ding S, Eggermont AM, Flaherty KT, Gimotty PA, Kirkwood JM, McMasters KM, Mihm MC Jr, Morton DL, Ross MI, Sober AJ, Sondak VK (2009b) Final version of 2009 AJCC melanoma staging and classification. J Clin Oncol 27:6199–6206

Banchereau J, Briere F, Caux C, Davoust J, Lebecque S, Liu YT, Pulendran B, Palucka K (2000) Immunobiology of dendritic cells. Annu Rev Immunol 18:767–811

Banchereau J, Palucka AK, Dhodapkar M, Burkeholder S, Taquet N, Rolland A, Taquet S, Coquery S, Wittkowski KM, Bhardwaj N, Pineiro L, Steinman R, Fay J (2001) Immune and clinical responses in patients with metastatic melanoma to CD34(+) progenitor-derived dendritic cell vaccine. Cancer Res 61:6451–6458

Barber DL, Wherry EJ, Masopust D, Zhu B, Allison JP, Sharpe AH, Freeman GJ, Ahmed R (2006) Restoring function in exhausted CD8 T cells during chronic viral infection. Nature 439:682–687

Bedoui S, Whitney PG, Waithman J, Eidsmo L, Wakim L, Caminschi I, Allan RS, Wojtasiak M, Shortman K, Carbone FR, Brooks AG, Heath WR (2009) Cross-presentation of viral and self antigens by skin-derived CD103+ dendritic cells. Nat Immunol 10:488–495

Bong AB, Bonnekoh B, Franke I, Schon MP, Ulrich J, Gollnick H (2002) Imiquimod, a topical immune response modifier, in the treatment of cutaneous metastases of malignant melanoma. Dermatology 205:135–138

Bonifaz L, Bonnyay D, Mahnke K, Rivera M, Nussenzweig MC, Steinman RM (2002) Efficient targeting of protein antigen to the dendritic cell receptor DEC-205 in the steady state leads to antigen presentation on major histocompatibility complex class I products and peripheral CD8+ T cell tolerance. J Exp Med 196:1627–1638

Bonifaz LC, Bonnyay DP, Charalambous A, Darguste DI, Fujii S, Soares H, Brimnes MK, Moltedo B, Moran TM, Steinman RM (2004) In vivo targeting of antigens to maturing dendritic cells via the DEC-205 receptor improves T cell vaccination. J Exp Med 199: 815–824

Bostick PJ, Morton DL, Turner RR, Huynh KT, Wang HJ, Elashoff R, Essner R, Hoon DS (1999) Prognostic significance of occult metastases detected by sentinel lymphadenectomy and reverse transcriptase-polymerase chain reaction in early-stage melanoma patients. J Clin Oncol 17:3238–3244

Bouwhuis MG, Suciu S, Collette S, Aamdal S, Kruit WH, Bastholt L, Stierner U, Sales F, Patel P, Punt CJ, Hernberg M, Spatz A, ten Hagen TL, Hansson J, Eggermont AM (2009) Autoimmune antibodies and recurrence-free interval in melanoma patients treated with adjuvant interferon. J Natl Cancer Inst 101:869–877

Brahmer JR, Drake CG, Wollner I, Powderly JD, Picus J, Sharfman WH, Stankevich E, Pons A, Salay TM, McMiller TL, Gilson MM, Wang C, Selby M, Taube JM, Anders R, Chen L, Korman AJ, Pardoll DM, Lowy I, Topalian SL (2010) Phase I study of single-agent anti-programmed death-1 (MDX-1106) in refractory solid tumors: safety, clinical activity, pharmacodynamics, and immunologic correlates. J Clin Oncol 28:3167–3175

Brand CU, Hunger RE, Yawalkar N, Gerber HA, Schaffner T, Braathen LR (1999) Characterization of human skin-derived CD1a-positive lymph cells. Arch Dermatol Res 291:65–72

Brandao JG, Scheper RJ, Lougheed SM, Curiel DT, Tillman BW, Gerritsen WR, van den Eertwegh AJ, Pinedo HM, Haisma HJ, de Gruijl TD (2003) CD40-targeted adenoviral gene transfer to dendritic cells through the use of a novel bispecific single-chain Fv antibody enhances cytotoxic T cell activation. Vaccine 21:2268–2272

Brody JR, Costantino CL, Berger AC, Sato T, Lisanti MP, Yeo CJ, Emmons RV, Witkiewicz AK (2009) Expression of indoleamine 2, 3-dioxygenase in metastatic malignant melanoma recruits regulatory T cells to avoid immune detection and affects survival. Cell Cycle 8: 1930–1934

Cecchi R, Buralli L, Innocenti S, De Gaudio C (2007) Sentinel lymph node biopsy in patients with thin melanomas. J Dermatol 34:512–515

Cesana GC, DeRaffele G, Cohen S, Moroziewicz D, Mitcham J, Stoutenburg J, Cheung K, Hesdorffer C, Kim-Schulze S, Kaufman HL (2006) Characterization of CD4+ CD25+ regulatory T cells in patients treated with high-dose interleukin-2 for metastatic melanoma or renal cell carcinoma. J Clin Oncol 24:1169–1177

Chang BA, Cross JL, Najar HM, Dutz JP (2009) Topical resiquimod promotes priming of CTL to parenteral antigens. Vaccine 27:5791–5799

Chaperot L, Blum A, Manches O, Lui G, Angel J, Molens JP, Plumas J (2006) Virus or TLR agonists induce TRAIL-mediated cytotoxic activity of plasmacytoid dendritic cells. J Immunol 176:248–255

Cheever MA (2008) Twelve immunotherapy drugs that could cure cancers. Immunol Rev 222:357–368

Chen L (2004) Co-inhibitory molecules of the B7-CD28 family in the control of T-cell immunity. Nat Rev Immunol 4:336–347

Chung EY, Liu J, Homma Y, Zhang Y, Brendolan A, Saggese M, Han J, Silverstein R, Selleri L, Ma X (2007) Interleukin-10 expression in macrophages during phagocytosis of apoptotic cells is mediated by homeodomain proteins Pbx1 and Prep-1. Immunity 27:952–964

Clark RA (2010) Skin-resident T cells: the ups and downs of on site immunity. J Invest Dermatol 130:362–370

Clive KS, Tyler JA, Clifton GT, Holmes JP, Mittendorf EA, Ponniah S, Peoples GE (2010) Use of GM-CSF as an adjuvant with cancer vaccines: beneficial or detrimental? Expert Rev Vaccines 9:519–525

Cochran AJ, Huang RR, Lee J, Itakura E, Leong SP, Essner R (2006) Tumour-induced immune modulation of sentinel lymph nodes. Nat Rev Immunol 6:659–670

Cochran AJ, Morton DL, Stern S, Lana AM, Essner R, Wen DR (2001) Sentinel lymph nodes show profound downregulation of antigen-presenting cells of the paracortex: implications for tumor biology and treatment. Mod Pathol 14:604–608

Combadiere B, Mahe B (2008) Particle-based vaccines for transcutaneous vaccination. Comp Immunol Microbiol Infect Dis 31:293–315

Crozat K, Guiton R, Contreras V, Feuillet V, Dutertre CA, Ventre E, Vu Manh TP, Baranek T, Storset AK, Marvel J, Boudinot P, Hosmalin A, Schwartz-Cornil I, Dalod M (2010) The XC chemokine receptor 1 is a conserved selective marker of mammalian cells homologous to mouse CD8alpha+ dendritic cells. J Exp Med 207:1283–1292

de Gruijl TD, Luykx-de Bakker SA, Tillman BW, van den Eertwegh AJ, Buter J, Lougheed SM, van der Bij GJ, Safer AM, Haisma HJ, Curiel DT, Scheper RJ, Pinedo HM, Gerritsen WR (2002) Prolonged maturation and enhanced transduction of dendritic cells migrated from human skin explants after in situ delivery of CD40-targeted adenoviral vectors. J Immunol 169:5322–5331

de Gruijl TD, Pinedo HM, Scheper RJ (2004) Immunotherapy of cancer through dendritic cell-targeted gene transfer. In: Curiel DT, Douglass JT (eds) Cancer gene therapy. Humana Press, Totowa, pp 143–172

de Gruijl TD, Sombroek CC, Lougheed SM, Oosterhoff D, Buter J, van den Eertwegh AJ, Scheper RJ, Pinedo HM (2006) A postmigrational switch among skin-derived dendritic cells to a macrophage-like phenotype is predetermined by the intracutaneous cytokine balance. J Immunol 176:7232–7242

Dranoff G (2003) GM-CSF-secreting melanoma vaccines. Oncogene 22:3188–3192

Dranoff G (2009) Targets of protective tumor immunity. Ann NY Acad Sci 1174:74–80

Dzionek A, Sohma Y, Nagafune J, Cella M, Colonna M, Facchetti F, Gunther G, Johnston I, Lanzavecchia A, Nagasaka T, Okada T, Vermi W, Winkels G, Yamamoto T, Zysk M, Yamaguchi Y, Schmitz J (2001) BDCA-2, a novel plasmacytoid dendritic cell-specific type II C-type lectin, mediates antigen capture and is a potent inhibitor of interferon alpha/beta induction. J Exp Med 194:1823–1834

Edele F, Molenaar R, Gutle D, Dudda JC, Jakob T, Homey B, Mebius R, Hornef M, Martin SF (2008) Cutting edge: instructive role of peripheral tissue cells in the imprinting of T cell homing receptor patterns. J Immunol 181:3745–3749

Egen JG, Kuhns MS, Allison JP (2002) CTLA-4: new insights into its biological function and use in tumor immunotherapy. Nat Immunol 3:611–618

Eggermont AM (2009) Immunostimulation versus immunosuppression after multiple vaccinations: the woes of therapeutic vaccine development. Clin Cancer Res 15:6745–6747

Engering A, van Vliet SJ, Hebeda K, Jackson DG, Prevo R, Singh SK, Geijtenbeek TB, van Krieken H, van Kooyk Y (2004) Dynamic populations of dendritic cell-specific ICAM-3 grabbing nonintegrin-positive immature dendritic cells and liver/lymph node-specific ICAM-3 grabbing nonintegrin-positive endothelial cells in the outer zones of the paracortex of human lymph nodes. Am J Pathol 164:1587–1595

Enk AH, Jonuleit H, Saloga J, Knop J (1997) Dendritic cells as mediators of tumor-induced tolerance in metastatic melanoma. Int J Cancer 73:309–316

Enk AH, Katz SI (1992) Identification and induction of keratinocyte-derived IL-10. J Immunol 149:92–95

Essner R, Kojima M (2002) Dendritic cell function in sentinel nodes. Oncology (Williston Park) 16:27–31

Fanning SL, George TC, Feng D, Feldman SB, Megjugorac NJ, Izaguirre AG, Fitzgerald-Bocarsly P (2006) Receptor cross-linking on human plasmacytoid dendritic cells leads to the regulation of IFN-alpha production. J Immunol 177:5829–5839

Faries MB, Hsueh EC, Ye X, Hoban M, Morton DL (2009) Effect of granulocyte/macrophage colony-stimulating factor on vaccination with an allogeneic whole-cell melanoma vaccine. Clin Cancer Res 15:7029–7035

Farrand KJ, Dickgreber N, Stoitzner P, Ronchese F, Petersen TR, Hermans IF (2009) Langerin+ CD8alpha+ dendritic cells are critical for cross-priming and IL-12 production in response to systemic antigens. J Immunol 183:7732–7742

Filipazzi P, Valenti R, Huber V, Pilla L, Canese P, Iero M, Castelli C, Mariani L, Parmiani G, Rivoltini L (2007) Identification of a new subset of myeloid suppressor cells in peripheral blood of melanoma patients with modulation by a granulocyte–macrophage colony-stimulation factor-based antitumor vaccine. J Clin Oncol 25:2546–2553

Flacher V, Tripp CH, Stoitzner P, Haid B, Ebner S, Del Frari B, Koch F, Park CG, Steinman RM, Idoyaga J, Romani N (2010) Epidermal Langerhans cells rapidly capture and present antigens from C-type lectin-targeting antibodies deposited in the dermis. J Invest Dermatol 130:755–762

Fourcade J, Kudela P, Sun Z, Shen H, Land SR, Lenzner D, Guillaume P, Luescher IF, Sander C, Ferrone S, Kirkwood JM, Zarour HM (2009) PD-1 is a regulator of NY-ESO-1-specific CD8+ T cell expansion in melanoma patients. J Immunol 182:5240–5249

Freeman GJ, Long AJ, Iwai Y, Bourque K, Chernova T, Nishimura H, Fitz LJ, Malenkovich N, Okazaki T, Byrne MC, Horton HF, Fouser L, Carter L, Ling V, Bowman MR, Carreno BM, Collins M, Wood CR, Honjo T (2000) Engagement of the PD-1 immunoinhibitory receptor by a novel B7 family member leads to negative regulation of lymphocyte activation. J Exp Med 192:1027–1034

Geissmann F, Dieu-Nosjean MC, Dezutter C, Valladeau J, Kayal S, Leborgne M, Brousse N, Saeland S, Davoust J (2002) Accumulation of immature Langerhans cells in human lymph nodes draining chronically inflamed skin. J Exp Med 196:417–430

Geissmann F, Manz MG, Jung S, Sieweke MH, Merad M, Ley K (2010) Development of monocytes, macrophages, and dendritic cells. Science 327:656–661

Gerlini G, Di Gennaro P, Mariotti G, Urso C, Chiarugi A, Pimpinelli N, Borgognoni L (2010) Indoleamine 2, 3-dioxygenase+ cells correspond to the BDCA2+ plasmacytoid dendritic cells in human melanoma sentinel nodes. J Invest Dermatol 130:898–901

Gerlini G, Mariotti G, Chiarugi A, Di Gennaro P, Caporale R, Parenti A, Cavone L, Tun-Kyi A, Prignano F, Saccardi R, Borgognoni L, Pimpinelli N (2008) Induction of CD83+ CD14+ nondendritic antigen-presenting cells by exposure of monocytes to IFN-alpha. J Immunol 181:2999–3008

Gerlini G, Tun-Kyi A, Dudli C, Burg G, Pimpinelli N, Nestle FO (2004) Metastatic melanoma secreted IL-10 down-regulates CD1 molecules on dendritic cells in metastatic tumor lesions. Am J Pathol 165:1853–1863

Gerlini G, Urso C, Mariotti G, Di Gennaro P, Palli D, Brandani P, Salvadori A, Pimpinelli N, Reali UM, Borgognoni L (2007) Plasmacytoid dendritic cells represent a major dendritic cell subset in sentinel lymph nodes of melanoma patients and accumulate in metastatic nodes. Clin Immunol 125:184–193

Gershenwald JE, Thompson W, Mansfield PF, Lee JE, Colome MI, Tseng CH, Lee JJ, Balch CM, Reintgen DS, Ross MI (1999) Multi-institutional melanoma lymphatic mapping experience: the prognostic value of sentinel lymph node status in 612 stage I or II melanoma patients. J Clin Oncol 17:976–983

Ghebeh H, Mohammed S, Al Omair A, Qattan A, Lehe C, Al Qudaihi G, Elkum N, Alshabanah M, Bin AS, Tulbah A, Ajarim D, Al Tweigeri T, Dermime S (2006) The B7–H1 (PD-L1) T lymphocyte-inhibitory molecule is expressed in breast cancer patients with infiltrating ductal carcinoma: correlation with important high-risk prognostic factors. Neoplasia 8:190–198

Ginhoux F, Collin MP, Bogunovic M, Abel M, Leboeuf M, Helft J, Ochando J, Kissenpfennig A, Malissen B, Grisotto M, Snoeck H, Randolph G, Merad M (2007) Blood-derived dermal langerin+ dendritic cells survey the skin in the steady state. J Exp Med 204:3133–3146

Glaspy J, Ribas A, Chmielowski B (2009) Interferon alfa in the postsurgical management of high-risk melanoma: is it worth it? J Clin Oncol 27:2896–2897

Gogas H, Ioannovich J, Dafni U, Stavropoulou-Giokas C, Frangia K, Tsoutsos D, Panagiotou P, Polyzos A, Papadopoulos O, Stratigos A, Markopoulos C, Bafaloukos D, Pectasides D, Fountzilas G, Kirkwood JM (2006) Prognostic significance of autoimmunity during treatment of melanoma with interferon. N Engl J Med 354:709–718

Granelli-Piperno A, Pritsker A, Pack M, Shimeliovich I, Arrighi JF, Park CG, Trumpfheller C, Piguet V, Moran TM, Steinman RM (2005) Dendritic cell-specific intercellular adhesion molecule 3-grabbing nonintegrin/CD209 is abundant on macrophages in the normal human lymph node and is not required for dendritic cell stimulation of the mixed leukocyte reaction. J Immunol 175:4265–4273

Green DS, Bodman-Smith MD, Dalgleish AG, Fischer MD (2007) Phase I/II study of topical imiquimod and intralesional interleukin-2 in the treatment of accessible metastases in malignant melanoma. Br J Dermatol 156:337–345

Green DS, Dalgleish AG, Belonwu N, Fischer MD, Bodman-Smith MD (2008) Topical imiquimod and intralesional interleukin-2 increase activated lymphocytes and restore the Th1/Th2 balance in patients with metastatic melanoma. Br J Dermatol 159:606–614

Gregor PD, Wolchok JD, Ferrone CR, Buchinshky H, Guevara-Patino JA, Perales MA, Mortazavi F, Bacich D, Heston W, Latouche JB, Sadelain M, Allison JP, Scher HI, Houghton AN (2004) CTLA-4 blockade in combination with xenogeneic DNA vaccines enhances T-cell responses, tumor immunity and autoimmunity to self antigens in animal and cellular model systems. Vaccine 22:1700–1708

Gursel M, Verthelyi D, Klinman DM (2002) CpG oligodeoxynucleotides induce human monocytes to mature into functional dendritic cells. Eur J Immunol 32:2617–2622

Haenssle H, Buhl T, Knudsen S, Krueger U, Rosenberger A, Reich K, Neumann C (2008) CD40 ligation during dendritic cell maturation reduces cell death and prevents interleukin-10-induced regression to macrophage-like monocytes. Exp Dermatol 17:177–187

Haining WN, Davies J, Kanzler H, Drury L, Brenn T, Evans J, Angelosanto J, Rivoli S, Russell K, George S, Sims P, Neuberg D, Li X, Kutok J, Morgan J, Wen P, Demetri G, Coffman RL, Nadler LM (2008) CpG oligodeoxynucleotides alter lymphocyte and dendritic cell trafficking in humans. Clin Cancer Res 14:5626–5634

Hangalapura BN, Oosterhoff D, Aggarwal S, Wijnands PGJTB, van de Ven R, Santegoets SJAM, van den Tol MP, Hooijberg E, Pereboev A, van den Eertwegh AJM, Curiel DT, Scheper RJ, de Gruijl TD (2010) Selective transduction of dendritic cells in human lymph nodes and superior induction of high-avidity melanoma-reactive cytotoxic T cells by a CD40-targeted adenovirus. J Immunother 33:706–715

Hartmann E, Wollenberg B, Rothenfusser S, Wagner M, Wellisch D, Mack B, Giese T, Gires O, Endres S, Hartmann G (2003) Identification and functional analysis of tumor-infiltrating plasmacytoid dendritic cells in head and neck cancer. Cancer Res 63:6478–6487

Hawiger D, Inaba K, Dorsett Y, Guo M, Mahnke K, Rivera M, Ravetch JV, Steinman RM, Nussenzweig MC (2001) Dendritic cells induce peripheral T cell unresponsiveness under steady state conditions in vivo. J Exp Med 194:769–779

Hedvat M, Huszar D, Herrmann A, Gozgit JM, Schroeder A, Sheehy A, Buettner R, Proia D, Kowolik CM, Xin H, Armstrong B, Bebernitz G, Weng S, Wang L, Ye M, McEachern K, Chen H, Morosini D, Bell K, Alimzhanov M, Ioannidis S, McCoon P, Cao ZA, Yu H, Jove R, Zinda M (2009) The JAK2 inhibitor AZD1480 potently blocks Stat3 signaling and oncogenesis in solid tumors. Cancer Cell 16:487–497

Hodi FS, Mihm MC, Soiffer RJ, Haluska FG, Butler M, Seiden MV, Davis T, Henry-Spires R, MacRae S, Willman A, Padera R, Jaklitsch MT, Shankar S, Chen TC, Korman A, Allison JP, Dranoff G (2003) Biologic activity of cytotoxic T lymphocyte-associated antigen 4 antibody blockade in previously vaccinated metastatic melanoma and ovarian carcinoma patients. Proc Natl Acad Sci USA 100:4712–4717

Hodi FS, O'Day SJ, McDermott DF, Weber RW, Sosman JA, Haanen JB, Gonzalez R, Robert C, Schadendorf D, Hassel JC, Akerley W, van den Eertwegh AJ, Lutzky J, Lorigan P, Vaubel JM, Linette GP, Hogg D, Ottensmeier CH, Lebbe C, Peschel C, Quirt I, Clark JI, Wolchok JD, Weber JS, Tian J, Yellin MJ, Nichol GM, Hoos A, Urba WJ (2010) Improved survival with ipilimumab in patients with metastatic melanoma. N Engl J Med 363:711–723

Hofmann MA, Kors C, Audring H, Walden P, Sterry W, Trefzer U (2008) Phase 1 evaluation of intralesionally injected TLR9-agonist PF-3512676 in patients with basal cell carcinoma or metastatic melanoma. J Immunother 31:520–527

Hornung V, Rothenfusser S, Britsch S, Krug A, Jahrsdorfer B, Giese T, Endres S, Hartmann G (2002) Quantitative expression of toll-like receptor 1–10 mRNA in cellular subsets of human peripheral blood mononuclear cells and sensitivity to CpG oligodeoxynucleotides. J Immunol 168:4531–4537

Huang D, Pereboev AV, Korokhov N, He R, Larocque L, Gravel C, Jaentschke B, Tocchi M, Casley WL, Lemieux M, Curiel DT, Chen W, Li X (2008) Significant alterations of biodistribution and immune responses in Balb/c mice administered with adenovirus targeted to CD40(+) cells. Gene Ther 15:298–308

Huang RR, Wen DR, Guo J, Giuliano AE, Nguyen M, Offodile R, Stern S, Turner R, Cochran AJ (2000) Selective modulation of paracortical dendritic cells and T-lymphocytes in breast cancer sentinel lymph nodes. Breast J 6:225–232

Hunter TB, Alsarraj M, Gladue RP, Bedian V, Antonia SJ (2007) An agonist antibody specific for CD40 induces dendritic cell maturation and promotes autologous anti-tumour T-cell responses in an in vitro mixed autologous tumour cell/lymph node cell model. Scand J Immunol 65:479–486

Ichikawa HT, Williams LP, Segal BM (2002) Activation of APCs through CD40 or Toll-like receptor 9 overcomes tolerance and precipitates autoimmune disease. J Immunol 169: 2781–2787

Ishigami S, Ueno S, Matsumoto M, Okumura H, Arigami T, Uchikado Y, Setoyama T, Arima H, Sasaki K, Kitazono M, Shinchi H, Kijima Y, Natsugoe S (2010) Prognostic value of CD208-positive cell infiltration in gastric cancer. Cancer Immunol Immunother 59:389–395

Iwai Y, Ishida M, Tanaka Y, Okazaki T, Honjo T, Minato N (2002) Involvement of PD-L1 on tumor cells in the escape from host immune system and tumor immunotherapy by PD-L1 blockade. Proc Natl Acad Sci USA 99:12293–12297

Iwamoto M, Shinohara H, Miyamoto A, Okuzawa M, Mabuchi H, Nohara T, Gon G, Toyoda M, Tanigawa N (2003) Prognostic value of tumor-infiltrating dendritic cells expressing CD83 in human breast carcinomas. Int J Cancer 104:92–97

Jakob T, Walker PS, Krieg AM, Udey MC, Vogel JC (1998) Activation of cutaneous dendritic cells by CpG-containing oligodeoxynucleotides: a role for dendritic cells in the augmentation of Th1 responses by immunostimulatory DNA. J Immunol 161:3042–3049

Jarrossay D, Napolitani G, Colonna M, Sallusto F, Lanzavecchia A (2001) Specialization and complementarity in microbial molecule recognition by human myeloid and plasmacytoid dendritic cells. Eur J Immunol 31:3388–3393

Jinushi M, Nakazaki Y, Dougan M, Carrasco DR, Mihm M, Dranoff G (2007) MFG-E8-mediated uptake of apoptotic cells by APCs links the pro- and anti-inflammatory activities of GM-CSF. J Clin Invest 117:1902–1913

Johnson TS, Mahnke K, Storn V, Schonfeld K, Ring S, Nettelbeck DM, Haisma HJ, Le Gall F, Kontermann RE, Enk AH (2008) Inhibition of melanoma growth by targeting of antigen to dendritic cells via an anti-DEC-205 single-chain fragment variable molecule. Clin Cancer Res 14:8169–8177

Jongbloed SL, Kassianos AJ, McDonald KJ, Clark GJ, Ju X, Angel CE, Chen CJ, Dunbar PR, Wadley RB, Jeet V, Vulink AJ, Hart DN, Radford KJ (2010) Human CD141+ (BDCA-3)+ dendritic cells (DCs) represent a unique myeloid DC subset that cross-presents necrotic cell antigens. J Exp Med 207:1247–1260

Jonuleit H, Schmitt E, Steinbrink K, Enk AH (2001) Dendritic cells as a tool to induce anergic and regulatory T cells. Trends Immunol 22:394–400

Kass E, Panicali DL, Mazzara G, Schlom J, Greiner JW (2001) Granulocyte/macrophage-colony stimulating factor produced by recombinant avian poxviruses enriches the regional lymph nodes with antigen-presenting cells and acts as an immunoadjuvant. Cancer Res 61: 206–214

Keir ME, Butte MJ, Freeman GJ, Sharpe AH (2008) PD-1 and its ligands in tolerance and immunity. Annu Rev Immunol 26:677–704

Kim YS, Kim YJ, Lee JM, Han SH, Ko HJ, Park HJ, Pereboev A, Nguyen HH, Kang CY (2010) CD40-targeted recombinant adenovirus significantly enhances the efficacy of DC and B cell-based anti-tumor vaccines. Hum Gene Ther 21:1697–1706

Kirkwood JM, Lorigan P, Hersey P, Hauschild A, Robert C, McDermott D, Marshall MA, Gomez-Navarro J, Liang JQ, Bulanhagui CA (2010) Phase II trial of tremelimumab (CP-675, 206) in patients with advanced refractory or relapsed melanoma. Clin Cancer Res 16: 1042–1048

Klechevsky E, Liu M, Morita R, Banchereau R, Thompson-Snipes L, Palucka AK, Ueno H, Banchereau J (2009) Understanding human myeloid dendritic cell subsets for the rational design of novel vaccines. Hum Immunol 70:281–288

Klechevsky E, Morita R, Liu M, Cao Y, Coquery S, Thompson-Snipes L, Briere F, Chaussabel D, Zurawski G, Palucka AK, Reiter Y, Banchereau J, Ueno H (2008) Functional specializations of human epidermal Langerhans cells and CD14+ dermal dendritic cells. Immunity 29: 497–510

Korokhov N, Noureddini SC, Curiel DT, Santegoets SJ, Scheper RJ, de Gruijl TD (2005) A single-component CD40-targeted adenovirus vector displays highly efficient transduction and activation of dendritic cells in a human skin substrate system. Mol Pharm 2:218–223

Kortylewski M, Kujawski M, Herrmann A, Yang C, Wang L, Liu Y, Salcedo R, Yu H (2009a) Toll-like receptor 9 activation of signal transducer and activator of transcription 3 constrains its agonist-based immunotherapy. Cancer Res 69:2497–2505

Kortylewski M, Swiderski P, Herrmann A, Wang L, Kowolik C, Kujawski M, Lee H, Scuto A, Liu Y, Yang C, Deng J, Soifer HS, Raubitschek A, Forman S, Rossi JJ, Pardoll DM, Jove R, Yu H (2009b) In vivo delivery of siRNA to immune cells by conjugation to a TLR9 agonist enhances antitumor immune responses. Nat Biotechnol 27:925–932

Koschella M, Voehringer D, Pircher H (2004) CD40 ligation in vivo induces bystander proliferation of memory phenotype CD8 T cells. J Immunol 172:4804–4811

Krieg AM (2001) Now I know my CpGs. Trends Microbiol 9:249–252

Krieg AM (2002) CpG motifs in bacterial DNA and their immune effects. Annu Rev Immunol 20:709–760

Krieg AM (2008) Toll-like receptor 9 (TLR9) agonists in the treatment of cancer. Oncogene 27:161–167

Lacelle MG, Jensen SM, Fox BA (2009) Partial CD4 depletion reduces regulatory T cells induced by multiple vaccinations and restores therapeutic efficacy. Clin Cancer Res 15:6881–6890

Ladanyi A, Kiss J, Somlai B, Gilde K, Fejos Z, Mohos A, Gaudi I, Timar J (2007) Density of DC-LAMP(+) mature dendritic cells in combination with activated T lymphocytes infiltrating primary cutaneous melanoma is a strong independent prognostic factor. Cancer Immunol Immunother 56:1459–1469

Lebre MC, van der Aar AM, van Baarsen L, van Capel TM, Schuitemaker JH, Kapsenberg ML, de Jong EC (2007) Human keratinocytes express functional Toll-like receptor 3, 4, 5, and 9. J Invest Dermatol 127:331–341

Lee JH, Torisu-Itakara H, Cochran AJ, Kadison A, Huynh Y, Morton DL, Essner R (2005) Quantitative analysis of melanoma-induced cytokine-mediated immunosuppression in melanoma sentinel nodes. Clin Cancer Res 11:107–112

Lee JR, Dalton RR, Messina JL, Sharma MD, Smith DM, Burgess RE, Mazzella F, Antonia SJ, Mellor AL, Munn DH (2003) Pattern of recruitment of immunoregulatory antigen-presenting cells in malignant melanoma. Lab Invest 83:1457–1466

Li B, VanRoey M, Wang C, Chen TH, Korman A, Jooss K (2009) Anti-programmed death-1 synergizes with granulocyte macrophage colony-stimulating factor-secreting tumor cell immunotherapy providing therapeutic benefit to mice with established tumors. Clin Cancer Res 15:1623–1634

Liu C, Lou Y, Lizee G, Qin H, Liu S, Rabinovich B, Kim GJ, Wang YH, Ye Y, Sikora AG, Overwijk WW, Liu YJ, Wang G, Hwu P (2008) Plasmacytoid dendritic cells induce NK cell-dependent, tumor antigen-specific T cell cross-priming and tumor regression in mice. J Clin Invest 118:1165–1175

Macagno A, Napolitani G, Lanzavecchia A, Sallusto F (2007) Duration, combination and timing: the signal integration model of dendritic cell activation. Trends Immunol 28:227–233

Mahnke K, Qian Y, Fondel S, Brueck J, Becker C, Enk AH (2005) Targeting of antigens to activated dendritic cells in vivo cures metastatic melanoma in mice. Cancer Res 65: 7007–7012

Mancuso G, Gambuzza M, Midiri A, Biondo C, Papasergi S, Akira S, Teti G, Beninati C (2009) Bacterial recognition by TLR7 in the lysosomes of conventional dendritic cells. Nat Immunol 10:587–594

Mathers AR, Janelsins BM, Rubin JP, Tkacheva OA, Shufesky WJ, Watkins SC, Morelli AE, Larregina AT (2009) Differential capability of human cutaneous dendritic cell subsets to initiate Th17 responses. J Immunol 182:921–933

Mathers AR, Larregina AT (2006) Professional antigen-presenting cells of the skin. Immunol Res 36:127–136

Melief CJ, Van Der Burg SH, Toes RE, Ossendorp F, Offringa R (2002) Effective therapeutic anticancer vaccines based on precision guiding of cytolytic T lymphocytes. Immunol Rev 188:177–182

Mellor AL, Munn DH (2008) Creating immune privilege: active local suppression that benefits friends, but protects foes. Nat Rev Immunol 8:74–80

Merad M, Ginhoux F, Collin M (2008) Origin, homeostasis and function of Langerhans cells and other langerin-expressing dendritic cells. Nat Rev Immunol 8:935–947

Meyer-Wentrup F, Benitez-Ribas D, Tacken PJ, Punt CJ, Figdor CG, de Vries IJ, Adema GJ (2008) Targeting DCIR on human plasmacytoid dendritic cells results in antigen presentation and inhibits IFN-alpha production. Blood 111:4245–4253

Mikszta JA, Laurent PE (2008) Cutaneous delivery of prophylactic and therapeutic vaccines: historical perspective and future outlook. Expert Rev Vaccines 7:1329–1339

Mitsui H, Okamoto T, Kanzaki M, Inozume T, Shibagaki N, Shimada S (2010) Intradermal injections of polyarginine-containing immunogenic antigens preferentially elicit Tc1 and Th1 activation and antitumour immunity. Br J Dermatol 162:29–41

Mohty M, Olive D, Gaugler B (2004) Plasmacytoid DCs and cancer: a new role for an enigmatic cell. Trends Immunol 25:397–398

Molenkamp BG, Sluijter BJR, van Leuwen PAM, Santegoets SJAM, Meijer S, Wijnands PGJT, Haanen JBAG, van den Eertwegh AJM, Scheper RJ, de Gruijl TD (2008) Local administration of PF-3512676 CpG-B instigates tumor-specific CD8(+) T-cell reactivity in melanoma patients. Clin Cancer Res 14:4532–4542

Molenkamp BG, van Leeuwen PAM, Meijer S, Sluijter BJR, Wijnands PGJT, Baars A, van den Eertwegh AJM, Scheper RJ, de Grujil TD (2007) Intradermal CpG-B activates both plasmacytoid and myeloid dendritic cells in the sentinel lymph node of melanoma patients. Clin Cancer Res 13:2961–2969

Molenkamp BG, van Leeuwen PAM, van den Eertwegh AJM, Sluijter BJR, Scheper RJ, Meijer S, de Gruijl TD (2006) Immunomodulation of the melanoma sentinel lymph node: A novel adjuvant therapeutic option. Immunobiology 211:651–661

Molenkamp BG, Vuylsteke RJCL, van Leeuwen PAM, Meijer S, Vos W, Wijnands PGJT, Scheper RJ, de Gruijl TD (2005) Matched skin and sentinel lymph node samples of melanoma patients reveal exclusive migration of mature dendritic cells. Am J Pathol 167:1301–1307

Mora JR, Cheng G, Picarella D, Briskin M, Buchanan N, von Andrian UH (2005) Reciprocal and dynamic control of CD8 T cell homing by dendritic cells from skin- and gut-associated lymphoid tissues. J Exp Med 201:303–316

Morelli AE, Rubin JP, Erdos G, Tkacheva OA, Mathers AR, Zahorchak AF, Thomson AW, Falo LD Jr, Larregina AT (2005) CD4+ T cell responses elicited by different subsets of human skin migratory dendritic cells. J Immunol 175:7905–7915

Morton DL, Cochran AJ, Thompson JF (2008) The rationale for sentinel-node biopsy in primary melanoma. Nat Clin Pract Oncol 5:510–511

Mouries J, Moron G, Schlecht G, Escriou N, Dadaglio G, Leclerc C (2008) Plasmacytoid dendritic cells efficiently cross-prime naive T cells in vivo after TLR activation. Blood 112:3713–3722

Munn DH, Mellor AL (2006) The tumor-draining lymph node as an immune-privileged site. Immunol Rev 213:146–158

Munn DH, Mellor AL (2007) Indoleamine 2, 3-dioxygenase and tumor-induced tolerance. J Clin Invest 117:1147–1154

Munn DH, Sharma MD, Hou D, Baban B, Lee JR, Antonia SJ, Messina JL, Chandler P, Koni PA, Mellor AL (2004a) Expression of indoleamine 2, 3-dioxygenase by plasmacytoid dendritic cells in tumor-draining lymph nodes. J Clin Invest 114:280–290

Munn DH, Sharma MD, Mellor AL (2004b) Ligation of B7-1/B7-2 by human CD4+ T cells triggers indoleamine 2, 3-dioxygenase activity in dendritic cells. J Immunol 172:4100–4110

Nagaraj S, Collazo M, Corzo CA, Youn JI, Ortiz M, Quiceno D, Gabrilovich DI (2009) Regulatory myeloid suppressor cells in health and disease. Cancer Res 69:7503–7506

Nestle FO, Di Meglio P, Qin JZ, Nickoloff BJ (2009) Skin immune sentinels in health and disease. Nat Rev Immunol 9:679–691

Nestle FO, Nickoloff BJ (2007) Deepening our understanding of immune sentinels in the skin. J Clin Invest 117:2382–2385

Nickoloff BJ, Fivenson DP, Kunkel SL, Strieter RM, Turka LA (1994) Keratinocyte interleukin-10 expression is upregulated in tape-stripped skin, poison ivy dermatitis, and Sezary syndrome, but not in psoriatic plaques. Clin Immunol Immunopathol 73:63–68

Ochoa MT, Loncaric A, Krutzik SR, Becker TC, Modlin RL (2008) "Dermal dendritic cells" comprise two distinct populations: CD1+ dendritic cells and CD209+ macrophages. J Invest Dermatol 128:2225–2231

Ohigashi Y, Sho M, Yamada Y, Tsurui Y, Hamada K, Ikeda N, Mizuno T, Yoriki R, Kashizuka H, Yane K, Tsushima F, Otsuki N, Yagita H, Azuma M, Nakajima Y (2005) Clinical significance of programmed death-1 ligand-1 and programmed death-1 ligand-2 expression in human esophageal cancer. Clin Cancer Res 11:2947–2953

Ouwehand K, Santegoets SJ, Bruynzeel DP, Scheper RJ, de Gruijl TD, Gibbs S (2008) CXCL12 is essential for migration of activated Langerhans cells from epidermis to dermis. Eur J Immunol 38:3050–3059

Ouwehand K, Scheper RJ, de Gruijl TD, Gibbs S (2010) Epidermis-to-dermis migration of immature Langerhans cells upon topical irritant exposure is dependent on CCL2 and CCL5. Eur J Immunol 40:2026–2034

Palm NW, Medzhitov R (2009) Pattern recognition receptors and control of adaptive immunity. Immunol Rev 227:221–233

Peguet-Navarro J, Sportouch M, Popa I, Berthier O, Schmitt D, Portoukalian J (2003) Gangliosides from human melanoma tumors impair dendritic cell differentiation from monocytes and induce their apoptosis. J Immunol 170:3488–3494

Pfeffer LM, Dinarello CA, Herberman RB, Williams BR, Borden EC, Bordens R, Walter MR, Nagabhushan TL, Trotta PP, Pestka S (1998) Biological properties of recombinant alpha-interferons: 40th anniversary of the discovery of interferons. Cancer Res 58:2489–2499

Phan GQ, Yang JC, Sherry RM, Hwu P, Topalian SL, Schwartzentruber DJ, Restifo NP, Haworth LR, Seipp CA, Freezer LJ, Morton KE, Mavroukakis SA, Duray PH, Steinberg SM, Allison JP, Davis TA, Rosenberg SA (2003) Cancer regression and autoimmunity induced by cytotoxic T lymphocyte-associated antigen 4 blockade in patients with metastatic melanoma. Proc Natl Acad Sci USA 100:8372–8377

Poulin LF, Salio M, Griessinger E, Anjos-Afonso F, Craciun L, Chen JL, Keller AM, Joffre O, Zelenay S, Nye E, Le Moine A, Faure F, Donckier V, Sancho D, Cerundolo V, Bonnet D, Reis e Sousa (2010) Characterization of human DNGR-1 + BDCA3 + leukocytes as putative equivalents of mouse CD8alpha + dendritic cells. J Exp Med 207:1261–1271

Rabinovich GA, Gabrilovich D, Sotomayor EM (2007) Immunosuppressive strategies that are mediated by tumor cells. Annu Rev Immunol 25:267–296

Randow F, Syrbe U, Meisel C, Krausch D, Zuckermann H, Platzer C, Volk HD (1995) Mechanism of endotoxin desensitization: involvement of interleukin 10 and transforming growth factor beta. J Exp Med 181:1887–1892

Ray CM, Kluk M, Grin CM, Grant-Kels JM (2005) Successful treatment of malignant melanoma in situ with topical 5% imiquimod cream. Int J Dermatol 44:428–434

Reddy ST, Swartz MA, Hubbell JA (2006) Targeting dendritic cells with biomaterials: developing the next generation of vaccines. Trends Immunol 27:573–579

Riboldi E, Daniele R, Cassatella MA, Sozzani S, Bosisio D (2009) Engagement of BDCA-2 blocks TRAIL-mediated cytotoxic activity of plasmacytoid dendritic cells. Immunobiology 214:868–876

Ridolfi L, Ridolfi R, Ascari-Raccagni A, Fabbri M, Casadei S, Gatti A, Trevisan G, Righini MG (2001) Intralesional granulocyte–monocyte colony-stimulating factor followed by subcutaneous interleukin-2 in metastatic melanoma: a pilot study in elderly patients. J Eur Acad Dermatol Venereol 15:218–223

Rieger R, Kipps TJ (2003) CpG oligodeoxynucleotides enhance the capacity of adenovirus-mediated CD154 gene transfer to generate effective B cell lymphoma vaccines. Cancer Res 63:4128–4135

Rivas JM, Ullrich SE (1992) Systemic suppression of delayed-type hypersensitivity by supernatants from UV-irradiated keratinocytes. An essential role for keratinocyte-derived IL-10. J Immunol 149:3865–3871

Robbins SH, Walzer T, Dembele D, Thibault C, Defays A, Bessou G, Xu H, Vivier E, Sellars M, Pierre P, Sharp FR, Chan S, Kastner P, Dalod M (2008) Novel insights into the relationships between dendritic cell subsets in human and mouse revealed by genome-wide expression profiling. Genome Biol 9:R17

Romani N, Clausen BE, Stoitzner P (2010) Langerhans cells and more: langerin-expressing dendritic cell subsets in the skin. Immunol Rev 234:120–141

Romero P, Cerottini JC, Speiser DE (2006) The human T cell response to melanoma antigens. Adv Immunol 92:187–224

Romero P, Dunbar PR, Valmori D, Pittet M, Ogg GS, Rimoldi D, Chen JL, Lienard D, Cerottini JC, Cerundolo V (1998) Ex vivo staining of metastatic lymph nodes by class I major histocompatibility complex tetramers reveals high numbers of antigen-experienced tumor-specific cytolytic T lymphocytes. Journal of Experimental Medicine 188:1641–1650

Rosenberg SA, Dudley ME (2009) Adoptive cell therapy for the treatment of patients with metastatic melanoma. Curr Opin Immunol 21:233–240

Salio M, Cella M, Vermi W, Facchetti F, Palmowski MJ, Smith CL, Shepherd D, Colonna M, Cerundolo V (2003) Plasmacytoid dendritic cells prime IFN-gamma-secreting melanoma-specific CD8 lymphocytes and are found in primary melanoma lesions. Eur J Immunol 33:1052–1062

Sancho D, Mourao-Sa D, Joffre OP, Schulz O, Rogers NC, Pennington DJ, Carlyle JR, Reis e Sousa (2008) Tumor therapy in mice via antigen targeting to a novel, DC-restricted C-type lectin. J Clin Invest 118:2098–2110

Santegoets SJ, Bontkes HJ, Stam AG, Bhoelan F, Ruizendaal JJ, van den Eertwegh AJ, Hooijberg E, Scheper RJ, de Gruijl TD (2008) Inducing antitumor T cell immunity: comparative functional analysis of interstitial versus Langerhans dendritic cells in a human cell line model. J Immunol 180:4540–4549

Santegoets SJ, Gibbs S, Kroeze K, Van de Van R, Scheper RJ, Borrebaeck CA, de Gruijl TD, Lindstedt M (2008b) Transcriptional profiling of human skin-resident Langerhans cells and CD1a+ dermal dendritic cells: differential activation states suggest distinct functions. J Leukoc Biol 84:143–151

Sarnaik AA, Weber JS (2009) Recent advances using anti-CTLA-4 for the treatment of melanoma. Cancer J 15:169–173

Schmidt C (2007) News: clinical setbacks for toll-like receptor 9 agonists in cancer. Nat Biotechnol 25:825–826

Schoenberger SP, Toes RE, van der Voort EI, Offringa R, Melief CJ (1998) T-cell help for cytotoxic T lymphocytes is mediated by CD40–CD40L interactions. Nature 393:480–483

Schon MP, Schon M (2008) TLR7 and TLR8 as targets in cancer therapy. Oncogene 27:190–199

Sen D, Forrest L, Kepler TB, Parker I, Cahalan MD (2010) Selective and site-specific mobilization of dermal dendritic cells and Langerhans cells by Th1- and Th2-polarizing adjuvants. Proc Natl Acad Sci USA 107:8334–8339

Serra P, Amrani A, Yamanouchi J, Han B, Thiessen S, Utsugi T, Verdaguer J, Santamaria P (2003) CD40 ligation releases immature dendritic cells from the control of regulatory CD4+ CD25+ T cells. Immunity 19:877–889

Sharma MD, Baban B, Chandler P, Hou DY, Singh N, Yagita H, Azuma M, Blazar BR, Mellor AL, Munn DH (2007) Plasmacytoid dendritic cells from mouse tumor-draining lymph nodes directly activate mature Tregs via indoleamine 2, 3-dioxygenase. J Clin Invest 117:2570–2582

Sharma MD, Hou DY, Liu Y, Koni PA, Metz R, Chandler P, Mellor AL, He Y, Munn DH (2009) Indoleamine 2, 3-dioxygenase controls conversion of Foxp3+ Tregs to TH17-like cells in tumor-draining lymph nodes. Blood 113:6102–6111

Simmons AD, Moskalenko M, Creson J, Fang J, Yi S, VanRoey MJ, Allison JP, Jooss K (2008) Local secretion of anti-CTLA-4 enhances the therapeutic efficacy of a cancer immunotherapy with reduced evidence of systemic autoimmunity. Cancer Immunol Immunother 57: 1263–1270

Skrzeczynska-Moncznik J, Wawro K, Stefanska A, Oleszycka E, Kulig P, Zabel BA, Sulkowski M, Kapinska-Mrowiecka M, Czubak-Macugowska M, Butcher EC, Cichy J (2009) Potential role of chemerin in recruitment of plasmacytoid dendritic cells to diseased skin. Biochem Biophys Res Commun 380:323–327

Slingluff CL Jr, Petroni GR, Olson WC, Smolkin ME, Ross MI, Haas NB, Grosh WW, Boisvert ME, Kirkwood JM, Chianese-Bullock KA (2009) Effect of granulocyte/macrophage colony-stimulating factor on circulating CD8+ and CD4+ T-cell responses to a multipeptide melanoma vaccine: outcome of a multicenter randomized trial. Clin Cancer Res 15: 7036–7044

Smalley KS (2010) PLX-4032, a small-molecule B-Raf inhibitor for the potential treatment of malignant melanoma. Curr Opin Investig Drugs 11:699–706

Sparber F, Tripp CH, Hermann M, Romani N, Stoitzner P (2010) Langerhans cells and dermal dendritic cells capture protein antigens in the skin: possible targets for vaccination through the skin. Immunobiology 215:770–779

Stanley MA (2002) Imiquimod and the imidazoquinolones: mechanism of action and therapeutic potential. Clin Exp Dermatol 27:571–577

Starz H, Balda BR (2007) Benefit of sentinel lymphadenectomy for patients with nonulcerated cutaneous melanomas in the Breslow range between 0.76 and 1 mm: a follow-up study of 148 patients. Int J Cancer 121:689–693

Statius Muller MG, Borgstein PJ, Pijpers R, van Leeuwen PA, van Diest PJ, Gupta A, Meijer S (2000) Reliability of the sentinel node procedure in melanoma patients: analysis of failures after long-term follow-up. Ann Surg Oncol 7:461–468

Stoitzner P, Green LK, Jung JY, Price KM, Tripp CH, Malissen B, Kissenpfennig A, Hermans IF, Ronchese F (2008) Tumor immunotherapy by epicutaneous immunization requires langerhans cells. J Immunol 180:1991–1998

Stoitzner P, Sparber F, Tripp CH (2010a) Langerhans cells as targets for immunotherapy against skin cancer. Immunol Cell Biol 88:431–437

Stoitzner P, Stingl G, Merad M, Romani N (2010b) Langerhans cells at the interface of medicine, science, and industry. J Invest Dermatol 130:331–335

Sun X, Hodge LM, Jones HP, Tabor L, Simecka JW (2002) Co-expression of granulocyte–macrophage colony-stimulating factor with antigen enhances humoral and tumor immunity after DNA vaccination. Vaccine 20:1466–1474

Tacken PJ, de Vries IJ, Torensma R, Figdor CG (2007) Dendritic-cell immunotherapy: from ex vivo loading to in vivo targeting. Nat Rev Immunol 7:790–802

Teunissen MBM, Koomen CW, Jansen J, de Waal MR, Schmitt E, Van den Wijngaard RM, Das PK, Bos JD (1997) In contrast to their murine counterparts, normal human keratinocytes and human epidermoid cell lines A431 and HaCaT fail to express IL-10 mRNA and protein. Clin Exp Immunol 107:213–223

Teunissen MBM, Haniffa M, Collin MP (2011) Insight into the immunobiology of human skin and functional specialization of skin dendritic cell subsets to innovate intradermal vaccination design. Curr Top Microbiol Immunol 351:25–76

Thacker EE, Nakayama M, Smith BF, Bird RC, Muminova Z, Strong TV, Timares L, Korokhov N, O'Neill AM, de Gruijl TD, Glasgow JN, Tani K, Curiel DT (2009) A genetically engineered adenovirus vector targeted to CD40 mediates transduction of canine dendritic cells and promotes antigen-specific immune responses in vivo. Vaccine 27:7116–7124

Tillman BW, de Gruijl TD, Luykx-de Bakker SA, Scheper RJ, Pinedo HM, Curiel TJ, Gerritsen WR, Curiel DT (1999) Maturation of dendritic cells accompanies high-efficiency gene transfer by a CD40-targeted adenoviral vector. J Immunol 162:6378–6383

Tillman BW, Hayes TL, DeGruijl TD, Douglas JT, Curiel DT (2000) Adenoviral vectors targeted to CD40 enhance the efficacy of dendritic cell-based vaccination against human papillomavirus 16-induced tumor cells in a murine model. Cancer Res 60:5456–5463

Timares L, Douglas JT, Tillman BW, Krasnykh V, Curiel DT (2004) Adenovirus-mediated gene delivery to dendritic cells. Methods Mol Biol 246:139–154

Toka FN, Gierynska M, Suvas S, Schoenberger SP, Rouse BT (2005) Rescue of memory CD8+ T cell reactivity in peptide/TLR9 ligand immunization by codelivery of cytokines or CD40 ligation. Virology 331:151–158

Toriyama K, Wen DR, Paul E, Cochran AJ (1993) Variations in the distribution, frequency, and phenotype of Langerhans cells during the evolution of malignant-melanoma of the skin. J Investig Dermatol 100:S269–S273

Tuve S, Chen BM, Liu Y, Cheng TL, Toure P, Sow PS, Feng Q, Kiviat N, Strauss R, Ni S, Li ZY, Roffler SR, Lieber A (2007) Combination of tumor site-located CTL-associated antigen-4 blockade and systemic regulatory T-cell depletion induces tumor-destructive immune responses. Cancer Res 67:5929–5939

van Broekhoven CL, Parish CR, Demangel C, Britton WJ, Altin JG (2004) Targeting dendritic cells with antigen-containing liposomes: a highly effective procedure for induction of antitumor immunity and for tumor immunotherapy. Cancer Res 64:4357–4365

van der Aar AMG, Sylva-Steenland RMR, Bos JD, Kapsenberg ML, de Jong EC, Teunissen MBM (2007) Loss of TLR2, TLR4, and TLR5 on Langerhans cells abolishes bacterial recognition. J Immunol 178:1986–1990

Vermi W, Bonecchi R, Facchetti F, Bianchi D, Sozzani S, Festa S, Berenzi A, Cella M, Colonna M (2003) Recruitment of immature plasmacytoid dendritic cells (plasmacytoid monocytes) and myeloid dendritic cells in primary cutaneous melanomas. J Pathol 200:255–268

Villadangos JA, Young L (2008) Antigen-presentation properties of plasmacytoid dendritic cells. Immunity 29:352–361

Vonderheide RH, Flaherty KT, Khalil M, Stumacher MS, Bajor DL, Hutnick NA, Sullivan P, Mahany JJ, Gallagher M, Kramer A, Green SJ, O'Dwyer PJ, Running KL, Huhn RD, Antonia SJ (2007) Clinical activity and immune modulation in cancer patients treated with CP-870, 893, a novel CD40 agonist monoclonal antibody. J Clin Oncol 25:876–883

Vuylsteke RJ, van Leeuwen PA, Meijer S, Wijnands PG, Statius Muller MG, Busch DH, Scheper RJ, de Gruijl TD (2002) Sampling tumor-draining lymph nodes for phenotypic and functional analysis of dendritic cells and T cells. Am J Pathol 161:19–26

Vuylsteke RJCL, Molenkamp BG, Gietema HA, van Leeuwen PAM, Wijnands PGJT, Vos W, van Diest PJ, Scheper RJ, Meijer S, de Gruijl TD (2004) Local administration of granulocyte/macrophage colony-stimulating factor increases the number and activation state of dendritic cells in the sentinel lymph node of early-stage melanoma. Cancer Research 64:8456–8460

Vuylsteke RJCL, Molenkamp BG, van Leeuwen PAM, Meijer S, Wijnands PGJT, Haanen JBAG, Scheper RJ, de Gruijl TD (2006) Tumor-specific CD8+ T cell reactivity in the sentinel lymph node of GM-CSF-treated stage I melanoma patients is associated with high myeloid dendritic cell content. Clin Cancer Res 12:2826–2833

Waller EK (2007) The role of sargramostim (rhGM-CSF) as immunotherapy. Oncologist 12 (Suppl 2):22–26

Wang W, Edington HD, Rao UN, Jukic DM, Land SR, Ferrone S, Kirkwood JM (2007) Modulation of signal transducers and activators of transcription 1 and 3 signaling in melanoma by high-dose IFNalpha2b. Clin Cancer Res 13:1523–1531

Wang W, Lau R, Yu D, Zhu W, Korman A, Weber J (2009) PD1 blockade reverses the suppression of melanoma antigen-specific CTL by CD4+ CD25(Hi) regulatory T cells. Int Immunol 21:1065–1077

Warren TL, Bhatia SK, Acosta AM, Dahle CE, Ratliff TL, Krieg AM, Weiner GJ (2000) APC stimulated by CpG oligodeoxynucleotide enhance activation of MHC class I-restricted T cells. J Immunol 165:6244–6251

Waterhouse P, Penninger JM, Timms E, Wakeham A, Shahinian A, Lee KP, Thompson CB, Griesser H, Mak TW (1995) Lymphoproliferative disorders with early lethality in mice deficient in Ctla-4. Science 270:985–988

Wei H, Wang S, Zhang D, Hou S, Qian W, Li B, Guo H, Kou G, He J, Wang H, Guo Y (2009) Targeted delivery of tumor antigens to activated dendritic cells via CD11c molecules induces potent antitumor immunity in mice. Clin Cancer Res 15:4612–4621

Wenzel J, Tormo D, Tuting T (2008) Toll-like receptor-agonists in the treatment of skin cancer: history, current developments and future prospects. Handb Exp Pharmacol 183:201–220

Wolf IH, Cerroni L, Kodama K, Kerl H (2005) Treatment of lentigo maligna (melanoma in situ) with the immune response modifier imiquimod. Arch Dermatol 141:510–514

Wolf IH, Kodama K, Cerroni L, Kerl H (2007) Nature of inflammatory infiltrate in superficial cutaneous malignancies during topical imiquimod treatment. Am J Dermatopathol 29: 237–241

Yoneyama H, Matsuno K, Zhang Y, Nishiwaki T, Kitabatake M, Ueha S, Narumi S, Morikawa S, Ezaki T, Lu B, Gerard C, Ishikawa S, Matsushima K (2004) Evidence for recruitment of plasmacytoid dendritic cell precursors to inflamed lymph nodes through high endothelial venules. Int Immunol 16:915–928

Yu H, Pardoll D, Jove R (2009) STATs in cancer inflammation and immunity: a leading role for STAT3. Nat Rev Cancer 9:798–809

Zaba LC, Fuentes-Duculan J, Steinman RM, Krueger JG, Lowes MA (2007) Normal human dermis contains distinct populations of CD11c+BDCA-1+ dendritic cells and CD163+FXIIIA+ macrophages. J Clin Invest 117:2517–2525

Zaba LC, Krueger JG, Lowes MA (2009) Resident and "inflammatory" dendritic cells in human skin. J Invest Dermatol 129:302–308

Zang X, Allison JP (2007) The B7 family and cancer therapy: costimulation and coinhibition. Clin Cancer Res 13:5271–5279

Zou W, Machelon V, Coulomb-L'Hermin A, Borvak J, Nome F, Isaeva T, Wei S, Krzysiek R, Durand-Gasselin I, Gordon A, Pustilnik T, Curiel DT, Galanaud P, Capron F, Emilie D, Curiel TJ (2001) Stromal-derived factor-1 in human tumors recruits and alters the function of plasmacytoid precursor dendritic cells. Nat Med 7:1339–1346

DNA Vaccines and Intradermal Vaccination by DNA Tattooing

K. Oosterhuis, J. H. van den Berg, T. N. Schumacher and J. B. A. G. Haanen

Abstract Over the past two decades, DNA vaccination has been developed as a method for the induction of immune responses. However, in spite of high expectations based on their efficacy in preclinical models, immunogenicity of first generation DNA vaccines in clinical trials was shown to be poor, and no DNA vaccines have yet been licensed for human use. In recent years significant progress has been made in the development of second generation DNA vaccines and DNA vaccine delivery methods. Here we review the key characteristics of DNA vaccines as compared to other vaccine platforms, and recent insights into the prerequisites for induction of immune responses by DNA vaccines will be discussed. We illustrate the development of second generation DNA vaccines with the description of DNA tattooing as a novel DNA delivery method. This technique has shown great promise both in a small animal model and in non-human primates and is currently under clinical evaluation.

Contents

K. Oosterhuis, J. H. van den Berg, T. N. Schumacher and J. B. A. G. Haanen (✉)
Division of Immunology, The Netherlands Cancer Institute, Plesmanlaan 121,
1066 CX Amsterdam, The Netherlands
e-mail: j.haanen@nki.nl

Current Topics in Microbiology and Immunology (2012) 351: 221–250
DOI: 10.1007/82_2010_117

Published Online: 24 November 2010

1 An Introduction on Two Decades of DNA Vaccination

It is now two decades ago since it was first demonstrated that injection of naked plasmid DNA into mouse muscle results in expression of the encoded protein (Wolff et al. 1990). Soon thereafter it was demonstrated that both cellular and humoral immune responses can be elicited against DNA vaccine-encoded proteins, when applied intradermally using a 'gene gun' (Tang et al. 1992) or upon intramuscular (IM) injection (Wang et al. 1993; Ulmer et al. 1993). Furthermore, these DNA vaccination-induced immune responses were shown to confer protection in various preclinical disease models, including models of viral, bacterial, and parasitic diseases and various tumor models [reviewed by Donnelly et al. (1997), Gurunathan et al. (2000)]. Based on these encouraging preclinical data and a number of perceived advantages of DNA-based vaccines (see below), a series of clinical trials was initiated during the late 1990s that evaluated the efficacy of DNA vaccines in the induction of immune responses against pathogen- (HIV, malaria, hepatitis B) and cancer-associated antigens (Donnelly et al. 2003; Liu and Ulmer 2005; Lu et al. 2008). While these trials provided overwhelming evidence for the overall safety of DNA vaccines (Donnelly et al. 2003; Liu and Ulmer 2005), immunogenicity of this first generation DNA vaccines was at best modest.

Following the observation of low immunogenicity of DNA vaccines in the early human trials, the field has taken two directions. (1) It has been argued that while DNA vaccines may not induce high-level immune responses as a single modality, these vaccines would nevertheless be valuable to provide low-level priming. Such low-level immune responses can then subsequently be amplified by administration of a virus-based vaccine (McConkey et al. 2003; Lu et al. 2008). Such DNA-prime viral vector-boost regimens can reduce the issue of vector-specific immune responses that are a common problem in viral vector-based vaccines. (2) As a second and more ambitious goal, a large effort has been made to develop (what we here will loosely call) "second generation DNA vaccines" that should be able to induce robust immune responses without a requirement for booster vaccination by virus-based vaccines. In these vaccines, optimization has either focused on (i) improvement of the expression vectors, (ii) improvement of the vaccine formulation, (iii) enhancement of the immunogenicity of the vaccine-encoded antigen, or (iv) the provision of molecular adjuvants in order to boost immunogenicity. A selected set of examples of such optimizations will be provided. Furthermore a large effort has been made to develop novel physical delivery methods that aim to increase DNA vaccine efficiency, of which intradermal (ID) DNA tattooing forms an example.

Is it plausible that DNA vaccines will become available for human use in the foreseeable future? The licensing of three different DNA vaccines in the field of veterinary medicine (against West Nile virus in horses, against infectious haematopoietic necrosis virus in salmon and for treatment of melanoma in dogs) (Redding and Weiner 2009), and a recent report showing DNA vaccination-mediated protection of human subjects against influenza challenge (Jones et al. 2009), both illustrate the therapeutic potential of DNA vaccines as single modalities. Owing to this, there is presently renewed optimism that DNA vaccines may within the next years be approved for applications in humans (Lu et al. 2008; Kutzler and Weiner 2008).

2 Advantages of DNA Vaccination Compared to Conventional Vaccine Platforms

DNA vaccines have a number of attractive properties that contribute to the strong interest in their development. Among these properties are the ease and speed of vaccine production, the ability to induce both cellular and humoral immunity and the favorable safety profile as compared to other gene-based vaccine platforms that are able to induce strong cellular immunity. These aspects are discussed in more detail below.

2.1 *Ease and Speed of Production*

Plasmid DNA is relatively easy to produce in small to large quantities in a generic way, with little if any need for adaptation of the production process for different individual plasmids. This is in sharp contrast to in particular protein-based vaccines, for which the production process needs to be specifically designed for each new vaccine. Moreover, since DNA vaccine-encoded proteins are synthesized by the host cells upon delivery, difficulties associated with recombinant protein-based vaccine production, such as protein folding and post translational modifications (e.g., glycosylation) are circumvented (Abdulhaqq and Weiner 2008; Jechlinger 2006). Another important advantage of DNA vaccines is the excellent stability of DNA as compared to other vaccine modalities, thereby likely circumventing the need for a ‘cold chain’ for vaccine distribution.

2.2 *Ability to Induce Cellular Immunity*

While direct experimental evidence is limited, there is some reason to assume that DNA vaccines are more suitable for the induction of $CD8^+$ (‘cytotoxic’) T cell immunity than recombinant peptide or protein vaccines (Gurunathan et al. 2000; Rice et al. 2008; Nagata et al. 2004; Liu 1997). Due to the fact that by definition, vaccination-induced antigen expression takes place by host cells, there is ample opportunity for the transfected cells to present peptide fragments of the antigen in MHC-class I molecules at the cell surface. In contrast, in many other vaccine formats such as protein, peptide, or inactivated pathogen-based vaccines, antigen is offered within the extracellular space. As extracellular antigens are mainly presented via MHC-class II molecules, induction of $CD4^+$ (‘helper’) T cell and antibody responses can be expected to predominate (Liu 1997). This discussion is somewhat complicated by the observation that induction of T cell responses upon DNA vaccination occurs at least in part by cross-priming rather than direct interaction between naive $CD8^+$ T cells and transfected skin or muscle cells (see below). However, as cross-priming is also more efficient for cell-associated than for soluble antigens (Li et al. 2001), the advantage of vaccine formats that induce intracellular antigen expression remains.

2.3 *Lack of Vector-Specific Immune Responses*

While the presumed advantage of DNA vaccines in the induction of $CD8^+$ T cell responses is shared with live attenuated viral vaccines or viral vector-based vaccines, the latter modalities bear greater risks in terms of production and safety (Draper and Heeney 2010; Robert-Guroff 2007). Furthermore, viral vector-based vaccines such as recombinant adenovirus or vaccinia virus can suffer from pre-existing immunity toward the vector or can induce vector-directed immunogenicity, thereby preventing repeated administration of these vectors (Limbach and Richie 2009). In the case of DNA vaccines the only immunogenic structure produced is the antigen itself, thereby allowing repeated administration.

2.4 Favorable Safety Profile

For the large-scale use of new vaccine formats in the general population their safety profile obviously needs to be well-established (Wilson and Marcuse 2001; O'Hagan and Rappuoli 2004). Because of their non-infectious and non-replicating nature, DNA vaccines are considered safer than live attenuated viruses or recombinant viral vectors. Furthermore, DNA vaccines have proven to be well tolerated and non-toxic in both preclinical- and clinical studies (Lu et al. 2008; Kutzler and Weiner 2008; Schalk et al. 2006; Parker et al. 2001; Parker et al. 1999). However, a few safety issues unique to plasmid DNA vaccines may potentially hamper their widespread use.

The main safety concern associated with DNA vaccines is the risk of genomic integration into the host genome. Genomic integration could potentially lead to activation of oncogenes, inactivation of tumor suppressor genes, or, when integrated into the chromosomal DNA of germ line cells, to vertical transmission. Several studies have examined the frequency of integration upon DNA vaccination. Collectively, these studies indicate that integration can occur but with a frequency that is manifold (around three orders of magnitude, depending on the system) lower than the spontaneous gene-inactivating mutation frequency of the genome. (Schalk et al. 2006; Ledwith et al. 2000; Wang et al. 2004). Vertical transmission due to genomic integration in germ line cells has been observed after direct injection of DNA into the gonads (Gao et al. 2009). However, genomic integration into germ line cells has not been observed after DNA vaccination at sites distant from the gonads (Parker et al. 1999; Manam et al. 2000). In conclusion, because of the low frequency of genomic integrations at the vaccination site and the absence of integrations in germ line cells, the risks associated with genomic integration upon DNA vaccination are at present considered negligible. An important exception to this is formed by DNA vaccines that encode proteins with known or suspected transforming activity (e.g., the HPV E6 and E7 oncoproteins). Proteins with transforming activity are attractive targets for vaccination as they can serve as unique tumor associated antigens. However, for such DNA vaccines, the survival advantage of cells that express the encoded proteins could conceivably lead to outgrowth of those (extremely) few cells in which genomic integration has occurred (Jeon et al. 1995). Because of this concern, the use of engineering strategies that abolish the transforming properties of the vaccine-encoded antigen should be considered essential.

A second potential safety concern in the use of DNA-based vaccines is the induction of anti-DNA antibodies and the subsequent development of autoimmune disease. This concern is increased by the fact that the bacterial derived DNA contains unmethylated phosphodiester-linked cytosine and guanine (CpG) motifs in the plasmid backbone that have an immunostimulatory activity via triggering of Toll-like receptor 9 (TLR9) (Krieg 2002), see also below. Anti-DNA antibodies are considered a hallmark of certain autoimmune diseases such as systemic lupus erythematosus (SLE), as most (but not all) patients manifest this characteristic of disease (Donnelly et al. 1997; Isenberg et al. 2007). Although induction of anti-DNA antibodies has been observed in some animal models after injection of plasmid DNA, thus far no evidence has been found that these antibodies are associated with the development of systemic autoimmune diseases, either in healthy animals or in animals that are at risk for the development of autoimmune disease [reviewed by Schalk et al. (2006), Smith and Klinman (2001)]. Furthermore, in human DNA vaccination trials no statistically significant increase in the presence of antinuclear antibodies and anti-DNA antibodies among vaccinees has been detected (Schalk et al. 2006).

In conclusion, all preclinical and clinical studies that have aimed to evaluate potential safety concerns of DNA vaccines have not provided any compelling evidence for substantial risks associated with the use of DNA vaccines. Because of this, we currently see no major obstacles for the application of DNA vaccines for therapeutic purposes, or for prophylaxis against high-risk disease. It is noted, however, that the potential toxicities of DNA vaccines would primarily concern long-term effects that may be difficult to address in the studies discussed above. Because of this, it would seem prudent to await the long-term outcome of clinical trials for high-risk indications before widespread application of DNA vaccination for low-risk disease is considered.

3 Mechanism of T cell Priming upon DNA Vaccination

At first glance, the general mechanism by which plasmid DNA vaccines induce immunity seems straightforward. Upon administration the plasmid DNA is taken up by host cells, leading to production of the antigen by these cells and to the release of 'danger' signals as dictated by the danger model. However, there is still substantial uncertainty about the antigen-presentation pathway that leads to the display of antigen-derived epitopes to naive T cells and also by which molecular mechanisms 'danger' is perceived upon DNA vaccination. Importantly, a better understanding of both of these factors is likely to result in more efficient DNA vaccine formats.

3.1 Direct- Versus Cross-priming

Through the use of bone marrow chimeras it has been demonstrated that the induction of cellular and humoral immune responses upon DNA vaccination is absolutely dependent on antigen presentation by bone marrow-derived professional antigen-presenting cells (APCs) (Iwasaki et al. 1997). On the other hand, for various routes of administration it has been demonstrated that antigen expression upon DNA vaccination primarily results in antigen expression in non-immune cells in peripheral tissues, such as myocytes in the muscle and keratinocytes in the skin (Dupuis et al. 2000; Porgador et al. 1998). An important question, therefore, is whether immune activation primarily occurs by the action of a small number of APCs that have become directly transfected, or whether antigen produced by the much larger number of non-immune cells serves as a source of antigen that is handed over to APCs that subsequently present the antigen (a process termed cross-presentation in the case of $CD8^{+}$ T cell activation). This issue is of more than academic interest as it has previously been demonstrated that the efficiency with which antigens are cross-presented can vary markedly depending on the context in which an epitope is provided (see also below) (Norbury et al. 2004; Wolkers et al. 2004).

Most DNA vaccination studies performed to address this question have used gene gun or IM needle injection as a delivery platform. From these studies there is clear evidence that both direct presentation of antigen by transfected APCs (Porgador et al. 1998; Condon et al. 1996; Chattergoon et al. 1998; Torres et al. 1997) and cross-presentation of antigen acquired from non-immune cells (Wolff et al. 1990; Cho et al. 2001; Ulmer et al. 1996) can occur in vivo after DNA vaccination. The design of most of these studies, however, does not allow a conclusion on the relative contribution of these two processes to $CD8^{+}$ T cell activation in vivo. An exception to this is formed by a study in which a DNA vaccine encoding the influenza A nucleoprotein (NP) under control of either the keratinocyte-specific K14 promoter or the APC-specific CD11b promoter was applied via gene gun (Cho et al. 2001). This study revealed that keratinocyte-directed transgene expression induced both higher cellular and humoral immune responses than APC-directed transgene expression, thus providing strong evidence for a dominant role for cross-presentation in $CD8^{+}$ T cell priming upon gene gun immunization. These data are in apparent contrast to a second study that—again using gene gun application—provided evidence for a dominant role for directly transfected APCs in $CD8^{+}$ T cell activation (Porgador et al. 1998). In this study, co-transfection, but not co-immunization of plasmids encoding co-stimulatory molecules was shown to restore the immunogenicity of an otherwise non-immunogenic nuclear protein (NP) variant. This observation seems most consistent with antigen presentation by directly transfected APCs, as cross-presentation would not be expected to result in cell surface expression of the vaccine-encoded costimulatory molecules on the APC. It is noted however, that the NP variant used in the latter study may form a poor substrate for cross-presentation, as the mutations within this antigen may prevent proper folding and thereby reduce antigen accumulation within the donor cell or by other means disrupt the transfer of antigen from the antigen-producing cells to specialized APCs (see below) (Iwasaki et al. 1997).

Taken together, to date no definitive answer exists regarding the exact mechanism of T cell priming upon DNA vaccination (Shedlock and Weiner 2000; Laddy and Weiner 2006), and it is plausible that the mechanism of immune induction will differ between different methods of immunization (Torres et al. 1997; Heath and Carbone 2001), between target tissues (e.g., skin vs. muscle) (Torres et al. 1997), and between different DNA vaccine designs.

3.2 Influencing Antigen Properties

Several strategies have been developed in which an antigen of interest is genetically fused to a 'carrier' protein. Carrier proteins that have been shown to (sometimes strongly) increase the immunogenicity of the fused antigen include tetanus toxin fragment C (TTFC), heat shock protein 70 (HSP 70), MHC-class II invariant chain (Ii), calreticulin (CRT), herpes simplex virus viral protein 22 (HSV VP 22) and *E. coli* β-glucuronidase (Table 1). The exact mechanism(s) by which these carrier proteins enhance the immunogenicity of the fused antigen remain largely unclear and may vary between different carrier molecules. However, based on our current understanding of DNA vaccines, two broad categories are likely to play dominant roles.

Provision of $CD4^+$ T cell help: There is abundant evidence that $CD8^+$ T cell responses induced by DNA vaccination are dependent on $CD4^+$ T cell help (Maecker et al. 1998). However, $CD4^+$ T cell responses are likely to be weak or lacking when using DNA vaccines that either encode self proteins or single $CD8^+$ T cell epitopes. In such cases, the provision of $CD4^+$ T cell help via carrier encoded helper epitopes is likely to be an important factor in the immune-enhancing effect of foreign carrier molecules, like TTFC and *E. coli* β-glucoronidase (Stevenson et al. 2004; Smahel et al. 2004).

Enhancement of antigen presentation: There is strong evidence that improvement of antigen stability enhances DNA vaccine immunogenicity. First, many of the above-mentioned fusions result in increased steady state antigen levels (Brulet et al. 2007; Smahel et al. 2004; Michel et al. 2002). Second, formal evidence for the notion that the stability of DNA vaccine-encoded antigens in the transfected cell contributes to vaccine immunogenicity has been provided using a set of engineered luciferase variants with a variable in vivo half-life (Bins et al. 2007). For this set of variants, immunogenicity was directly correlated to antigen stability. Also the observation that covalent linkage of an epitope toward a carrier protein, but not the simultaneous expression of the epitope and the carrier using a bicistronic vector, improves vaccine immunogenicity is consistent with the notion that carrier proteins can influence vaccine immunogenicity by increasing antigen half-life (Wolkers et al. 2002). At present, the most straightforward explanation for the observed effect of antigen stability on vaccine immunogenicity is that it would enhance cross-presentation, although a direct analysis of epitope density on APCs would be required to provide formal evidence for this model. Genetic fusion to carrier proteins may also influence antigen presentation through other mechanisms. For VP-22 it has been proposed that it enhances antigen spreading to neighboring cells (Michel et al. 2002). For HSP-70 it has been proposed that it increases uptake of the antigen by APCs via a HSP specific receptor (Wu 2007). Finally, some carrier molecules such as Ii (Brulet et al. 2007) and calreticulin (Cheng et al. 2001) alter the subcellular localization of an antigen and might thereby improve the immunogenicity of the DNA encoded antigen. This is in line with the finding that the sole addition of signals influencing subcellular localization

Table 1 Selection of methods to enhance DNA vaccine potency

Type of optimization	Method	Proposed mode of action[a]	Reference
Improvement of the vector	Gene optimization	Stabilization of RNA; more efficient translation of RNA	Liu et al. (2002), Lin et al. (2006)
	Addition of viral post-transcriptional regulatory elements	Increased cytoplasmic mRNA levels	Sun et al. (2009), Garg et al. (2004)
Improvement of vaccine formulation	Formulation of naked DNA into nano/micro particles	Increased cellular uptake of DNA	van den Berg et al. (2010a, b) Hedley et al. (1998), Klencke et al. (2002)
Improvement of antigen immunogenicity	TTFC fusion	Provision of CD4$^+$ help	Stevenson et al. (2004)
	HSP-70 fusion	Improved cross-presentation of antigen	Chen et al. (2000)
	Calreticulin fusion	Targeting of antigen for antigen processing and presentation	Cheng et al. (2001)
	Invariant chain fusion	Enhanced stability/changed subcellular localization	Brulet et al. (2007)
	E. coli β-glucoronidase fusion	Changed subcellular localization of antigen, provision of CD4$^+$ help	Smahel et al. (2004)
	HSV VP 22 fusion	Improved antigen spreading	Kim et al. (2004), Michel et al. (2002)
Enhancement of immune activation by addition of adjuvants	Co-delivery of pro-inflammatory cytokines (GM-CSF, IL-2, IL-12)	Recruitment, expansion and activation of APCs	Scheerlinck (2001), Barouch et al. (2004), Abdulhaqq and Weiner (2008)
	Co-delivery of chemokines (CCL-21, CCL27, CCL-28, CCL-5)	Attraction of immune cells to the site of vaccination	Kutzler et al. (2010), Yamano et al. (2006), Calarota and Weiner (2004)
	Co-delivery of co-stimulatory genes (CD80, CD86)	Improvement of co-stimulation	Calarota and Weiner (2004), Iwasaki et al. (1997)
	HMGB-1 co-delivery	Recruitment, expansion and activation of APCs	Muthumani et al. (2009)
	TLR agonists (imiquimod,CpG)	Activation of APCs	Thomsen et al. (2004), Schneeberger et al. (2004)

[a] For most of these methods, evidence that the increase in vaccine immunogenicity is indeed due to the proposed mechanism is at best circumstantial. Furthermore, only for selected strategies their added value has been confirmed in independent studies

(such as ER targeting signals) to DNA vaccine-encoded antigens can improve their immunogenicity (Michel et al. 2002; Boyle et al. 1997; Kim et al. 2006; Rice et al. 1999). Also in this case, enhanced immunogenicity may be due to increased cross-presentation, but again, formal evidence is lacking. Clearly, improved insight into the mechanisms by which different carrier influence vaccine immunogenicity will enable more rational DNA vaccine optimization and should be an important area of future research.

4 Origin of the "Danger Signal" in DNA Vaccines

Although the addition of various adjuvants (Table 1) can enhance their immunogenicity, DNA vaccines are also able to induce strong immune responses in animal models without the addition of adjuvants that provide inflammatory signals. As the induction of adaptive immune responses requires not only the presence of antigen, but also the presence of signals that induce APC activation (something often referred to as the danger model) (Heath and Carbone 2001; Matzinger 2002; Pulendran and Ahmed 2006), this implies that either DNA vaccines themselves or the DNA vaccination procedure provides elements that result in a sense of danger.

4.1 Danger in 'Naked' DNA

For many years it has been assumed that unmethylated CpG motifs were the primary source of danger in DNA vaccine preparations. Unmethylated CpG motifs form one of the so called 'pathogen-associated molecular patterns' (PAMP) that are recognized by pattern recognition receptors (PRR), in the case of CpG the TLR9. TLR9 is expressed in the endocytic pathway, providing endocytosing cells with the ability to detect CpG motifs within ingested material. Triggering of TLR9 initiates a cascade of signaling events that leads to NF-κB and activator protein 1 (AP-1) activation, and the subsequent induction of a pro-inflammatory response characterized by the release of cytokines and chemokines, e.g., type I interferons (IFNs), interleukin (IL)-6, IL-12 and tumor necrosis factor (TNF)-α (Tang and Pietersz 2009). In early work, the inclusion of additional CpG motifs within the plasmid backbone was shown to improve DNA vaccine efficiency after ID vaccination in a murine melanoma model (Schneeberger et al. 2004). As TLR9 is differentially expressed between mice (all dendritic cell subsets) and men (only plasmacytoid dendritic cells) (Iwasaki and Medzhitov 2004), it has been suggested that a reduced ability to initiate a CpG-dependent danger response could explain the poor track record of DNA vaccines in humans. However, several studies have shown that both the induction of cellular as well as humoral immune responses is unaffected in TLR9-deficient mice (Babiuk et al. 2004; Spies et al. 2003).

Assuming that TLR9 forms the sole receptor for CpG, these data suggest that danger in DNA vaccination must (also) be sensed by other means.

Recently, evidence has been provided indicating that double stranded DNA (dsDNA) in the B form (right-handed helical structure) functions as an intrinsic adjuvant in DNA vaccines [reviewed by Tang and Pietersz (2009), Coban et al. (2008)]. Two dsDNA sensors have been identified thus far, namely DAI (DNA-dependent activator of IFN-regulatory factors) and AIM 2 (absent in melanoma-2). Contrary to TLR9, these dsDNA sensors are expressed within the cytosol, providing transfected cells with the ability to detect incoming DNA. DAI-induced immune activation is mediated through the activation of IFN-regulatory factor 3 (IRF3) and NF-κB and results in the production of type I IFNs (Takaoka et al. 2007). AIM 2 has recently been described as the cytosolic DNA sensor that is responsible for activation of the inflammasome, thereby resulting in the production of active IL-1β, IL-18 and IL-33 (Schroder et al. 2009). However, as optimal DNA vaccine immunogenicity requires type I IFNs (Ishii et al. 2008) and AIM2 is not required for type I IFN production, it is considered to have a secondary role in the DNA-induced adjuvant response (Tang and Pietersz 2009). An important study by Ishii et al. has demonstrated a pivotal role for TANK-binding kinase 1 (TBK-1), a non-canonical IκB kinase, in mediating the adjuvant effect of DNA vaccines. In the presence of dsDNA, TBK-1 activates IRF3 and IRF7, leading to the production of type I IFNs. Notably, TBK-1 deficient mice were unable to generate antigen-specific humoral and cellular immune responses upon vaccination with a DNA vaccine delivered by IM injection followed by electroporation (Ishii et al. 2008). In contrast, DNA vaccine-induced immune responses were not affected by DAI deficiency and from this observation it was concluded that TBK-1 but not DAI is essential to the DNA vaccine mediated adjuvant response. Recently evidence was provided for the involvement of another signaling component named stimulator of IFN genes (STING) in TBK-1 mediated dsDNA sensing (Ishikawa et al. 2009). STING assembles with TBK-1 after dsDNA stimulation (Saitoh et al. 2009) and TBK-1 trafficking is blocked in the absence of STING (Ishikawa et al. 2009). Morever STING is essential for intracellular DNA-mediated type I IFN production and STING deficient mice showed an almost complete inhibition of both humoral and cellular immune responses upon DNA vaccination. Notably, despite the increasing knowledge on the signaling route that controls cellular responses upon cytosolic DNA encounter, the critical element recognizing dsDNA in this pathway still needs to be identified. Our current knowledge on intracellular DNA sensors is summarized in Table 2.

4.2 Administration-Induced Danger

While recognition of the introduced DNA forms one route through which DNA vaccination results in a danger response, the physical damage induced by the administration procedure itself is likely to be a second factor. Sensing of physical

Table 2 Cellular DNA sensing elements and their importance in DNA vaccination-induced immune responses

Pattern recognized	DNA recognizing element	Signaling components involved	Mediators released	Relevance for DNA vaccination	Reference
CpG motifs	TLR9	MyD88	IL-6, IL-12, TNF-α, type 1 IFN	Little/ moderate	Krieg (2002), Babiuk et al. (2004), Spies et al. (2003)
dsDNA	AIM2	Inflammasome	IL-1β, IL-18, IL-33	Little	Schroder et al. (2009)
	DAI	TBK-1/IRF3	Type 1 IFN	Little	Takaoka et al. (2007)
	Unknown	TBK-1/ STING/ IRF3	Type 1 IFN	High	Ishii et al. (2008), Ishikawa et al. (2009)

damage seems likely to be of particular importance for ID delivered DNA vaccines, as the skin has an important barrier function in host defense and is densely populated with immune cells. Therefore, administration procedure-induced local skin injury is likely to result in an inflammatory response that can boost vaccine immunogenicity (Nestle et al. 2009). This notion is supported by a recent report demonstrating that epidermal injury during poxvirus immunization is crucial for the generation of protective T cell mediated immunity (Liu et al. 2010). Furthermore, delivery-induced damage has also been suggested to play a role following electroporation-mediated IM delivery (Chiarella et al. 2008; Peng et al. 2007) and even following simple IM injection in mice, as the injection volume used (usually about 50 μl) exceeds the fluid capacity of the muscle resulting in local tissue damage (Rice et al. 2008; Dupuis et al. 2000).

What are the molecular mediators of the inflammatory response that is induced by physical damage? First, cell death that occurs during vaccination may lead to the release of intracellular molecules (with high-mobility group protein B1 (HMGB-1) as a prototype) that can be recognized by neighboring cells, or can result in the formation of uric acid crystals. This class of endogenous indicators of danger, sometimes referred to as alarmins [reviewed by Matzinger (2002), Pulendran (2004)] is likely to grow further in coming years, and it seems plausible that the role of individual alarmins as indicators of danger will depend on the strategy used for DNA vaccine delivery. In the case of ID DNA vaccine delivery, the vaccination-induced damage may also result in a danger response through an indirect mechanism. Specifically, the disruption of the skin barrier will create opportunities for pathogens/skin-resident microorganisms to locally invade the epidermal or dermal layer. As a consequence, immune activation can be expected to occur via the sensing of one of the many identified PAMPs, such as LPS, peptidoglycans, flagellin, etc. (Pulendran and Ahmed 2006).

While there is increasing interest in the role of adjuvant signals provided by the DNA itself, little attention has thus far been given to the contribution of the DNA vaccination procedure-induced damage to vaccine immunogenicity. Furthermore, our understanding of the contribution of different danger signals (be they either DNA- or damage-induced) to different types of adaptive immune responses (humoral, Th1, Th2, Th17, cytotoxic) is still limited.

5 Optimizing DNA Vaccination by Intradermal Tattooing

Given the poor performance of DNA vaccines (mostly IM delivered) in non-human primates and early clinical trials we set out to develop an improved strategy for DNA vaccine delivery. First, we postulated that a strategy in which DNA vaccines are introduced into the skin by a multitude of needle injections rather than a single injection would be superior. This method, in which DNA is delivered to the epidermal skin layer by many thousands of injections using a permanent make-up or tattoo device has been named DNA tattooing (Bins et al. 2005). Secondly, by measuring DNA vaccination-induced antigen expression in vivo using a firefly luciferase-encoding DNA, the kinetics of antigen expression could be followed. Notably, despite the fact that antigen expression after ID tattoo was approximately 10- to 100-fold lower and of much shorter duration than after IM injection, presentation of the vaccine-encoded epitope to $CD8^+$ T cells was shown to be markedly better. Based on the observation that DNA tattoo-induced antigen expression was restricted to approximately 96 h, a vaccination schedule was developed in which DNA is applied three times with 2 day intervals. Using this short-interval ID DNA delivery schedule, robust $CD8^+$ T cell responses that can readily be measured directly ex vivo could be induced within 2 weeks. In contrast, IM vaccination with this short-interval regimen did not lead to detectable T cell responses. Furthermore, in comparison to IM DNA vaccination, DNA tattooing was shown to mediate substantially better protection in mouse models of influenza A infection and HPV 16-associated cancer. A likely explanation for the higher immunogenicity of DNA tattoo vaccination is that skin is a better equipped for the induction of immune responses. In contrast to muscle, skin is rich in APCs (Zaba et al. 2009) and is the body's first line of defense against many pathogens (Nestle et al. 2009). Also, since the tattoo procedure inflicts thousands of skin perforations it is likely to result in the release of many more danger signals than simple IM or ID injection, thereby serving as a potent adjuvant (see below).

Interestingly, ID tattoo vaccination has also been applied to other vaccine modalities. For peptide-based vaccines it was shown that ID tattooing was more efficient than a subcutaneous (SC) injection (Pokorna et al. 2009). Also adenoviral vectors have been administered via ID tattoo in a side-by-side comparison with SC injection. In contrast to the results obtained with DNA vaccines, delivery of adenovirus via ID tattoo immunization did not provide any obvious advantage over delivery via ID injection (Potthoff et al. 2009). A possible explanation for this lack of superiority of ID tattoo vaccination is that the uptake of the adenovirus into host cells is much more efficient obviating the need for a more sophisticated delivery procedure and/or that viral particles themselves serve as a strong adjuvant, thereby making the tattoo procedure redundant.

6 Mechanism of Immune Induction upon DNA Tattooing

6.1 Antigen Expression and Priming

How does ID DNA tattooing induce $CD8^+$ T cell responses? Upon ID DNA tattoo vaccination, antigen expression is largely confined to cells within the epidermal layer, as revealed by beta-Gal staining (Bins et al. 2005). Furthermore, by flow cytometric analysis of single cell suspensions of tattooed ex vivo human skin (see below for more details on this model) it was shown that the vast majority of transfected cells consists of keratinocytes. Sporadic transfection of Langerhans cells (LCs) in the epidermis could also be observed (approximately 1% of transfected cells, more or less proportional to their frequency in human skin cell preparations) (van den Berg et al. 2009). Notably, the fact that only few antigen-expressing LCs could be recovered from human skin could not be explained by rapid migration of these cells after DNA administration. Does the fact that antigen expression upon DNA tattoo is largely restricted to keratinocytes indicate a dominant role for this cell type in the induction of immune responses? When vaccination-induced antigen expression is restricted to keratinocytes by the use of the K14 promoter, $CD8^+$ T cell responses could still be induced by this strategy for DNA vaccination in a murine model (Bins et al. 2007). As there is no evidence for migration of keratinocytes to the skin-draining lymph nodes, nor for na T cell priming at the site of vaccination, these data strongly suggest that the induction of a vaccine-specific $CD8^+$ T cell response upon DNA tattooing is at least partially due to cross-priming. A schematic representation of the different possibilities that lead to $CD8^+$ T cell priming upon DNA tattooing is provided in Fig. 1.

6.2 Provision of Danger Signals

As discussed above, recognition of danger signals upon DNA vaccination may either involve the direct recognition of the introduced DNA, or the detection of physical damage caused by DNA introduction. Thus far, only the role of TLR9 in sensing unmethylated CpG motifs upon DNA tattoo has been evaluated. Consistent with data from studies that have evaluated the role of TLR9 in other DNA vaccination modalities, the magnitude of $CD8^+$ T cell responses induced by DNA tattoo in wild type and in $TLR9^{-/-}$ mice were identical, demonstrating that—at least in mice—TLR9 mediated signaling is not essential for the induction of immune responses by DNA tattoo vaccination (Bins et al. 2005). Evidence for or against a role for different cytosolic dsDNA sensing systems in DNA tattoo vaccination-induced immunity is at present lacking. However, as this DNA vaccination strategy relies on the generation of thousands of skin perforations, a contribution of vaccination-induced skin damage to the immunogenicity of DNA tattooing, therefore, seems plausible. Support for the notion that inflammatory signals inflicted by tissue damage contribute to the immunogenicity of DNA tattoo

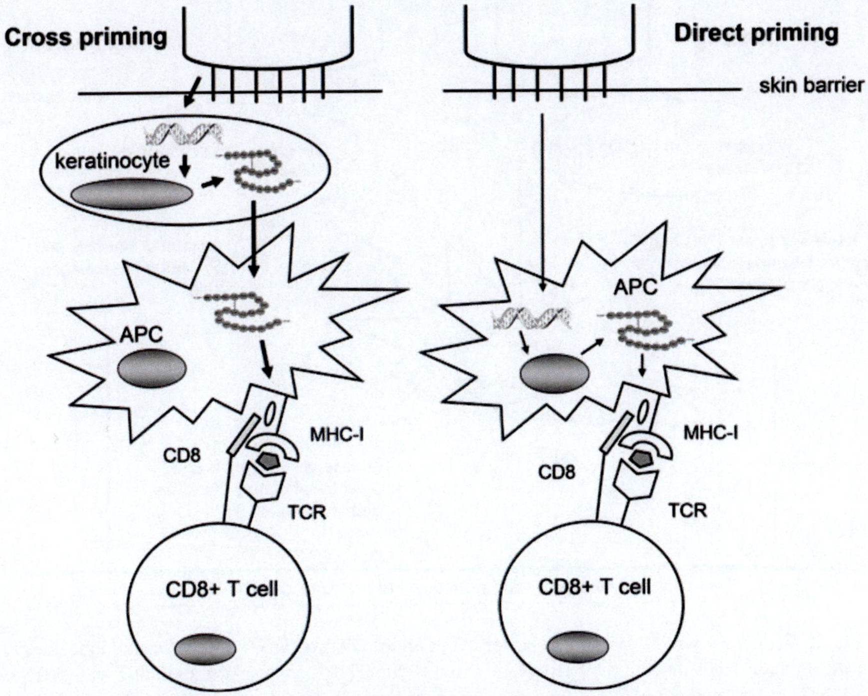

Fig. 1 Possible routes for the priming of CD8+ cytotoxic T cells upon ID DNA tattoo vaccination. Upon DNA tattooing mainly keratinocytes are transfected and produce antigen that is acquired by professional APCs, leading to cross-presentation to CD8+ cytotoxic T cells. As an alternative, APCs can become directly transfected, leading to direct priming of CD8+cytotoxic T cells. Based on available evidence, cross-presentation is considered the predominant route (see text)

is provided by a study in which we measured serum IL-6 levels upon tattoo application of either DNA or water-for-injections (WFI). Notably, systemic IL-6 levels were increased to the same extent in both groups of mice and exceeded those seen upon intraperitoneal delivery of 100 IU of LPS [a known inducer of IL-6 (Harden et al. 2006)]. These data suggest that administration-induced danger signals form a major factor in the immunogenicity of DNA tattoo (van den Berg et al. 2010c). A schematic representation of the different routes by which danger can be sensed upon DNA tattooing is provided in Fig. 2.

7 DNA Tattoo Versus Other DNA Delivery Techniques

To date, a large number of different delivery methods for DNA vaccines have been developed. In the following section a selection of these methods is discussed and their pros and cons relative to DNA tattooing are evaluated.

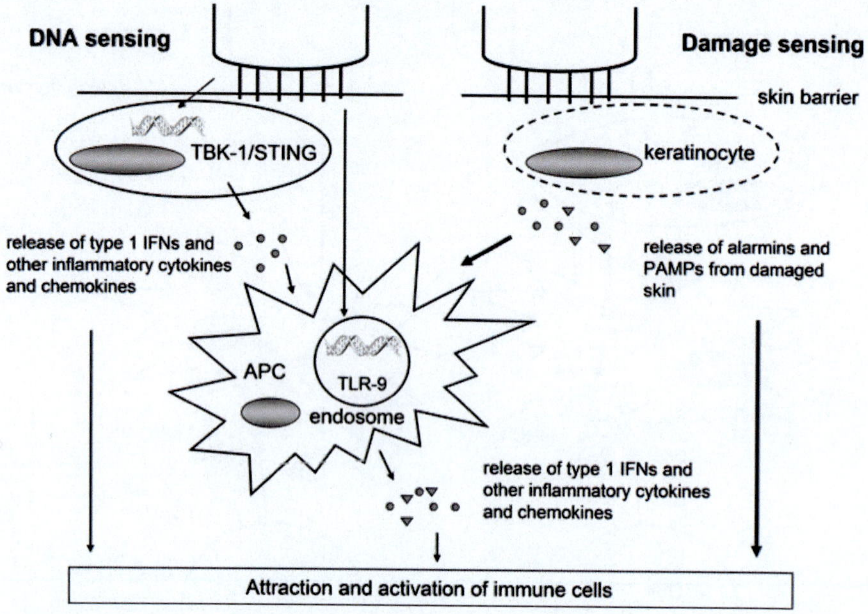

Fig. 2 Routes by which danger can be sensed upon intradermal DNA tattoo vaccination. Danger can be sensed via detection of dsDNA by cytosolic DNA sensors and signaling via TBK-1/STING, or via detection of CpG motifs by endosomal TLR9 (although the latter route is not critical). On the other hand, the tattoo procedure can induce damage to the skin leading to the release of PAMPs and alarmins. The thus released mediators can activate skin-resident APCs and attract/activate other immune cells. The fact that tattooing without any DNA already results in strong immune activation as measured by serum IL-6 levels (see text) suggests that damage-induced danger signals may play a dominant role

7.1 Intramuscular Injection

IM injection is one of the first routes of administration used for the delivery of naked plasmid DNA (Wolff et al. 1990) and the ease and simplicity of the method are particularly attractive for large-scale use. Although the method has proven effective in small animal models, the results obtained in studies in non-human primates and clinical trials have been disappointing even when doses up to 5 mg plasmid were used (Lu et al. 2008; Dean et al. 2003; Johnston et al. 2002). This translational block has been referred to as the "simian barrier" (Johnston et al. 2002) and is possibly explained by the impossibility to scale-up the injection volume used in mice (50 μl) to non-human primates and humans. Based on the difference in body weight (20 g vs. 80 kg) an injection volume of about 200 ml would be needed for a linear scale-up. Inability to perform such scale-up may be a particularly important factor as it has been suggested that the tissue damage inflicted by injection of a large volume of DNA relative to the volume of the injection site contributes to the immunogenicity of IM DNA vaccination in mice (Rice et al. 2008; Dupuis et al. 2000).

As described above we have performed an extensive comparison of the efficiency of ID tattoo vaccination and classical IM DNA vaccination in murine models. These data demonstrated that DNA tattoo outperformed IM DNA vaccination both with respect to the speed of $CD8^+$ T cell induction and with respect to the magnitude of this immune response. The superiority of DNA tattoo in mice has since then been confirmed in a study by Pokorna et al., in which previously described strategies to enhance the potency of IM DNA vaccination (cardiotoxin pretreatment or GM-CSF DNA co-delivery) were also included. In this study, ID DNA tattooing elicited significantly higher L1 specific humoral and cellular immune responses as compared to all IM conditions evaluated, even if the number of IM injections exceeded the number of tattoo administrations (Pokorna et al. 2008).

Having demonstrated the superiority of DNA tattoo in small animal models we set out to determine if the translational block described for IM delivery would also apply to DNA tattoo. To this end we performed a study in rhesus macaques, in which we delivered an HIV clade C DNA vaccine via ID DNA tattooing and compared the results with a prior study using exactly the same vaccine and vaccine dose but delivered by IM injection. This study demonstrated a 10- to 100-fold increase in the magnitude of vaccine-specific T cell responses in peripheral blood from rhesus macaques vaccinated by DNA tattoo, as compared to T cell responses in animals immunized via the IM route. Furthermore an increase in the fraction of animals responding to the immunogens was also observed. In conclusion, DNA tattoo outperforms IM DNA vaccination in both small and large animal models, warranting its further testing in humans (Verstrepen et al. 2008).

7.2 Particle-Mediated Epidermal Delivery

Particle-mediated epidermal delivery (PMED) comprises the bombardment of the skin with gold particles coated with DNA and is often referred to as 'gene gun' vaccination. Gene gun-mediated gene transfer is the first method that was successfully used for DNA vaccination in murine models (Tang et al. 1992). The method, which was originally developed for the transfection of cells in vitro, has been extensively studied in human subjects. Within these studies, both cellular and humoral vaccine-specific responses have been demonstrated and—even though a side-by-side comparison has to our knowledge not been performed in clinical trials—the method is generally considered more efficient than IM injection (Dean et al. 2003; Dean et al. 2005). A comparison of the efficiency of gene gun and ID tattoo vaccination (using the same short-interval administration schedule) has demonstrated that the two methods are equipotent in $CD8^+$ T cell activation in a murine model.

The doses of DNA required to induce immune responses by gene gun administration are surprisingly low, about 1 μg/dose, being approximately 100–1,000 fold lower than that used for IM injection, and this holds true for both murine and larger animal models (Dean et al. 2003; Dean et al. 2005). Moreover, also in human clinical trials, immune responses have been detected with doses below 10 μg (Dean et al. 2005). A possible explanation for this high efficiency is that gene gun is believed to directly deliver the DNA into the intracellular environment, in contrast to any other DNA delivery method (Dean et al. 2003). However, as the capacity of the current delivery devices is also low (1–2 μg of DNA per 'shot') the scaling of gun vaccination from mice to human application may still form an issue (Jechlinger 2006; Dean et al. 2005). Specifically, taking into account the difference in body surface (0.0075 vs. 1.85 m^2), approximately 250 vaccinations would be required to achieve the same dose per body surface. A second drawback is that the costs per immunization may be substantial (in particular when such scaling is performed), because of the need for formulating the DNA onto gold particles (Jechlinger 2006).

7.3 Electroporation-Mediated Gene Transfer

Electroporation (EP) is successfully used as a strategy for the transfection of cells in vitro (Bodles-Brakhop et al. 2009). EP uses short electrical pulses to destabilize cell membranes. While the precise mechanism is unclear, EP is thought to promote cellular uptake of DNA through permeabilizing cell membranes and driving DNA entry via an electrophoretic process (Mir 2008). As it is believed that the poor performance of DNA vaccines in larger animals and humans can at least in part be explained by the low transfection efficiency upon needle mediated delivery of naked DNA (Babiuk et al. 2002; Nishikawa and Huang 2001), EP has been extensively evaluated for its potential to increase in vivo transfection. Several devices for EP-assisted DNA vaccination have been developed and EP has been shown to result in an increase in antigen expression and vaccine immunogenicity in murine models when combined with either IM (Dupuis et al. 2000; Widera et al. 2000) or ID DNA injection (Roos et al. 2006; Roos et al. 2009). In a direct comparison, the combination of IM injection and EP was shown to be more efficient than gene gun-mediated DNA administration (Best et al. 2009). EP mediated DNA vaccination has also been shown to increase antigen expression levels and vaccine immunogenicity in large animals (Babiuk et al. 2002; Hirao et al. 2008). Based on these highly promising preclinical data EP is now also being evaluated in clinical trials [reviewed by Bodles-Brakhop et al. (2009)].

A slight complication of this technique is that there are many variables such as pulse duration, pulse strength and the number of pulses that need to be optimized. It has been demonstrated that EP settings that result in high expression levels are not necessarily those that induce the highest immune responses (Roos et al. 2006).

Furthermore, the optimal settings may also differ depending on the array used and the targeted tissue (Mir 2008; Rabussay 2008).

A safety concern that has been associated with the improved transfection efficiency upon EP is a possible increase of the number of chromosomal integrations (Schalk et al. 2006; Smith and Klinman 2001). In one study by Wang et al. (2004), it was observed that EP markedly increased the amount of plasmid associated with high molecular weight (i.e., genomic) DNA. Furthermore, using a newly developed PCR method, four independent integration events were detected in electroporated muscle, providing direct proof for genomic integration upon DNA vaccination. However, other studies have shown no increase in the amount of plasmid DNA associated with high-molecular-weight DNA after EP in combination with IM delivery (Luckay et al. 2007). More importantly, it seems plausible that the risk of genomic integration will scale proportionally with any improvement in DNA vaccine delivery strategies and this risk is, therefore, unlikely to be unique to EP.

7.4 Jet Injection

Jet injection is a needle-free technique in which fluid is injected under high pressure and this technique is suitable for both IM and ID administration. Jet injectors have successfully been used for immunizing humans with live attenuated vaccines against measles and smallpox, as well as inactivated life vaccines against cholera, hepatitis B, influenza and polio (Mitragotri 2005). Advantages of the method are that it avoids the use of sharps and its compatibility with existing vaccine formulations that have been developed for needle-based administration. Disadvantages of the method include higher levels of pain and more frequent side reactions than observed with needle-based vaccine delivery (Mitragotri 2005). In a report by Trimble et al., $CD8^+$ T cell responses and antitumor effects generated by a DNA vaccine administered ID via gene gun or Biojector® (a jet injector suitable for ID delivery) and IM via needle injection were directly compared in a murine model (Trimble et al. 2003). In this comparison, gene gun vaccination formed the most potent method of immunization. Furthermore, in non-human primates IM jet injection with the Biojector® or Mini-Ject™ was not more efficient than simple IM injection with respect to the induction of both cellular and humoral immune responses (Rao et al. 2006). Based on these data it can be concluded that jet injection does not significantly improve the immunogenicity of IM administered DNA vaccines.

7.5 Microneedle-Assisted Gene Transfer

Microneedles are small needles with a size between 200 and 400 μm that have been designed to deliver drugs to the epidermal layer of the skin, without stimulating the pain receptors that populate the underlying dermis (Birchall et al. 2005). Microneedles have been shown to be useful for the delivery of protein-based vaccines in clinical trials as delivery of the seasonal influenza vaccine via microneedles has been shown to be more effective than simple IM delivery (Arnou et al. 2009; Van Damme et al. 2009). A recent study by Zhou et al. demonstrated that microneedle-based delivery of a hepatitis B virus DNA vaccine in mice resulted in higher levels of humoral and cellular immune responses when compared to IM injection with the same DNA construct (Zhou et al. 2010). However, protein expression levels upon DNA application with microneedles are also reported to be unpredictable and difficult to control, and because of this, further optimization is likely to be required for the future development of this strategy into a robust DNA vaccination platform (Birchall et al. 2005).

7.6 Concluding Remarks on the Different DNA Vaccine Delivery Methods

Compared to the above-mentioned administration techniques (summarized in Table 3), DNA tattoo stands out by its simplicity. There is no need for formulation of the DNA as is the case for PMED. As compared to jet injection, EP and PMED, the required equipment is relatively simple and cheap. More importantly, linear scale-up from mice to man can simply be done by vaccination of larger skin areas. This notion is supported by the promising results of DNA tattoo in non-human primates (Verstrepen et al. 2008). Furthermore, as the tattoo procedure causes substantial damage to the skin requirement for the inclusion of adjuvants may not be needed, making clinical translation relatively straightforward. By the same token, it is noted, however, that the invasiveness of the method and also the requirement for repeated administration are likely to limit the current DNA tattoo strategy to high-risk diseases.

8 Clinical Translation of Intradermal DNA Tattooing

8.1 Ex Vivo Human Skin Model

On the basis of the promising preclinical data both in mice and in non-human primates an effort has been made to translate DNA tattoo vaccination into clinical application. However, before initiation of studies in humans it was important to determine the optimal settings for DNA tattoo in human skin, in particular because the physiology of human skin has obvious differences compared to that of furred murine and non-human primate skin (Godin and Touitou 2007). To address this issue we have analyzed the parameters that result in optimal expression of

Table 3 Advantages and limitations of different DNA delivery methods

Gene transfer method	Advantages	Limitations	Ref.
IM injection	Ease of the method, low costs of equipment	Poor track record in larger animals and human subjects	Wolff et al. (1990), Johnston et al. (2002), Verstrepen et al. (2008), McCluskie et al. (1999)
PMED ('gene gun')	High potency in relation to dose, extensive preclinical and clinical experience	Complex gold particle-based formulation/ high cost of the equipment, dose limitation to microgram range	Jechlinger (2006), Dean et al. (2005), Mitragotri (2005)
Electroporation	Extensive preclinical and clinical experience, can be combined with other delivery methods	High cost of the equipment	Wang et al. (2004), Bodles-Brakhop et al. (2009)
Jet injection	Needle-free method, ability to work with existing formulations, and success with many forms of vaccines	High cost of the device, higher levels of pain than with needles No evidence for superior performance relative to IM DNA vaccination	Mitragotri (2005), Ren et al. (2002)
Microneedle-based application	Favorable patient acceptability, possibility for self administration	Limited experience in DNA vaccination, low protein expression levels	Birchall et al. (2005)
DNA tattoo	Linear scale-up from mice to men possible, relatively cheap/ portable instrument	Invasiveness of the method may limit patient acceptability	Bins et al. (2005), Verstrepen et al. (2008)

vaccine-encoded antigens applied to human skin by DNA tattoo (van den Berg et al. 2009). For this purpose, we have developed an ex vivo human skin, in which DNA vaccines encoding reporter proteins are applied via ID tattoo. These studies revealed that gene expression upon ID DNA tattoo of human skin is almost exclusively restricted to the epidermal layer. Furthermore, consistent with the data obtained in mice, the vast majority of transfected cells consisted of keratinocytes. In order to optimize variables that we considered likely to influence the efficiency of DNA vaccination we have tattooed a total of 428 skin areas with luciferase-encoding DNA, thereby examining the effect of variations in (1) DNA concentration, (2) the duration of tattooing, (3) needle depth and (4) the type of tattoo machine. From these experiments, analyzed in a linear mixed effects model, it was concluded that DNA concentration is the most important factor influencing antigen expression in human skin. Furthermore, it was shown that also tattoo time and tattoo depth had significant effects on antigen expression. These data have been instrumental for the design of the first clinical trial of DNA tattoo and we speculate that this in vitro model will also be of value for the preclinical optimization of other DNA vaccine delivery strategies.

8.2 *Ongoing and Planned Clinical Trials*

Currently a first phase I clinical trial is ongoing to evaluate the safety and tolerability of ID DNA tattoo for the treatment of HLA-A2 positive advanced stage melanoma patients. Melanoma forms an interesting target for therapeutic vaccination as there is evidence to suggest that cellular immune responses contribute to the spontaneous regressions that are sporadically observed (van Oijen et al. 2004). Furthermore, a large number of melanoma-associated antigens (such as MART-1, tyrosinase, and gp100) have been identified and a substantial number of cytotoxic T cell epitopes from these antigens have been mapped. The DNA vaccine that is being used within this first trial encodes a modified (affinity-enhanced) MART-1 epitope fused to tetanus toxin fragment C. The plasmid DNA for this trial was manufactured in our in-house GMP production facility (Quaak et al. 2008), illustrating that clinical translation of DNA vaccines is relatively straightforward as compared to most other vaccine formats. Thus far, the tattoo procedure is well tolerated and no obvious toxicity has been observed. MART-1-specific T cell immunity will be assayed in peripheral blood samples and on skin biopsies from the vaccination site, using both MHC-tetramer staining and IFN-γ ELISPOT. Furthermore, serum antitetanus toxin antibody titers will be measured in order to monitor the induction of humoral immune responses by the vaccine.

In the near future we will also initiate a phase I clinical trial to evaluate DNA tattoo for the treatment of HPV-16 positive penile- and cervical cancer. HPV-induced malignancies form an excellent target for immunotherapy as the transformed cells express viral proteins, thereby enabling recognition of malignant cells without the danger of targeting healthy cells (Frazer 2004). For this trial we have developed two DNA vaccines directed against the HPV 16 E6 and E7 oncogenes and clinical grade production of these plasmids is currently ongoing.

9 Opinion on Usefulness of Intradermal DNA Vaccination, Large-Scale Use of DNA Tattoo, and Future Perspectives

As mentioned above, disadvantages of DNA tattoo are the invasiveness of the method, the fact that the tattoo procedure is more time-consuming than simple injection and that multiple administrations are required in order to induce high-level immune responses. Owing to this we consider the method currently well suitable for the development of therapeutic vaccines for high-risk diseases, but not for (prophylactic) mass vaccination. However, when tattoo time can be shortened and/or the number of administrations can be reduced, for example, by improving transfection efficiency and construct immunogenicity, the method may become more suitable for large-scale application. One of the strategies to further improve the efficiency of DNA tattoo vaccination, which is currently under evaluation, is briefly discussed below.

Thus far, most of our studies have focused on the use of naked DNA. However, from studies in the ex vivo human skin model, it has been calculated that the transfection efficiency of naked DNA upon tattooing is extremely low: estimated between 1 out of 1×10^{-6} to 1×10^{-9} copies applied (van den Berg et al. 2009). Therefore, there is ample room for improving the transfection efficiency of DNA vaccines applied by DNA tattoo. In a recent study we have evaluated the use of cationic nanoparticles as synthetic delivery vehicles for DNA vaccines (van den Berg et al. 2010a). Interestingly, these studies revealed that the positive charge of such particles that dramatically enhances transfection efficiency in cell culture systems essentially prevents transfection in human skin. Only when the cationic surface charge of these particles was shielded with polyethylene glycol (PEG), transfection in human skin was apparent. Delivery of a model vaccine using these PEGylated nanoparticles resulted in an increase in transfection efficiency as compared to naked DNA both in ex vivo human skin and in mice (in the latter about two- to fivefold depending on the type of nanoparticle). Unfortunately, for this first variant DNA formulation that we have analyzed, no significant increase in immunogenicity was observed in spite of these higher expression levels. These data do, however, illustrate the value of the combined use of these two models for preclinical DNA vaccine delivery optimization. First, the human skin model allows one to rapidly identify vaccine formulations that yield substantial antigen expression (going from the reasonable assumption that in the absence of substantial antigen expression immunogenicity will be poor). Second, those selected formulations that yield substantial antigen expression in human skin can subsequently be analyzed for immunogenicity within the murine model. As an example, skin electroporation-mediated DNA delivery has shown great promise in both small and large animal models (Roos et al. 2009), and the combined use of DNA tattoo and electroporation may well be evaluated by combining these two models.

10 Conclusion

DNA tattoo has progressed from the first preclinical evaluation to clinical testing in a period of approximately 5 years, and based on its preclinical track record ID DNA tattoo can be considered a promising strategy for DNA vaccination. At present the two main priorities will be to evaluate the current strategy for DNA tattoo in clinical trials, while at the same time developing optimized strategies in preclinical models that can be evaluated in follow-up trials.

Acknowledgments This study was in part supported by the Netherlands organization for health research and development (ZonMw) grant 432-00-001.

References

Abdulhaqq SA, Weiner DB (2008) DNA vaccines: developing new strategies to enhance immune responses. Immunol Res 42:219–232

Arnou R, Icardi G, De Decker M, Ambrozaitis A, Kazek MP, Weber F, Van Damme P (2009) Intradermal influenza vaccine for older adults: a randomized controlled multicenter phase III study. Vaccine 27:7304–7312

Babiuk S, Baca-Estrada ME, Foldvari M, Storms M, Rabussay D, Widera G, Babiuk LA (2002) Electroporation improves the efficacy of DNA vaccines in large animals. Vaccine 20: 3399–3408

Babiuk S, Mookherjee N, Pontarollo R, Griebel P, van Drunen Littel-van den Hurk S, Hecker R, Babiuk L (2004) $TLR9^{-/-}$ and $TLR9^{+/+}$ mice display similar immune responses to a DNA vaccine. Immunology 113:114–120

Barouch DH, Letvin NL, Seder RA (2004) The role of cytokine DNAs as vaccine adjuvants for optimizing cellular immune responses. Immunol Rev 202:266–274

Best SR, Peng S, Juang CM, Hung CF, Hannaman D, Saunders JR, Wu TC, Pai SI (2009) Administration of HPV DNA vaccine via electroporation elicits the strongest $CD8^+$ T cell immune responses compared to intramuscular injection and intradermal gene gun delivery. Vaccine 27:5450–5459

Bins AD, Jorritsma A, Wolkers MC, Hung CF, Wu TC, Schumacher TN, Haanen JB (2005) A rapid and potent DNA vaccination strategy defined by in vivo monitoring of antigen expression. Nat Med 11:899–904

Bins AD, Wolkers MC, van den Boom MD, Haanen JB, Schumacher TN (2007) In vivo antigen stability affects DNA vaccine immunogenicity. J Immunol 179:2126–2133

Birchall J, Coulman S, Pearton M, Allender C, Brain K, Anstey A, Gateley C, Wilke N, Morrissey A (2005) Cutaneous DNA delivery and gene expression in ex vivo human skin explants via wet-etch micro-fabricated micro-needles. J Drug Target 13:415–421

Bodles-Brakhop AM, Heller R, Draghia-Akli R (2009) Electroporation for the delivery of DNA-based vaccines and immunotherapeutics: current clinical developments. Mol Ther 17:585–592

Boyle JS, Koniaras C, Lew AM (1997) Influence of cellular location of expressed antigen on the efficacy of DNA vaccination: cytotoxic T lymphocyte and antibody responses are suboptimal when antigen is cytoplasmic after intramuscular DNA immunization. Int Immunol 9: 1897–1906

Brulet JM, Maudoux F, Thomas S, Thielemans K, Burny A, Leo O, Bex F, Hallez S (2007) DNA vaccine encoding endosome-targeted human papillomavirus type 16 E7 protein generates $CD4^+$ T cell-dependent protection. Eur J Immunol 37:376–384

Calarota SA, Weiner DB (2004) Enhancement of human immunodeficiency virus type 1-DNA vaccine potency through incorporation of T-helper 1 molecular adjuvants. Immunol Rev 199:84–99

Chattergoon MA, Robinson TM, Boyer JD, Weiner DB (1998) Specific immune induction following DNA-based immunization through in vivo transfection and activation of macrophages/antigen-presenting cells. J Immunol 160:5707–5718

Chen CH, Wang TL, Hung CF, Yang Y, Young RA, Pardoll DM, Wu TC (2000) Enhancement of DNA vaccine potency by linkage of antigen gene to an HSP70 gene. Cancer Res 60: 1035–1042

Cheng WF, Hung CF, Chai CY, Hsu KF, He L, Ling M, Wu TC (2001) Tumor-specific immunity and antiangiogenesis generated by a DNA vaccine encoding calreticulin linked to a tumor antigen. J Clin Invest 108:669–678

Chiarella P, Massi E, De Robertis M, Sibilio A, Parrella P, Fazio VM, Signori E (2008) Electroporation of skeletal muscle induces danger signal release and antigen-presenting cell recruitment independently of DNA vaccine administration. Expert Opin Biol Ther 8: 1645–1657

Cho JH, Youn JW, Sung YC (2001) Cross-priming as a predominant mechanism for inducing CD8(+) T cell responses in gene gun DNA immunization. J Immunol 167:5549–5557

Coban C, Koyama S, Takeshita F, Akira S, Ishii KJ (2008) Molecular and cellular mechanisms of DNA vaccines. Hum Vaccin 4:453–456

Condon C, Watkins SC, Celluzzi CM, Thompson K, Falo LD, Jr (1996) DNA-based immunization by in vivo transfection of dendritic cells. Nat Med 2:1122–1128

Dean HJ, Fuller D, Osorio JE (2003) Powder and particle-mediated approaches for delivery of DNA and protein vaccines into the epidermis. Comp Immunol Microbiol Infect Dis 26: 373–388

Dean HJ, Haynes J, Schmaljohn C (2005) The role of particle-mediated DNA vaccines in biodefense preparedness. Adv Drug Deliv Rev 57:1315–1342

Donnelly JJ, Ulmer JB, Shiver JW, Liu MA (1997) DNA vaccines. Annu Rev Immunol 15: 617–648

Donnelly J, Berry K, Ulmer JB (2003) Technical and regulatory hurdles for DNA vaccines. Int J Parasitol 33:457–467

Draper SJ, Heeney JL (2010) Viruses as vaccine vectors for infectious diseases and cancer. Nat Rev Microbiol 8:62–73

Dupuis M, Denis-Mize K, Woo C, Goldbeck C, Selby MJ, Chen M, Otten GR, Ulmer JB, Donnelly JJ, Ott G, McDonald DM (2000) Distribution of DNA vaccines determines their immunogenicity after intramuscular injection in mice. J Immunol 165:2850–2858

Frazer IH (2004) Prevention of cervical cancer through papillomavirus vaccination. Nat Rev Immunol 4:46–54

Gao YS, Huang TH, Wang D, Xie QD, Kang XJ (2009) In vivo study on vertical transmission of the HIV-1 gag gene via mouse oocytes. Curr HIV Res 7:562–568

Garg S, Oran AE, Hon H, Jacob J (2004) The hybrid cytomegalovirus enhancer/chicken beta-actin promoter along with woodchuck hepatitis virus posttranscriptional regulatory element enhances the protective efficacy of DNA vaccines. J Immunol 173:550–558

Godin B, Touitou E (2007) Transdermal skin delivery: predictions for humans from in vivo, ex vivo and animal models. Adv Drug Deliv Rev 59:1152–1161

Gurunathan S, Klinman DM, Seder RA (2000) DNA vaccines: immunology, application, and optimization. Annu Rev Immunol 18:927–974

Harden LM, du Plessis I, Poole S, Laburn HP (2006) Interleukin-6 and leptin mediate lipopolysaccharide-induced fever and sickness behavior. Physiol Behav 89:146–155

Heath WR, Carbone FR (2001) Cross-presentation, dendritic cells, tolerance and immunity. Annu Rev Immunol 19:47–64

Hedley ML, Curley J, Urban R (1998) Microspheres containing plasmid-encoded antigens elicit cytotoxic T-cell responses. Nat Med 4:365–368

Hirao LA, Wu L, Khan AS, Satishchandran A, Draghia-Akli R, Weiner DB (2008) Intradermal/subcutaneous immunization by electroporation improves plasmid vaccine delivery and potency in pigs and rhesus macaques. Vaccine 26:440–448

Isenberg DA, Manson JJ, Ehrenstein MR, Rahman A (2007) Fifty years of anti-ds DNA antibodies: are we approaching journey's end? Rheumatology (Oxford) 46:1052–1056

Ishii KJ, Kawagoe T, Koyama S, Matsui K, Kumar H, Kawai T, Uematsu S, Takeuchi O, Takeshita F, Coban C, Akira S (2008) TANK-binding kinase-1 delineates innate and adaptive immune responses to DNA vaccines. Nature 451:725–729

Ishikawa H, Ma Z, Barber GN (2009) STING regulates intracellular DNA-mediated, type I interferon-dependent innate immunity. Nature 461:788–792

Iwasaki A, Medzhitov R (2004) Toll-like receptor control of the adaptive immune responses. Nat Immunol 5:987–995

Iwasaki A, Stiernholm BJ, Chan AK, Berinstein NL, Barber BH (1997) Enhanced CTL responses mediated by plasmid DNA immunogens encoding costimulatory molecules and cytokines. J Immunol 158:4591–4601

Iwasaki A, Torres CA, Ohashi PS, Robinson HL, Barber BH (1997) The dominant role of bone marrow-derived cells in CTL induction following plasmid DNA immunization at different sites. J Immunol 159:11–14

Jechlinger W (2006) Optimization and delivery of plasmid DNA for vaccination. Expert Rev Vaccines 5:803–825

Jeon S, Allen-Hoffmann BL, Lambert PF (1995) Integration of human papillomavirus type 16 into the human genome correlates with a selective growth advantage of cells. J Virol 69: 2989–2997

Johnston SA, Talaat AM, McGuire MJ (2002) Genetic immunization: what's in a name? Arch Med Res 33:325–329

Jones S, Evans K, McElwaine-Johnn H, Sharpe M, Oxford J, Lambkin-Williams R, Mant T, Nolan A, Zambon M, Ellis J, Beadle J, Loudon PT (2009) DNA vaccination protects against an influenza challenge in a double-blind randomised placebo-controlled phase 1b clinical trial. Vaccine 27:2506–2512

Kim TW, Hung CF, Kim JW, Juang J, Chen PJ, He L, Boyd DA, Wu TC (2004) Vaccination with a DNA vaccine encoding herpes simplex virus type 1 VP22 linked to antigen generates long-term antigen-specific CD8-positive memory T cells and protective immunity. Hum Gene Ther 15:167–177

Kim SA, Liang CM, Cheng IC, Cheng YC, Chiao MT, Tseng CJ, Lee F, Jong MH, Tao MH, Yang NS, Liang SM (2006) DNA vaccination against foot-and-mouth disease via electroporation: study of molecular approaches for enhancing VP1 antigenicity. J Gene Med 8:1182–1191

Klencke B, Matijevic M, Urban RG, Lathey JL, Hedley ML, Berry M, Thatcher J, Weinberg V, Wilson J, Darragh T, Jay N, Da Costa M, Palefsky JM (2002) Encapsulated plasmid DNA treatment for human papillomavirus 16-associated anal dysplasia: a phase I study of ZYC101. Clin Cancer Res 8:1028–1037

Krieg AM (2002) CpG motifs in bacterial DNA and their immune effects. Annu Rev Immunol 20:709–760

Kutzler MA, Weiner DB (2008) DNA vaccines: ready for prime time? Nat Rev Genet 9:776–788

Kutzler MA, Kraynyak KA, Nagle SJ, Parkinson RM, Zharikova D, Chattergoon M, Maguire H, Muthumani K, Ugen K, Weiner DB (2010) Plasmids encoding the mucosal chemokines CCL27 and CCL28 are effective adjuvants in eliciting antigen-specific immunity in vivo. Gene Ther 17:72–82

Laddy DJ, Weiner DB (2006) From plasmids to protection: a review of DNA vaccines against infectious diseases. Int Rev Immunol 25:99–123

Ledwith BJ, Manam S, Troilo PJ, Barnum AB, Pauley CJ, Griffiths TG, Harper LB, Beare CM, Bagdon WJ, Nichols WW (2000) Plasmid DNA vaccines: investigation of integration into host cellular DNA following intramuscular injection in mice. Intervirology 43:258–272

Li M, Davey GM, Sutherland RM, Kurts C, Lew AM, Hirst C, Carbone FR, Heath WR (2001) Cell-associated ovalbumin is cross-presented much more efficiently than soluble ovalbumin in vivo. J Immunol 166:6099–6103

Limbach KJ, Richie TL (2009) Viral vectors in malaria vaccine development. Parasite Immunol 31:501–519

Lin CT, Tsai YC, He L, Calizo R, Chou HH, Chang TC, Soong YK, Hung CF, Lai CH (2006) A DNA vaccine encoding a codon-optimized human papillomavirus type 16 E6 gene enhances CTL response and anti-tumor activity. J Biomed Sci 13:481–488

Liu MA (1997) The immunologist's grail: vaccines that generate cellular immunity. Proc Natl Acad Sci USA 94:10496–10498

Liu MA, Ulmer JB (2005) Human clinical trials of plasmid DNA vaccines. Adv Genet 55:25–40

Liu WJ, Gao F, Zhao KN, Zhao W, Fernando GJ, Thomas R, Frazer IH (2002) Codon modified human papillomavirus type 16 E7 DNA vaccine enhances cytotoxic T-lymphocyte induction and anti-tumour activity. Virology 301:43–52

Liu L, Zhong Q, Tian T, Dubin K, Athale SK, Kupper TS (2010) Epidermal injury and infection during poxvirus immunization is crucial for the generation of highly protective T cell-mediated immunity. Nat Med 16:224–227

Lu S (2008) Immunogenicity of DNA vaccines in humans: it takes two to tango. Hum Vaccin 4:449–452

Lu S, Wang S, Grimes-Serrano JM (2008) Current progress of DNA vaccine studies in humans. Expert Rev Vaccines 7:175–191

Luckay A, Sidhu MK, Kjeken R, Megati S, Chong SY, Roopchand V, Garcia-Hand D, Abdullah R, Braun R, Montefiori DC, Rosati M, Felber BK, Pavlakis GN, Mathiesen I, Israel ZR, Eldridge JH, Egan MA (2007) Effect of plasmid DNA vaccine design and in vivo electroporation on the resulting vaccine-specific immune responses in rhesus macaques. J Virol 81:5257–5269

Maecker HT, Umetsu DT, DeKruyff RH, Levy S (1998) Cytotoxic T cell responses to DNA vaccination: dependence on antigen presentation via class II MHC. J Immunol 161:6532–6536

Manam S, Ledwith BJ, Barnum AB, Troilo PJ, Pauley CJ, Harper LB, Griffiths TG, Niu Z, Denisova L, Follmer TT, Pacchione SJ, Wang Z, Beare CM, Bagdon WJ, Nichols WW (2000) Plasmid DNA vaccines: tissue distribution and effects of DNA sequence, adjuvants and delivery method on integration into host DNA. Intervirology 43:273–281

Matzinger P (2002) The danger model: a renewed sense of self. Science 296:301–305

McCluskie MJ, Brazolot Millan CL, Gramzinski RA, Robinson HL, Santoro JC, Fuller JT, Widera G, Haynes JR, Purcell RH, Davis HL (1999) Route and method of delivery of DNA vaccine influence immune responses in mice and non-human primates. Mol Med 5:287–300

McConkey SJ, Reece WH, Moorthy VS, Webster D, Dunachie S, Butcher G, Vuola JM, Blanchard TJ, Gothard P, Watkins K, Hannan CM, Everaere S, Brown K, Kester KE, Cummings J, Williams J, Heppner DG, Pathan A, Flanagan K, Arulanantham N, Roberts MT, Roy M, Smith GL, Schneider J, Peto T, Sinden RE, Gilbert SC, Hill AV (2003) Enhanced T-cell immunogenicity of plasmid DNA vaccines boosted by recombinant modified vaccinia virus Ankara in humans. Nat Med 9:729–735

Michel N, Osen W, Gissmann L, Schumacher TN, Zentgraf H, Muller M (2002) Enhanced immunogenicity of HPV 16 E7 fusion proteins in DNA vaccination. Virology 294:47–59

Mir LM (2008) Application of electroporation gene therapy: past, current, and future. Methods Mol Biol 423:3–17

Mitragotri S (2005) Immunization without needles. Nat Rev Immunol 5:905–916

Muthumani G, Laddy DJ, Sundaram SG, Fagone P, Shedlock DJ, Kannan S, Wu L, Chung CW, Lankaraman KM, Burns J, Muthumani K, Weiner DB (2009) Co-immunization with an optimized plasmid-encoded immune stimulatory interleukin, high-mobility group box 1 protein, results in enhanced interferon-gamma secretion by antigen-specific CD8 T cells. Immunology 128:e612–e620

Nagata T, Aoshi T, Uchijima M, Suzuki M, Koide Y (2004) Cytotoxic T-lymphocyte-, and helper T-lymphocyte-oriented DNA vaccination. DNA Cell Biol 23:93–106

Nestle FO, Di Meglio P, Qin JZ, Nickoloff BJ (2009) Skin immune sentinels in health and disease. Nat Rev Immunol 9:679–691

Nishikawa M, Huang L (2001) Nonviral vectors in the new millennium: delivery barriers in gene transfer. Hum Gene Ther 12:861–870

Norbury CC, Basta S, Donohue KB, Tscharke DC, Principtta MF, Berglund P, Gibbs J, Bennink JR, Yewdell JW (2004) $CD8^{+}$ T cell cross-priming via transfer of proteasome substrates. Science 304:1318–1321

O'Hagan DT, Rappuoli R (2004) The safety of vaccines. Drug Discov Today 9:846–854

Parker SE, Borellini F, Wenk ML, Hobart P, Hoffman SL, Hedstrom R, Le T, Norman JA (1999) Plasmid DNA malaria vaccine: tissue distribution and safety studies in mice and rabbits. Hum Gene Ther 10:741–758

Parker SE, Monteith D, Horton H, Hof R, Hernandez P, Vilalta A, Hartikka J, Hobart P, Bentley CE, Chang A, Hedstrom R, Rogers WO, Kumar S, Hoffman SL, Norman JA (2001) Safety of a GM-CSF adjuvant-plasmid DNA malaria vaccine. Gene Ther 8:1011–1023

Peng B, Zhao Y, Xu L, Xu Y (2007) Electric pulses applied prior to intramuscular DNA vaccination greatly improve the vaccine immunogenicity. Vaccine 25:2064–2073

Pokorna D, Rubio I, Muller M (2008) DNA-vaccination via tattooing induces stronger humoral and cellular immune responses than intramuscular delivery supported by molecular adjuvants. Genet Vaccines Ther 6:4.

Pokorna D, Polakova I, Kindlova M, Duskova M, Ludvikova V, Gabriel P, Kutinova L, Muller M, Smahel M (2009) Vaccination with human papillomavirus type 16-derived peptides using a tattoo device. Vaccine 27:3519–3529

Porgador A, Irvine KR, Iwasaki A, Barber BH, Restifo NP, Germain RN (1998) Predominant role for directly transfected dendritic cells in antigen presentation to $CD8^+$ T cells after gene gun immunization. J Exp Med 188:1075–1082

Potthoff A, Schwannecke S, Nabi G, Hoffmann D, Grunwald T, Wildner O, Brockmeyer NH, Uberla K, Tenbusch M (2009) Immunogenicity and efficacy of intradermal tattoo immunization with adenoviral vector vaccines. Vaccine 27:2768–2774

Pulendran B (2004) Immune activation: death, danger and dendritic cells. Curr Biol 14:R30–R32

Pulendran B, Ahmed R (2006) Translating innate immunity into immunological memory: implications for vaccine development. Cell 124:849–863

Quaak SG, van den Berg JH, Toebes M, Schumacher TN, Haanen JB, Beijnen JH, Nuijen B (2008) GMP production of pDERMATT for vaccination against melanoma in a phase I clinical trial. Eur J Pharm Biopharm 70:429–438

Rabussay D (2008) Applicator and electrode design for in vivo DNA delivery by electroporation. Methods Mol Biol 423:35–59

Rao SS, Gomez P, Mascola JR, Dang V, Krivulka GR, Yu F, Lord CI, Shen L, Bailer R, Nabel GJ, Letvin NL (2006) Comparative evaluation of three different intramuscular delivery methods for DNA immunization in a nonhuman primate animal model. Vaccine 24:367–373

Redding L, Weiner DB (2009) DNA vaccines in veterinary use. Expert Rev Vaccines 8: 1251–1276

Ren S, Li M, Smith JM, DeTolla LJ, Furth PA (2002) Low-volume jet injection for intradermal immunization in rabbits. BMC Biotechnol 2:10

Rice J, King CA, Spellerberg MB, Fairweather N, Stevenson FK (1999) Manipulation of pathogen-derived genes to influence antigen presentation via DNA vaccines. Vaccine 17:3030–3038

Rice J, Ottensmeier CH, Stevenson FK (2008) DNA vaccines: precision tools for activating effective immunity against cancer. Nat Rev Cancer 8:108–120

Robert-Guroff M (2007) Replicating and non-replicating viral vectors for vaccine development. Curr Opin Biotechnol 18:546–556

Roos AK, Moreno S, Leder C, Pavlenko M, King A, Pisa P (2006) Enhancement of cellular immune response to a prostate cancer DNA vaccine by intradermal electroporation. Mol Ther 13:320–327

Roos AK, Eriksson F, Timmons JA, Gerhardt J, Nyman U, Gudmundsdotter L, Brave A, Wahren B, Pisa P (2009) Skin electroporation: effects on transgene expression, DNA persistence and local tissue environment. PLoS One 4:e7226.

Saitoh T, Fujita N, Hayashi T, Takahara K, Satoh T, Lee H, Matsunaga K, Kageyama S, Omori H, Noda T, Yamamoto N, Kawai T, Ishii K, Takeuchi O, Yoshimori T, Akira S (2009) Atg9a controls dsDNA-driven dynamic translocation of STING and the innate immune response. Proc Natl Acad Sci USA 106:20842–20846

Schalk JA, Mooi FR, Berbers GA, van Aerts LA, Ovelgonne H, Kimman TG (2006) Preclinical and clinical safety studies on DNA vaccines. Hum Vaccin 2:45–53

Scheerlinck JY (2001) Genetic adjuvants for DNA vaccines. Vaccine 19:2647–2656

Schneeberger A, Wagner C, Zemann A, Luhrs P, Kutil R, Goos M, Stingl G, Wagner SN (2004) CpG motifs are efficient adjuvants for DNA cancer vaccines. J Invest Dermatol 123:371–379

Schroder K, Muruve DA, Tschopp J (2009) Innate immunity: cytoplasmic DNA sensing by the AIM2 inflammasome. Curr Biol 19:R262–R265

Shedlock DJ, Weiner DB (2000) DNA vaccination: antigen presentation and the induction of immunity. J Leukoc Biol 68:793–806

Smahel M, Pokorna D, Mackova J, Vlasak J (2004) Enhancement of immunogenicity of HPV16 E7 oncogene by fusion with E. coli beta-glucuronidase. J Gene Med 6:1092–1101

Smith HA, Klinman DM (2001) The regulation of DNA vaccines. Curr Opin Biotechnol 12: 299–303

Spies B, Hochrein H, Vabulas M, Huster K, Busch DH, Schmitz F, Heit A, Wagner H (2003) Vaccination with plasmid DNA activates dendritic cells via Toll-like receptor 9 (TLR9) but functions in TLR9-deficient mice. J Immunol 171:5908–5912

Stevenson FK, Rice J, Ottensmeier CH, Thirdborough SM, Zhu D (2004) DNA fusion gene vaccines against cancer: from the laboratory to the clinic. Immunol Rev 199:156–180

Sun J, Li D, Hao Y, Zhang Y, Fan W, Fu J, Hu Y, Liu Y, Shao Y (2009) Posttranscriptional regulatory elements enhance antigen expression and DNA vaccine efficacy. DNA Cell Biol 28:233–240

Takaoka A, Wang Z, Choi MK, Yanai H, Negishi H, Ban T, Lu Y, Miyagishi M, Kodama T, Honda K, Ohba Y, Taniguchi T (2007) DAI (DLM-1/ZBP1) is a cytosolic DNA sensor and an activator of innate immune response. Nature 448:501–505

Tang CK, Pietersz GA (2009) Intracellular detection and immune signaling pathways of DNA vaccines. Expert Rev Vaccines 8:1161–1170

Tang DC, DeVit M, Johnston SA (1992) Genetic immunization is a simple method for eliciting an immune response. Nature 356:152–154

Thomsen LL, Topley P, Daly MG, Brett SJ, Tite JP (2004) Imiquimod and resiquimod in a mouse model: adjuvants for DNA vaccination by particle-mediated immunotherapeutic delivery. Vaccine 22:1799–1809

Torres CA, Iwasaki A, Barber BH, Robinson HL (1997) Differential dependence on target site tissue for gene gun and intramuscular DNA immunizations. J Immunol 158:4529–4532

Trimble C, Lin CT, Hung CF, Pai S, Juang J, He L, Gillison M, Pardoll D, Wu L, Wu TC (2003) Comparison of the $CD8^+$ T cell responses and antitumor effects generated by DNA vaccine administered through gene gun, biojector, and syringe. Vaccine 21:4036–4042

Ulmer JB, Donnelly JJ, Parker SE, Rhodes GH, Felgner PL, Dwarki VJ, Gromkowski SH, Deck RR, DeWitt CM, Friedman A et al (1993) Heterologous protection against influenza by injection of DNA encoding a viral protein. Science 259:1745–1749

Ulmer JB, Deck RR, DeWitt CM, Donnhly JI, Liu MA (1996) Generation of MHC class I-restricted cytotoxic T lymphocytes by expression of a viral protein in muscle cells: antigen presentation by non-muscle cells. Immunology 89:59–67

Van Damme P, Oosterhuis-Kafeja F, Van der Wielen M, Almagor Y, Sharon O, Levin Y (2009) Safety and efficacy of a novel microneedle device for dose sparing intradermal influenza vaccination in healthy adults. Vaccine 27:454–459

van den Berg JH, Nujien B, Beijnen JH, Vincent A, van Tinteren H, Kluge J, Woerdeman LA, Hennink WE, Storm G, Schumacher TN, Haanen JB (2009) Optimization of intradermal vaccination by DNA tattooing in human skin. Hum Gene Ther 20:181–189

van den Berg JH, Oosterhuis K, Hennink WE, Storm G, van der Aa LJ, Engbersen JF, Haanen JB, Beijnen JH, Schumacher TN, Nuijen B (2010a) Shielding the cationic charge of nanoparticle-formulated dermal DNA vaccines is essential for antigen expression and immunogenicity. J Control Release 141:234–240

van den Berg JH, Nuijen B, Schumacher TN, Haanen JB, Storm G, Beijnen JH, Hennink WE (2010b) Synthetic vehicles for DNA vaccination. J Drug Target 18:1–14 van den Berg JH, Quaak SG, Beijnen JH, Hennink WE, Storm G, Schumacher TN, Haanen JB, Nuijen B (2010c) Lipopolysaccharide contamination in intradermal DNA vaccination: Toxic impurity or adjuvant? Int J Pharm 390:32–36

van Oijen M, Bins A, Elias S, Sein J, Weder P, de Gast G, Mallo H, Gallee M, van Tinteren H, Schumacher T, Haanen J (2004) On the role of melanoma-specific $CD8^+$ T-cell immunity in disease progression of advanced-stage melanoma patients. Clin Cancer Res 10:4754–4760

Verstrepen BE, Bins AD, Rollier CS, Mooij P, Koopman G, Sheppard NC, Sattentau Q, Wagner R, Wolf H, Schumacher TN, Heeney JL, Haanen JB (2008) Improved HIV-1 specific T-cell responses by short-interval DNA tattooing as compared to intramuscular immunization in non-human primates. Vaccine 26:3346–3351

Wang B, Ugen KE, Srikantan V, Agadjanyan MG, Dang K, Refaeli Y, Sato AI, Boyer J, Williams WV, Weiner DB (1993) Gene inoculation generates immune responses against human immunodeficiency virus type 1. Proc Natl Acad Sci USA 90:4156–4160

Wang Z, Troilo PJ, Wang X, Griffiths TG, Pacchione SJ, Barnum AB, Harper LB, Pauley CJ, Niu Z, Denisova L, Follmer TT, Rizzuto G, Ciliberto G, Fattori E, Monica NL, Manam S, Ledwith BJ (2004) Detection of integration of plasmid DNA into host genomic DNA following intramuscular injection and electroporation. Gene Ther 11:711–721

Widera G, Austin M, Rabussay D, Goldbeck C, Barnett SW, Chen M, Leung L, Otten GR, Thudium K, Selby MJ, Ulmer JB (2000) Increased DNA vaccine delivery and immunogenicity by electroporation in vivo. J Immunol 164:4635–4640

Wilson CB, Marcuse EK (2001) Vaccine safety–vaccine benefits: science and the public's perception. Nat Rev Immunol 1:160–165

Wolff JA, Malone RW, Williams P, Chong W, Acsadi G, Jani A, Felgner PL (1990) Direct gene transfer into mouse muscle in vivo. Science 247:1465–1468

Wolkers MC, Toebes M, Okabe M, Haanen JB, Schumacher TN (2002) Optimizing the efficacy of epitope-directed DNA vaccination. J Immunol 168:4998–5004

Wolkers MC, Brouwenstijn N, Bakker AH, Toebes M, Schumacher TN (2004) Antigen bias in T cell cross-priming. Science 304:1314–1317

Wu TC (2007) Therapeutic human papillomavirus DNA vaccination strategies to control cervical cancer. Eur J Immunol 37:310–314

Yamano T, Kaneda Y, Huang S, Hiramatsu SH, Hoon DS (2006) Enhancement of immunity by a DNA melanoma vaccine against TRP2 with CCL21 as an adjuvant. Mol Ther 13:194–202

Zaba LC, Krueger JG, Lowes MA (2009) Resident and "inflammatory" dendritic cells in human skin. J Invest Dermatol 129:302–308

Zhou Q, Wang F, Yang F, Wang Y, Zhang X, Sun S (2010) Augmented humoral and cellular immune response of hepatitis B virus DNA vaccine by micro-needle vaccination using Flt3L as an adjuvant. Vaccine 28:1357–1362

Index

Current Topics in Microbiology and Immunology (2012) 351: 251–253
DOI: 10.1007/978-3-642-23690-7